Rethinking Social Epidemiology

Patricia O'Campo • James R. Dunn
Editors

Rethinking Social Epidemiology

Towards a Science of Change

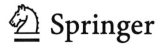 Springer

Editors
Patricia O'Campo
Alma and Baxter Ricard Chair in Inner
City Health
Professor, Dalla Lana School of Public
Health, University of Toronto
Director, Centre for Research on Inner City
Health part of the Keenan Research Centre
of the Li Ka Shing Knowledge Institute
St. Michael's Hospital
Bond Street 30
Toronto, ON M5B 1W8
Canada
pat.ocampo@utoronto.ca

James R. Dunn
Department of Health, Aging and Society
McMaster University
Kenneth Taylor Hall 226
Main Street West 1280
Hamilton, ON L8S 4L8
Canada
jim.dunn@mcmaster.ca

ISBN 978-94-007-2137-1   e-ISBN 978-94-007-2138-8
DOI 10.1007/978-94-007-2138-8
Springer Dordrecht Heidelberg London New York

Library of Congress Control Number: 2011939065

Springer is part of Springer Science+Business Media (www.springer.com)

Foreword

To illustrate the probabilistic nature of causation in epidemiology, a well-known lecturer in epidemiology used the example of a medieval archer defending a castle. The defender, high up there on the ramparts, is safe from the archers on the ground, provided he hides behind the battlements. But to shoot his arrows he has to appear in the space. If his timing is unlucky, he cops an arrow. Random. Bad luck of the draw. Play of chance.

Except that, of course, it is anything but random. First, at the individual level, we know that "accidents" are not randomly distributed – psychology, training and experience, tiredness and nutrition all play a role. Going beyond the individual level, the environment matters – the design of weapons, or castles, or houses or cars – and so do regulations. Give the archer a litre of wine before he goes on duty and his risk will be changed – as will his aim. Social structures condition risk: aristocrats rarely man battlements, except in movies. The leaders are safe, while expendable troops, battle fodder, are on the front line. The relative strengths of the attacking and defending armies will play a role. But why is there a war happening in the first place? What are the political processes that have led to two armies facing off at the castle?

In the end, my colleague's point may be correct: there is an element of randomness in disease causation, whether it is the susceptibility to a mediaeval arrow, the likelihood of the renegade cell becoming cancerous or the likelihood of the atheromatous plaque in the coronary arteries rupturing with catastrophic effects on the heart. But this randomness is at the end of the process. If we want to do something about death from arrow wound, there are layers of psychological, social, economic and political causes that must be addressed. So it is with all health and disease.

The Commission on Social Determinants of Health (2008) used the phrase "the causes of the causes" to capture this concept. The dominant perspective in epidemiology has been a focus on individual risk factors. Even when analyzing social inequalities in health, policy focus has been on behaviour of individuals. One colleague who contributed to the English review of health inequalities used the term "lifestyle drift" (Marmot Review 2010); it is all too easy for policy makers to focus on aspects of lifestyle as being the causes of health inequalities while ignoring the causes of the causes.

When, in 1971, having finished conventional medical training, I went to Berkeley to do a PhD with Len Syme, I was not aware there was such a thing as social epidemiology. There were Len Syme and John Cassel studying how various social aspects related to health. There was also, of course, the British tradition of social medicine, going back at least to William Farr, the great Victorian observer of things medical and statistical. The most active practitioner of social medicine, then current, was Jerry Morris, who said: "Society largely determines health; ill-health is not a personal misfortune due often to personal inadequacy but a social misfortune due, more commonly, to social mismanagement and social failure." Not a bad starting credo for social epidemiology, alongside Virchow's famous phrase, quoted in this volume.

Studying epidemiology in the United States in the 1970s, social class was at best a variable to be controlled for in analyses, not an object of study. There were exceptions (Syme and Berkman 1976; Cassel 1971), but investigation of *explanations* for social class differences in rates of disease occurrence was scarcely in view. My own investigation of explanations for the social gradient in mortality in the first Whitehall study (Marmot et al. 1976, 1984) was initially limited to the role of individual risk factors as mediators. By the time I started to ask the broader question of why we had such social differentiation in society in Britain and elsewhere, the government of the day thought that social inequality in health was not a legitimate question for enquiry.

This brings us to the question of values, which is admirably discussed in the present volume (see Chap. 3). We read an illustration of the importance of values daily in our newspapers. No economist, I observe the current (2011) debates over economic policy with frustration and puzzlement. There was a global credit crunch that led to severe economic difficulties in many countries with large government debt and structural budget deficits. Everyone is agreed there is a problem, but proposed solutions differ markedly. Crudely speaking, there are two sides. One says that in order to get economic growth we need to cut the deficit; the other says that in order to cut the deficit we need to get economic growth. These are radically different. The first says government should cut spending to reduce the deficit, including reducing public-sector employment and private-sector dependence on government spending. The other side, more Keynesian, says that in a depressed economy with high unemployment, government should increase spending to stimulate demand and create jobs. For the moment, I am leaving out the third side, the green one, that asks why we want to go back to economic growth.

Naively, I would have thought that the data would settle the argument – what do all those macroeconomists do? But it would appear not. The deficit cutters seem to be to the political right and the Keynesians to the political left – although Keynes himself was a Liberal, in the British sense. Paul Krugman, a Keynesian, draws attention to salt water and fresh water economists in the United States. The saltwater Keynesians are on the coasts at such intellectually doubtful places as Princeton, Columbia and Berkeley; the freshwater types at places of rigour, such as Chicago. (Please, I am being ironic!)

What should be a debate about economic science turns out to be a debate about values, the outcome of which has absolutely profound consequences for the well-being, and hence, the health of populations. One, of course, has the suspicion that social distributions are the subtext of the argument. Reducing welfare, cutting public services and reducing public sector employment all, demonstrably, affect the lower ends of the income distribution. A stimulus, via tax cuts for the wealthy, benefits the rich. Values are affecting scientific conclusions and policy implications.

I have had my own disagreements with economists (Marmot 2009). I proposed a screening test for economists. Show someone the social gradient in health. If he/she concludes that health leads to social position then he/she is an economist. As with any screening test, there are false positives and false negatives, but the starting position for economists seems to be that health determines your social conditions; social epidemiologists' starting position is that social conditions determine health. Both sides justify their arguments with "evidence." But the starting position, which may well include values, determines how the evidence is collected and analyzed. What purports to be a debate about empirical evidence is actually a debate about how different disciplines view the world (Marmot et al. 2010).

It is then tempting to wonder if there is an intellectual connection between being a deficit cutter and believing that social conditions are *not* responsible for the social gradient in health. The intellectual tussle between having a coherent set of values and yet sticking close to the evidence is well brought out in this volume. Given that people who deny the importance of values in empirical research are ignoring the empirical evidence, such as that to which I have just alluded, it is well to be explicit about the values that guide our intellectual enquiry, particularly because epidemiology in general, and social epidemiology in particular, has an action focus as well as needing to be conducted at the highest intellectual level.

Social epidemiologists want a more just distribution of health. The Commission on Social Determinants of Health (2008) said that health inequity results from the conditions in which people are born, grow, live, work and age, and the structural drivers of those conditions. We said that inequities in power, money and resources are at the heart of health inequity and concluded that social injustice is killing on a grand scale. Carles Muntaner, in this volume (see Chap. 9), picks up Vincente Navarro's response to this call and says that what is needed is a more explicitly political level of analysis, in addition to the social, economic, cultural and environmental. Muntaner shows impressively and persuasively how this can be done with rigour.

The starting position for the present volume is that the reality of people's lives matters for their health. Their lived reality and the conditions that lead to it are responsible for the health of populations, provide explanations for health inequity and suggest solutions. Such a starting point is greatly welcome. Further, this volume both presents much-needed discussion of the intellectual and ethical basis for social epidemiology and can be seen as a rallying call for research in the best interests of improving population health. We called our English review of health inequalities *Fair Society, Healthy Lives*. Put fairness at the heart of all decision making and population health will improve and avoidable health inequalities will diminish. The present volume is very much in that tradition and takes thinking a very large step forward.

Michael Marmot
Professor of Epidemiology and Public Health
University College London
(Chair of WHO Commission on Social Determinants
of Health 2005–2008; and Marmot Review Team,
University College London)
e-mail: m.marmot@ucl.ac.uk

References

Cassel J (1971) Incidence of coronary heart diseases by ethnic group, social class, and sex. Arch Intern Med 128:901–906

Commission on Social Determinants of Health (2008) Closing the gap in a generation: health equity through action on the social determinants of health. Final report of the Commission on Social Determinants of Health. World Health Organization, Geneva

Marmot MG (2009) Commentary: a continued affair with science and judgements. Int J Epidemiol 38:908–910

Marmot M, Allen J, Goldblatt P (2010) A social movement, based on evidence, to remove social inequalities in health. Soc Sci Med 71:1254–1258

Marmot MG, Rose G, Shipley M et al (1978) Employment grade and coronary heart disease in British civil servants. J Epidemiol Community Health 32:244–249

Marmot MG, Shipley MJ, Rose G (1984) Inequalities in death – specific explanations of a general pattern? Lancet 323:1003–1006

Marmot Review (2010) Fair society, healthy lives: strategic review of health inequalities in England post-2010. Marmot Review, London

Syme SL, Berkman LF (1976) Social class, susceptibility, and sickness. Am J Epidemiol 104:1–8

Contents

1 Introduction 1
Patricia O'Campo and James R. Dunn

Part I   Foundations

2 **"Explanation," Philosophy and Theory in Health Inequalities
Research: Towards a Critical Realist Approach** 23
James R. Dunn

3 **Values and Social Epidemiologic Research** 43
Ahmed M. Bayoumi and Adrian Guta

4 **Population-Based Data and Community Empowerment** 67
Janet Smylie, Aisha Lofters, Michelle Firestone,
and Patricia O'Campo

5 **Differences That Matter** 93
Aisha Lofters and Patricia O'Campo

Part II   Context

6 **Place-Based Stress and Chronic Disease: A Systems View
of Environmental Determinants** 113
Ketan Shankardass

7 **How Goes the Neighbourhood? Rethinking Neighbourhoods
and Health Research in Social Epidemiology** 137
Ketan Shankardass and James R. Dunn

8 **Application of Two Schools of Social Theory to Neighbourhood,
Place and Health Research** 157
Irene H. Yen, Janet K. Shim, and Airín D. Martínez

9   Locating Politics in Social Epidemiology 175
    Carles Muntaner, Carme Borrell, Edwin Ng, Haejoo Chung,
    Albert Espelt, Maica Rodriguez-Sanz, Joan Benach,
    and Patricia O'Campo

Part III   Research Tools in Action

10 Structural Violence and Structural Vulnerability Within
    the Risk Environment: Theoretical and Methodological
    Perspectives for a Social Epidemiology of HIV Risk
    Among Injection Drug Users and Sex Workers 205
    Tim Rhodes, Karla Wagner, Steffanie A. Strathdee, Kate Shannon,
    Peter Davidson, and Philippe Bourgois

11 Realist Review Methods for Complex Health Problems 231
    Maritt Kirst and Patricia O'Campo

12 Addressing Health Equities in Social Epidemiology: Learning
    from Evaluation(s) 247
    Sanjeev Sridharan, James R. Dunn, and April Nakaima

Part IV   Making a Difference

13 Knowledge Translation and Social Epidemiology:
    Taking Power, Politics and Values Seriously 267
    Kelly Murphy and Patrick Fafard

14 Community-Academic Partnerships and Social Change 285
    Peter Schafer

15 Producing More Relevant Evidence: Applying a Social
    Epidemiology Research Agenda to Public Health Practice 305
    David Mowat and Catharine Chambers

16 Conclusions 327
    James R. Dunn and Patricia O'Campo

Index 335

Chapter 1
Introduction

Patricia O'Campo and James R. Dunn

Contents

1.1	Rethinking Social Epidemiology: An Introduction	2
1.2	An Expanded Vision of Social Epidemiology	4
1.3	Going Beyond the Need for Social Theory	9
1.4	Making Social Epidemiology Matter	14
1.5	Conclusions	15
References		15

Abstract Social epidemiology is now widely accepted as a legitimate area of inquiry, with a vast number of practicing social epidemiologists in universities, public health departments and other venues throughout the world. Social epidemiologists have focused on demonstrating the impact of growing social and health inequalities worldwide and have repeatedly demonstrated that health status is not distributed equally in society. Yet an almost exclusive focus on the existence and growth of gaps in income or health alone will not inform effective solutions. Social epidemiology risks exclusion from contributing to the formulation of solutions if our field continues to simply emphasize empirical studies demonstrating the existence of a variety of different health inequalities. We seek to challenge social epidemiology to "rethink its current practice" and adopt a greater focus on generating evidence required to "take action" to alleviate conditions of marginalization and

P. O'Campo (✉)
Centre for Research on Inner City Health, St. Michael's Hospital, 30 Bond Street,
Toronto M5B 1W8, ON, Canada
e-mail: O'CampoP@smh.ca

J.R. Dunn
Department of Health, Aging and Society, McMaster University, Kenneth Taylor
Hall 226, 1280 Main Street West, Hamilton L8S 4L8, ON, Canada
e-mail: jim.dunn@mcmaster.ca

P. O'Campo and J.R. Dunn (eds.), *Rethinking Social Epidemiology:*
Towards a Science of Change, DOI 10.1007/978-94-007-2138-8_1,
© Springer Science+Business Media B.V. 2012

poverty (i.e., solution-focused research). We review a number of challenges facing the field that prevent social epidemiologists from participating in the formulation of solutions to these growing social problems and health inequities. We provide an overview of the topics of the chapters in this volume intended to provide a vision of social epidemiology as a science of change.

Abbreviations

CIHR   Canadian Institutes of Health Research
TANF   Temporary Assistance for Needy Families
WHO   World Health Organization

1.1   Rethinking Social Epidemiology: An Introduction

Epidemiology is the study of the patterns of health and illness in populations, while *social* epidemiology focuses on the social determinants that shape the risk and occurrence of poor health in these populations (Berkman and Kawachi 2000; James 2009). Since the late 1970s, social epidemiology has grown rapidly as a subdiscipline within epidemiology. It has reached a level of maturity to the extent that among mainstream epidemiology journals and funding agencies it is widely accepted as a legitimate area of inquiry. There are now a large number of practicing social epidemiologists in universities, public health departments and other institutions throughout the world. Courses, clusters, centres and degree programs in social epidemiology, while rare a decade ago, are now widespread throughout North America and Europe.

Over the past few decades, thousands of studies and several books (e.g., Berkman and Kawachi 2000; Oakes and Kaufman 2006; Cwikel 2006) have identified a range of individual and, more recently, contextual characteristics that are associated with a wide variety of health status measures and disease processes. Social epidemiology is now known for its ability to demonstrate that there are large differences in health status among identifiable social groups, and for the implication that these differences are unjust and avoidable (Commission on Social Determinants of Health 2008; Braveman 2006). As such, social epidemiologists in the last decades have built a large empirical base for an expanding set of potentially deleterious and hazardous exposures emanating from the social, cultural, political and economic environments (Acevedo-Garcia et al. 2003; Sorensen et al. 2004; Bernstein et al. 2007; Goldberg et al. 2002; Kasl and Jones 2002; Matheson et al. 2008; O'Campo et al. 1995).

At the start of the twenty first century, we continue to experience the enormous social problems contributing to poor health in individuals and in populations. Examples include poverty, wealth inequities, unemployment, oppression and, more recently, financial strain resulting from the recent global economic crisis (Hacker and Pierson 2010; Seabrook 2007; Ellwood 2006). In most countries (even prior to the recent global economic recession), various sectors including labour, housing, transportation, health, justice, environment and education, to name a few, are not meeting the needs of all individuals equally. This statement is true even for countries that have the financial resources to meet the basic needs of their entire population. These economic and resource problems are not confined within the borders of nation-states. Overconsumption of valuable natural resources by high-income countries impacts the well-being of populations in lower-income countries where the resources are located. Production efficiencies in the affluent countries are achieved at the expense of labour and human rights of people in other parts of the globe. While natural hazards seem to be on the rise, including geological (e.g., hurricanes, earthquakes), hydrological (e.g., floods, tsunamis), meteorological (e.g., tornados, droughts, heat waves) and health (e.g., pandemics) disasters, it is the *social* circumstances that shape population vulnerability to their impacts (e.g., excess mortality rates among low- versus high-income populations experiencing earthquakes worldwide, highest mortality among the poor in recent heat waves, or the heavy health and social burden placed on the poor as a result of the Katrina hurricane in New Orleans) (Chou et al. 2004; Atkins and Moy 2005; Fothergill et al. 1999; Borrell et al. 2006; Naughton et al. 2002; Kruk et al. 2011; Bambra 2011; Elliott and Pais 2006; Centre for Research on the Epidemiology of Disasters 2011).

In almost any one of the aforementioned circumstances, whether regarding the consequences of economic downturns or of a geological disaster such as an earthquake, social forces determine who bears the greatest health burden (Ellwood 2006). Not surprisingly, there has been an exponential growth in studies focused on documenting the longstanding and increasing social and health inequalities worldwide (Commission on Social Determinants of Health 2008; Asthana and Halliday 2006; Braveman 2007; Macinko et al. 2003; Phelan et al. 2004; Starfield 2007; Syme 2008; Wilkinson 2007). Yet a focus on the existence and growth of gaps in income or health alone will not inform effective solutions. As others before us have noted, social epidemiology has reached a critical turning point in its development (Braveman et al. 2011; Schwartz et al. 1999; Oakes 2005; Rychetnik et al. 2002; Venkatapuram and Marmot 2009; Kaplan 2004). Throughout this book, we seek to challenge the field of social epidemiology. We aim to advance and accelerate our field's efforts to the next logical phase, during which epidemiologists will be prepared to address key questions on the causes of social inequalities in health (i.e., *problem-focused research*) and more critically generate the epidemiologic evidence required for the design of effective interventions to alleviate conditions of marginalization and poverty (i.e., *solution-focused research*). Too much of social epidemiology, we argue, currently focuses on problem identification, including describing the magnitude of problems, identifying risk factors and establishing associations between risk factors or markers and health outcomes. If social epidemiology continues on its current path, we are likely to see a continued growth of empirical studies demonstrating the existence of a variety of different health inequalities, with relatively little contribution to studies that characterize and inform solutions to those inequities.

One epidemiologist recently noted that while our field faces "a feast of descriptive studies of socio-economic causes of ill health we still face a famine of evaluative intervention studies" (Bonneux 2007). Solution-focused research includes identifying causal mechanisms that have intervention potential for contributing to health outcomes. This type of research might include program evaluations, evidence syntheses (e.g., systematic reviews of interventions), policy analyses or syntheses and even tailored programs for subpopulations (Muntaner et al. 2010; O'Campo et al. 2009, 2011; O'Campo and Rojas-Smith 1998; Edwards et al. 2010; Gómez-Olmedo et al. 1996). And while there is evidence of some movement towards such a research program already in other fields (e.g., Smedslund et al. 2006; Welsh and Farrington 2008), there is no evidence of it in social epidemiology. Continuation with the *status quo* increases the probability of our field becoming complacent (Kaplan 2004; Berkman 2004), with social epidemiologists making little to no contributions in the formulation of solutions to growing social problems and health inequities.

In this chapter and throughout this book we highlight some of the barriers to fostering a discipline capable of investigating both the nature of and the remedy to social inequalities in health. If social epidemiology does in fact have unique domains of investigation related to the social influences on population well-being, it should also have unique approaches and mandates that shape its practice. We are by no means suggesting that the new directions we are promoting in this book are the only changes that would enable our young subdiscipline to progress. We are, however, suggesting that the research areas we are highlighting are a critical and necessary advancement of our field. In this chapter, we review the challenges facing social epidemiology while reviewing the themes of the book and specific chapters.

1.2 An Expanded Vision of Social Epidemiology

As modern social epidemiology has gained momentum over the last few decades, explanatory models of health have increasingly included social factors and contextual social processes (Berkman and Kawachi 2000; Oakes and Kaufman 2006). What holds this large body of mostly problem-focused research together is the repeated finding that health status is not distributed equally in society and that persistent differences exist between groups along a number of axes of social differentiation, including gender, income, education, race, ethnicity, immigration status and housing status, to name a few. With but few exceptions, these health inequalities can be characterized as situations in which the less powerful experience poorer health outcomes. Understanding the problem, describing its magnitude, trends and risk factors, however, is not the same as generating the necessary evidence on effective interventions needed to solve the problem (Brownson et al. 2009a, b). Generating epidemiologic evidence to inform solutions around the social determinants of health requires that we resolve the question of whether a focus on solutions or the policy implications of our research is a legitimate mandate for social epidemiologists and should be pursued more vigorously.

Many social epidemiologists are motivated to study the social determinants of health out of concern for the injustice of growing health and social disparities or out of the desire to alleviate the misery of those experiencing oppression and deprivation. Applied epidemiology has a longstanding history of generating evidence to promote positive social change (Mackenbach 2009; Wallerstein and Duran 2010). However, not all epidemiologists agree that the purview of our field should include a focus on the uses of the evidence that we generate (Savitz et al. 1999; Rothman et al. 1998; Epstein 2003). This position is in part fueled by the idea that being concerned about the uses and implications of epidemiologic research for policy, practice or advocacy can threaten the perceived objectivity of the scientific process. Yet, others feel strongly that our scientific activities must include a focus on the means to solving these longstanding and seemingly intractable social problems (Krieger 1999; Ruffin 2010; Mackenbach 2009). This focus on solutions can take the form of studying the ways in which interventions and policies can improve population well-being, or even adopting an advocacy position either individually or as part of a coalition or interest group to promote positive social change (Mackenbach 2009; Wallerstein and Duran 2010). Thacker and Buffington (2001), in arguing for an applied epidemiology for the twenty first Century, note that an

> applied epidemiologist is by definition an activist, moving rapidly from findings to policy, putting epidemiological knowledge to good use. Skills in communication must be an integral part of an epidemiologist's repertoire, as must the ability to work in multi-disciplinary coalitions. The 21st century epidemiologist must do all these things in addressing public concerns while maintaining a foundation of high quality epidemiologic research and practice.

Nancy Krieger (1999), in commenting over a decade ago on the two extremes of this debate, proposed that we move from our current position of presenting this issue as an "either/or" situation and adopt the stance that "epidemiology is, like any science, at once objective (using defined, rigorous, and replicable methods to assess refutable propositions) and partisan (reflecting underlying values and assumptions guiding conceptualization, choice, and analysis of research problems)." Like Krieger, we support the idea that, in directly engaging these seemingly opposing positions, social epidemiologists should utilize this inherent tension to reconcile differences in these views and further advance the field.

To meet this challenge, social epidemiology must recognize the legitimacy of different audiences and scientific methods for our research, as well as different goals for this research (Krieger 1999; Schwartz and Carpenter 1999; Rothman et al. 1998; Morabia 2009). Right now, there are broad audiences, from our colleagues and students to policy makers, program planners and the public, interested in the abundant problem-focused research that social epidemiologists generate, which establishes associations between social factors or processes and health outcomes. A subset of these audiences – program planners, policy and decision makers – might closely follow, be engaged in or partner with epidemiologists in generating applied social epidemiologic research. Yet another audience, advocates, might seek to engage scientists in gaining access to existing or new scientific knowledge concerning problems facing the public (Altevogt et al. 2008; Brown 1992; Fuchs 1996; Morgan 2005). Michael Burawoy (2004), a professor at University of California, Berkeley, while describing a disciplinary division of labour within sociology, identifies four types of sociological research, each of which has its own primary audience, approach to generating knowledge, legitimacy and accountability. This framework, Burawoy argues, can be applied to any discipline. Such a typology, if applied to social epidemiology, might facilitate the recognition of a myriad of forms of research that should be present within any applied field. Table 1.1 applies Burawoy's typology to social epidemiology.

Two approaches, *professional-* and *policy-focused research*, derive from what Burawoy calls *technically rational* or *instrumental knowledge*. Originating from positivism a few centuries ago, during a time when science and technology were thought to drive progress in society, technically rational approaches to science, especially among professional scientists, were considered deterministic, specialized, quantitative, reliable and objective (Broom and Willis 2007). Thus, the focus on quantitative methods, reliability, generaliziblity and their accurate implementation is one of the defining characteristics of professional knowledge generation using a positivist paradigm. Much of the training, research and publication in epidemiology adhere to these standards (Bhopal 1997). *Policy-focused research* is the application of such methods to specific problems that are defined by the end users of that knowledge. For social epidemiologic research, these end users include decision makers and those involved in policy making within organizations and at varying levels of government, or even advocates in coalitions concerned with improving the social conditions that impact upon health (Boulton et al. 2009; Walke and Simone 2009).

In contrast to those types of knowledge that are informed by positivist paradigms, the two types of *reflexive knowledge* in the typology explicitly recognize values inherent in the scientific process and encourage critical reflection and dialogue between those who generate and those who use this knowledge. Buroway argues that *critical science* is needed to challenge those engaged in professional scientific activities to improve and advance the discipline. A number of examples of such efforts within epidemiology can be found, including the arguments over the last two decades for explicitly including contextual data and variables in research studies (O'Campo et al. 1995, 1997; Diez-Roux 1998), and debates about the status of randomized clinical trials for epidemiologic research (Rychetnik et al. 2002; Sanson-Fisher et al. 2007). *Popular epidemiology*, as has been argued by several authors (Wallerstein and Duran 2010; Leung et al. 2004; Brown 1987, 1992; Morgan 2005; San Sebastián and Hurtig 2005), is critical to ensuring that epidemiologic evidence and knowledge are relevant for informing and solving contemporary social problems that impact on population health. This approach to epidemiology is undertaken with and for those who are concerned with and affected by the issues under study. Initiation of research by affected communities (Brown 1987, 1992; Fuchs 1996) and formation of scientific-community partnerships with communities, a method that is increasingly utilized in epidemiologic research, are but two examples of this approach (Leung et al. 2004; Yen 2005; Minkler 2005; Wallerstein and Duran 2010).

In exploring this framework as it applies to epidemiology, policy and popular approaches are currently underrepresented, which in part explains the imbalance in problem- versus solution-focused social epidemiologic research. Popular epidemiology may be particularly important for ensuring that the social problems of interest are accurately captured in our research and that solutions, once identified, are

Table 1.1 Types of knowledge generation in social epidemiology

Approach to social epidemiology	Professional epidemiology	Critical epidemiology	Policy epidemiology	Popular epidemiology
Type of knowledge	Technically rational knowledge: theoretical/empirical	Reflexive knowledge: foundational	Technically rational knowledge: concrete	Reflexive knowledge: engaged
Audience	Academic audience	Academic audience	Extra-academic audience	Extra-academic audience
Legitimacy	Scientific norms	Moral vision	Effectiveness	Relevance to addressing social determinants of health
Accountability	Peers	Critical intellectuals	Clients/decision makers	Designated publics
Politics	Disciplinary self-interest	Internal debate	Policy intervention	Public
Examples	Population-based studies on the social determinants of health	Disciplinary discussions and debates about role of individual versus social determinants in epidemiologic research	Assessment of the health impacts or benefits of social or economic policies	Community-based participatory health research

Adapted from Burawoy (2004)

feasible and acceptable to affected populations. While examples of epidemiological research involving community-based participatory research are growing in number (Leung et al. 2004; Yen 2005; Minkler 2005; Wallerstein and Duran 2010), new research approaches to academic-community partnerships, defined and controlled by affected communities, are also emerging. An example is the set of principles put forth by Canadian Indigenous populations to guide research undertaken about their communities and populations, called OCAP – Ownership (community ownership of cultural knowledge, information or data), Control (communities control and are involved in all aspects of the research project), Access (communities must have access to the research information and data) and Possession (communities should be able to hold information in their possession). In addition to requiring meaningful engagement between the researchers and community, these principles support self-governance and self-determination of research concerning Indigenous populations in Canada. While this approach may challenge the way research is traditionally undertaken in academic settings (e.g., the principal investigator is the owner of research data), these practices were developed in response to the observation of the outright failure of past research to improve the well-being of Canadian Aboriginal populations. OCAP is therefore "a political response to colonialism and the role of knowledge production in reproducing colonial relations" (Schnarch 2004). In practice these principles enable Indigenous communities to gain control over which researchers they collaborate with. They also yield several benefits to the research process and outcomes, including but not limited to: building and restoring community trust in research; improving the quality, accuracy and relevance of research; and building capacity of community as well as among researchers (Schnarch 2004). These principles, reflecting an approach to community-controlled popular epidemiology, have been adopted by the national health research funding agency, the Canadian Institutes to Health Research (CIHR), to be adhered to when conducting research on or with Canadian Aboriginal populations.

Although applying Buroway to epidemiology is not the only way to examine our discipline, his framework facilitates a greater understanding of the current strengths and limitations of our field. We immediately recognize that there is a preponderance of professional epidemiology and perhaps critical epidemiology (Table 1.1). Yet, if social epidemiologists seek a greater focus on informing, designing and evaluating the programs and policies that will address growing inequities, our discipline needs to engage in more policy and public epidemiology.

To remedy the current imbalance, we must move beyond the simplistic debates about whether epidemiologists should stay within the bounds of professional epidemiology, on the one hand, or, on the other, become a discipline of scientists engaged in public epidemiology. Those engaged in policy or practice and public epidemiology fields would primarily, but not exclusively, undertake the solution-focused research that we are encouraging. Yet, to ensure appropriate methods and legitimacy of the research, such knowledge generation should draw from professional and critical epidemiologic research activity approaches. Moreover, epidemiologists could, as Buroway notes, engage in more than one type of approach in their own research programs.

1.3 Going Beyond the Need for Social Theory

Recent calls for more social theory to inform social epidemiologic research should be heeded (Krieger 2011; Carpiano and Daley 2006; Dunn 2006). Currently, much of social epidemiology focuses on the downstream determinants of health, and too few studies examine the macrosocial determinants of health (Schwartz et al. 1999; House 2002; Putnam and Galea 2008; Berkman 2004; Williams 2003; Woodcock and Aldred 2008; Whitehead 2007). Any cursory exposure to the media reveals the critical contemporary social issues of our day that, because of their direct and indirect impacts upon population well-being, should be the subject of our social epidemiologic inquiries. Examples of contemporary social problems with implications for population health include: national policies that enable rapid concentration of power and wealth; overconsumption of valuable global resources by those in developed countries; "structural adjustment" policies that lead to widespread deprivation of basic necessities of life (e.g., shelter, food, water); revolutions against contemporary oppressive governments; and even the adverse consequences of increasingly popular programs such as micro lending (Roy 2010). These examples offer a small view of a growing list of global social problems at the start of the twenty first century. These global issues are, no doubt, at the root of the local social problems contributing to the growth in the very health inequities that comprise an increasing focus of social epidemiologic research. Yet where are these social determinants within the body of research that we are so rapidly generating?

Part of the explanation stems from the dominant explanatory model traditionally used in epidemiologic inquiry, the biomedical or "disease-specific model," which seeks to identify mostly individual-based risk markers and risk factors for specified health conditions. This model is consistent with the increasing specialization in health research, through which those concerned with particular conditions (e.g., diabetes, unintentional injury) seek specific models that apply to their area of inquiry. Consequently, social epidemiologists continue this tradition by researching a narrow range of social questions concerning health that primarily focus on downstream social health determinants.

It may be of little comfort to know that this problem is not specific to epidemiology. The social sciences, the basis for much of social epidemiology, experienced a similar misplaced focus on individual risks for poverty and welfare participation at the end of the last century with detrimental consequences to key national poverty-related policies in the United States. Alice O'Connor (2001), Professor at the University of California Santa Barbara, while writing about the multimillion-dollar "poverty knowledge" industry, demonstrated that social scientists failed to study and recognize the role of macrosocial labour and economic factors that were major contributors, if not causes, of growing long-term poverty. She notes "how completely the energies of the poverty research industry, with all its advanced technology, were being channeled into a very narrowly defined set of issues revolving around the characteristics, behaviour, and attitudes of poor people," resulting in policy solutions being focused on individual factors. Given that individual characteristics were the focus of the analyses informing the policy recommendations concerning poor families and families receiving welfare, it should not be surprising that the major features of the federal act that ended "welfare as we know it" and created the Temporary Assistance for Needy Families (TANF) in 1996 emphasized remedial solutions to the flaws of individuals (i.e., failure to be gainfully employed) and proposed increasing marriage rates (in 2002 with newer federal legislation) as means for addressing deep poverty. Of the type of research that was informing policy formulation, O'Conner notes that the "problem was with what was being left out. Poverty analysts at that time rarely incorporated institutional practices, political decisions, or structural economic changes into their research; the focus was on individuals and families, not society." This legislation permanently eliminated a long-standing guaranteed income for women and families in deep poverty, and the misguided focus of the evidence being generated to inform policy options supported the new controversial policies (O'Connor 2001).

Lest we repeat such experiences in social epidemiology, solution-focused research must expand beyond individual and proximal social risk factors and markers. Recent frameworks more explicitly and more appropriately identify the macrosocial determinants of health that should be included in the focus of our work, especially when conducting solution-focused research. For example, in 2008 the World Health Organization (WHO) Commission on Social Determinants of Health put forth a framework that builds upon several existing frameworks and ideas and explicitly identifies the role of macrosocial as well as proximal social determinants of health (Fig. 1.1).

Although social inequality has become a major focus of social epidemiologic research and of many major, authoritative reports (Commission on Social Determinants of Health 2008) in the last two decades, and has even been implicated as a major cause of morbidity and mortality, there are others who feel as Navarro (2009) does when he claims that "it is not *inequalities* that kill, but *those who benefit from the inequalities* that kill" (emphasis in original). There are also those who argue that macrosocial interventions might be less effective than proximal interventions (Rothman et al. 1998), but we disagree. Macrosocial policies and processes are efficient ways of both increasing and curtailing social and health inequalities and should be a greater focus of our work, both in terms of identifying how they contribute to inequalities and how they can be modified to bring about positive social change (Goldberg et al. 2002; House 2002; Muntaner and Chung 2008; Putnam and Galea 2008; Stuckler 2008). This is not to say that we should not focus at all on proximal social determinants, but rather that the focus on macrosocial factors has been too sparse to date and should receive greater emphasis if our research is to inform policies and programs to address social inequities.

A number of chapters in this book illustrate how social epidemiologists can and do incorporate macrosocial factors into frameworks and research studies. Not surprisingly, some (but not all) of this research involves qualitative methods or mixed qualitative and quantitative approaches – methods that do not typically appear in epidemiology textbooks or get taught in epidemiology training programs. In this volume, Shankardass (Chap. 6) presents a conceptual framework for the mediating

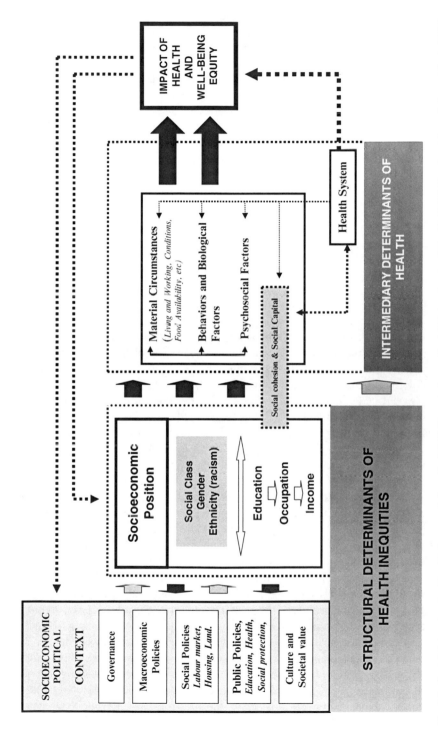

Fig. 1.1 Social determinants of health framework from the WHO Commission on Social Determinants of Health, 2007 (Reprinted from Solar and Irwin 2007)

role of place-based stress on chronic disease disparities. Drawing on sociological, psychological and psychoneuroimmunological research, and integrating notions of geographical "place," the chapter presents a multidisciplinary narrative review of the stress discourse and adopts a systems view to describe the macrosocial environmental determinants of chronic stress and its impact on chronic disease. Yen, Shim and Martínez (Chap. 8) apply two sociological paradigms – conflict theory and interactionist theory – to neighbourhood-health research, using Eric Klinenberg's *Heat Wave* as an illustrative example. They also discuss how these social theories can be used to expand upon the proposed mechanisms, namely social capital and physical disorder, connecting neighbourhoods, place and health. Rhodes and colleagues (Chap. 10) apply the concepts of "structural violence" and "structural vulnerability" to the social epidemiology of HIV risks among marginalized populations. Using four illustrative case studies of sex trade workers and injection drug users, they consider how methods and concepts in the social and epidemiologic sciences can be used to understand HIV risk as an effect of social, cultural and political conditions. Muntaner and colleagues (Chap. 9) discuss the role of politics in social epidemiology. Using political economy of health and welfare regimes frameworks, they present the results of a systematic literature review of 73 empirical and comparative studies on politics and health. Through this review, they show that political and welfare state variables are salient determinants of population health and health inequalities and that absolute and relative health differences exist across countries along a range of political variables. The chapter also takes into account important considerations regarding comparative political studies in social epidemiology. Shankardass and Dunn (Chap. 7) provide a discussion of space, geography and neighbourhoods. They argue that despite a longstanding focus on neighbourhoods, social epidemiology has failed to identify the social mechanisms of causation that result in inequalities. In particular, they critique the treatment of neighbourhoods as "containers" and argue for a more diverse use of theory to capture and explain complexity in neighbourhood processes.

Social epidemiologists will not generate critical evidence needed to inform the solutions to the most pressing social problems unless we use frameworks and theories that tap into the macrosocial determinants of health (Kaplan 2004; Schwartz and Carpenter 1999; Krieger 2008; Morabia 2009; Putnam and Galea 2008). A major barrier to studying the influence of macrosocial factors on health is the absence of appropriate data and research methods to operationalize the study of these frameworks. As can be seen in the WHO Commission on Social Determinants of Health framework (Fig. 1.1), macrosocial determinants have complex relationships to the proximal determinants of health inequities or health outcomes. Not only are macrosocial and economic factors at a different level of analysis than individual-based health outcomes, but the interaction between macrosocial factors and individual-level risks and outcomes (i.e., cross-level interactions) complicate their study. Currently, most research on inequities relies primarily on individual-level, cross-sectional and (more rarely) longitudinal data sets that are not ideally suited for the study of macrosocial determinants of health (Crone 2011; Dahlgren and Whitehead 1991; Wallace 2008; Westley et al. 2006). Even when newer methods for complex, multilevel social determinants of health are proposed (Galea et al. 2009), methodological issues present ongoing challenges. As noted previously, databases of individuals, while useful for understanding proximal contributors to health, cannot reveal the key pathways of macrosocial and economic processes that influence individual well-being. Two chapters in this book address issues surrounding data and the systems that generate relevant data for social epidemiology. Smylie, Lofters, Firestone and O'Campo (Chap. 4) offer strategies for the transformation of population-based data and data systems currently used in social epidemiology into social resources that actively contribute to social, economic and political solutions to reduce health inequities. They argue that population health data collection, management, analysis and use systems are too often disconnected from communities. In order for data to become a tool for social empowerment and social change, the social structuring of data governance and management must transform from systems that reinforce social exclusion to systems in which communities are fully and centrally involved in data collection decision making. Lofters and O'Campo (Chap. 5) explore how the practice of stratification based on variables or indicators such as race, ethnicity, gender and socioeconomic position can evolve from simply demonstrating social inequalities to identifying underlying causes of gaps in health status. Through a discussion of theories about casual mechanisms, societal and contextual factors, and the heterogeneity of experiences within socially-defined groups, they offer key recommendations for how stratification in social epidemiologic analyses can be used to go beyond just describing inequalities and gaps to generating evidence to inform interventions – and evaluations of interventions – that target identified health inequities.

One issue that deserves much more explicit attention in our field is the role of values in informing social epidemiologic research. Bayoumi and Guta (Chap. 3) use theories of ethics – including deontological ethics, consequentialism, rights theory, virtue ethics, communitarianism and the capability approach – to show how core values can inform social epidemiology research. Using two illustrative examples from harm reduction and obesity research, the authors demonstrate that social epidemiology research is inherently value-laden. They draw upon critical theory and sociological models to develop a value-based vision of social epidemiology that is critical, engaged and relevant.

Another area where methods are being refined and developed to generate strong evidence for solutions draws from realist philosophy (Chap. 2). Realist philosophy is fruitful for what we hope is a forthcoming theoretical turn in social epidemiology, as it provides an alternative to positivism for conducting causal analysis and explanation. This alternative framework reflects the reality that social phenomena, like social inequalities in health, are open systems, and require theoretical explanations. Two other chapters in this volume draw explicitly upon realist philosophy, focusing on evidence synthesis and evaluation of interventions, respectively. Kirst and O'Campo (Chap. 11) apply realist philosophy to systematic literature review methods and offer these methods as a critical research tool that can be used by social epidemiologists to evaluate interventions for complex health problems. Using the example of a realist-informed review of universal intimate partner violence screening programs in health care settings, they use these methods to identify key intervention mechanisms and contextual effects associated with successful programs. Sridharan, Dunn and Nakaima (Chap. 12) discuss realism as it applies to the evaluation of social programs and interventions to address health inequities. The authors emphasize the importance of understanding the contexts and mechanisms needed for interventions to work in addressing health inequities and focus on the time-dependent dynamics of interventions and their implications for evaluation of complex population-based programs.

1.4   Making Social Epidemiology Matter

Social epidemiologists should be strongly committed to generating actionable evidence for the solutions to the problems under study. As such, we must not only refocus the topics of our research to generate evidence to inform solutions, but we must also become more effective at disseminating our existing research, and, perhaps more importantly, we must ensure that we generate evidence and explanations that can be used to inform and support positive social change. While the topics of policy-relevant research and knowledge translation have been addressed previously, we seek to extend those discussions by incorporating the perspective of those engaged in designing programs and/or disseminating research findings. The final section of our book explores how social epidemiology can make a difference to policy and practice in terms of knowledge translation, community-academic partnerships and public health practice. Murphy and Fafard (Chap. 13) review the applicability of conventional knowledge translation strategies and argue that increased recognition of the complex social, political and value-based dimensions of policy and research is required for social epidemiology research to have practical and political impacts. Drawing on Jürgen Habermas' "knowledge constitutive interests" framework, they discuss how taking power, politics and values seriously can ensure that social epidemiology research plays a significant role in advancing social change. Schafer (Chap. 14) looks at how social epidemiologists who train and work in academic institutions can collaborate with program planners and policy makers in the community to address health problems. Interspersed within this chapter are excerpts from a conversation between its author, Peter Schafer (a community-based program planner), and Patricia O'Campo (an academic social epidemiologist) about the successes and challenges of their longstanding community-academic partnership for the Baltimore Healthy Start Program in Maryland. Finally, Mowat and Chambers (Chap. 15) discuss how social epidemiologists can produce evidence that is more relevant to public health policy and practice. Based on Dr. Mowat's experiences as the Medical Officer of Health for the Region of Peel in Ontario, Canada, they examine the challenges associated with integrating social epidemiology research into practice and offer guidance for how a social epidemiology research agenda can be implemented.

1.5   Conclusions

This volume is intended to be a constructive contribution to help guide the future of social epidemiology, a field that has much to contribute to the reduction of health inequities among many groups in many parts of the world. Yet at this stage of its development, the very things that helped social epidemiologists gain legitimacy in mainstream epidemiology (e.g., a strong focus and attention to scientific rigour, generalizability, etc.), may be what inhibit its wider impact in redressing health inequalities. That it not to say that we are promoting weaker studies; the same kinds of scientific activity that have been the cornerstones of social epidemiology must continue, but they must be supplemented by more theoretical research, a more pluralistic approach to methods and, ultimately, a more solution-focused emphasis that embraces the needs of decision makers. The purpose of this book is to assist in broadening the focus of social epidemiology from analysis to action. Although many will disagree with the premise of the book, we hope that all social epidemiologists can take something from it for their work. The health of many could be profoundly affected by evidence that directly informs greater action.

References

Acevedo-Garcia D, Lochner KA, Osypuk TL et al (2003) Future directions in residential segregation and health research: a multilevel approach. Am J Public Health 93:215–221

Altevogt BM, Hanson S, Leshner A (2008) Autism and the environment: challenges and opportunities for research. Pediatrics 121:1225–1229

Asthana S, Halliday J (2006) Inequalities in the health behaviour of children and youth: policy and practice. In: Asthana S, Halliday J (eds) What works in tackling health inequalities? Pathways, policies and practice through the lifecourse. The Policy Press, Bristol

Atkins D, Moy E (2005) Left behind: the legacy of hurricane Katrina. BMJ 331:916–918

Bambra C (2011) Work, worklessness and the political economy of health inequalities. J Epidemiol Community Health:jech.2009.102103Published Online First: 30 January 2011

Berkman LF (2004) Seeing the forest and the trees: new visions in social epidemiology. Am J Epidemiol 160:1–2

Berkman LF, Kawachi I (2000) Social epidemiology. Oxford University Press, New York

Bernstein K, Galea S, Ahern J et al (2007) The built environment and alcohol consumption in urban neighborhoods. Drug Alcohol Depend 91:244–252

Bhopal R (1997) Which book? A comparative review of 25 introductory epidemiology textbooks. J Epidemiol Community Health 51:612–622

Bonneux L (2007) From evidence based bioethics to evidence based social policies. Eur J Epidemiol 22:483–485

Borrell C, Marí-Dell'Olmo M, Rodríguez-Sanz M et al (2006) Socioeconomic position and excess mortality during the heat wave of 2003 in Barcelona. Eur J Epidemiol 21:633–640

Boulton ML, Lemmings J, Beck AJ (2009) Assessment of epidemiology capacity in state health departments, 2001–2006. J Public Health Manag Pract 15:328–336

Braveman PA (2006) Health disparities and health equity: concepts and measurement. Annu Rev Public Health 27:167–194

Braveman PA (2007) We also need bold experiments: a response to Starfield's "Commentary: pathways of influence on equity in health". Soc Sci Med 64:1363–1366

Braveman PA, Egerter SA, Mockenhaupt RE (2011) Broadening the focus: the need to address the social determinants of health. Am J Prev Med 40:S4–18

Broom A, Willis E (2007) Competing paradigms and health research. In: Saks M, Allsop J (eds) Researching health: qualitative, quantitative and mixed methods. Sage, London

Brown P (1987) Popular epidemiology: community response to toxic waste-induced disease in Woburn, Massachusetts. Sci Technol Hum Values 12:78–85

Brown P (1992) Popular epidemiology and toxic waste contamination: lay and professional ways of knowing. J Health Soc Behav 33:267–281

Brownson RC, Chriqui JF, Stamatakis KA (2009a) Understanding evidence-based public health policy. Am J Public Health 99:1576–1583

Brownson RC, Fielding JE, Maylahn CM (2009b) Evidence-based public health: a fundamental concept for public health practice. Annu Rev Public Health 30:175–201

Burawoy M (2004) Public sociologies: contradictions, dilemmas, and possibilities. Soc Forces 82:1603–1618

Carpiano RM, Daley DM (2006) A guide and glossary on postpositivist theory building for population health. J Epidemiol Community Health 60:564–570

Centre for Research on the Epidemiology of Disasters (CRED) (2011) 2010 disasters in numbers. http://www.preventionweb.net/files/17615_confpress2010.pdf. Accessed 25 Apr 2011

Chou YJ, Huang N, Lee CH et al (2004) Who is at risk of death in an earthquake. Am J Epidemiol 160:688–695

Commission on Social Determinants of Health (2008) Closing the gap in a generation: health equity through action on the social determinants of health. Final report of the Commission on Social Determinants of Health. World Health Organization, Geneva

Crone J (2011) How can we solve our social problems? 2nd edn. Pine Forge Press, Thousand Oaks

Cwikel J (2006) Social epidemiology: strategies for public health activism. Columbia University Press, New York

Dahlgren G, Whitehead M (1991) Policies and strategies to promote social equity in health. Institute for Futures Studies, Stockholm

Diez-Roux AV (1998) Bringing context back into epidemiology: variables and fallacies in multilevel analysis. Am J Public Health 88:216–222

Dunn JR (2006) Speaking theoretically about population health. J Epidemiol Community Health 60:572–573

Edwards KL, Clarke GP, Ransley JK et al (2010) The neighbourhood matters: studying exposures relevant to childhood obesity and the policy implications in Leeds, UK. J Epidemiol Community Health 64:194–201

Elliott JR, Pais J (2006) Race, class and Hurricane Katrina: social differences in human responses to disaster. Soc Sci Res 35:295–321

Ellwood W (2006) The no-nonsense guide to globalization, 2nd edn. New Internationalist Publications, Oxford

Epstein RA (2003) Let the shoemaker stick to his last: a defense of the "old" public health. Perspect Biol Med 46:S138–159

Fothergill A, Maestas EG, Darlington JD (1999) Race, ethnicity and disasters in the United States: a review of the literature. Disasters 23:156–173

Fuchs M (1996) Woburn's burden of proof: corporate social responsibility and public health. J Undergrad Sci 3:165–170

Galea S, Hall C, Kaplan GA (2009) Social epidemiology and complex system dynamic modelling as applied to health behaviour and drug use research. Int J Drug Policy 20:209–216

Goldberg M, Melchoir M, Leclerc A et al (2002) Social factors in health: recent contributions from social epidemiology and the social sciences of health. Sci Soc Sante 20:75–128

Gómez-Olmedo M, Delgado-Rodriguez M, Bueno-Cavanillas A et al (1996) Prenatal care and prevention of preterm birth. A case-control study in southern Spain. Eur J Epidemiol 12:37–44

Hacker J, Pierson P (2010) Winner-take-all politics: public policy, political organization and the precipitous rise of top incomes in the United States. Polit Soc 38:152–204

House JS (2002) Understanding social factors and inequalities in health: 20th century progress and 21st century prospects. J Health Soc Behav 43:125–142

James SA (2009) Epidemiologic research on health disparities: some thoughts on history and current developments. Epidemiol Rev 31:1–6

Kaplan GA (2004) What's wrong with social epidemiology, and how can we make it better? Epidemiol Rev 26:124–135

Kasl SV, Jones BA (2002) Social epidemiology: towards a better understanding of the field. Int J Epidemiol 31:1094–1097

Krieger N (1999) Questioning epidemiology: objectivity, advocacy, and socially responsible science. Am J Public Health 89:1151–1153

Krieger N (2008) Proximal, distal, and the politics of causation: what's level got to do with it? Am J Public Health 98:221–230

Krieger N (2011) Epidemiology and the people's health: theory and context. Oxford University Press, New York

Kruk M, Prescott M, de Pinho H et al (2011) Equity and the child health Millennium Development Goal: the role of pro-poor health policies. J Epidemiol Community Health 65:327–333

Leung MW, Yen IH, Minkler M (2004) Community based participatory research: a promising approach for increasing epidemiology's relevance in the 21st century. Int J Epidemiol 33:499–506

Macinko JA, Shi L, Starfield B et al (2003) Income inequality and health: a critical review of the literature. Med Care Res Rev 60:407–452

Mackenbach JP (2009) Politics is nothing but medicine at a larger scale: reflections on public health's biggest idea. J Epidemiol Community Health 63:181–184

Matheson FI, Moineddin R, Glazier RH (2008) The weight of place: a multilevel analysis of gender, neighborhood material deprivation, and body mass index among Canadian adults. Soc Sci Med 66:675–690

Minkler M (2005) Community-based research partnerships: challenges and opportunities. J Urban Health 82:ii3–12

Morabia A (2009) Is epidemiology nothing but politics at a different level? J Epidemiol Community Health 63:188–190

Morgan G (2005) Highlighting the importance of "popular epidemiology". J Epidemiol Community Health 59:254

Muntaner C, Chung H (2008) Macrosocial determinants, epidemiology, and health policy: should politics and economics be banned from social determinants of health research? J Public Health Policy 29:299–306

Muntaner C, Sridharan S, Chung H et al (2010) The solution space: developing research and policy agendas to eliminate employment-related health inequalities. Int J Health Serv 40:309–314

Naughton MP, Henderson A, Mirabelli MC et al (2002) Heath-related mortality during 1999 heat wave in Chicago. Am J Prev Med 22:221–227

Navarro V (2009) What we mean by social determinants of health. Glob Health Promot 16:5–16

O'Campo P, Rojas-Smith L (1998) Welfare reform and women's health: review of the literature and implications for state policy. J Public Health Policy 19:420–446

O'Campo P, Gielen AC, Faden RR et al (1995) Violence by male partners against women during the childbearing year: a contextual analysis. Am J Public Health 85:1092–1097

O'Campo P, Xue X, Wang MC et al (1997) Neighborhood risk factors for low birthweight in Baltimore: a multilevel analysis. Am J Public Health 87:1113–1118

O'Campo P, Kirst M, Schaefer-McDaniel N et al (2009) Community-based services for homeless adults experiencing concurrent mental health and substance use disorders: a realist approach to synthesizing evidence. J Urban Health 86:985–989

O'Campo P, Kirst M, Tsamis C et al (2011) Implementing successful intimate partner violence screening programs in health care settings: evidence generated from a realist-informed systematic review. Soc Sci Med 72:855–866

O'Connor A (2001) Poverty knowledge: social science, social policy, and the poor in twentieth century U.S. history. Princeton University Press, Princeton

Oakes JM (2005) An analysis of American Journal of Epidemiology citations with special reference to statistics and social science. Am J Epidemiol 161:494–500

Oakes JM, Kaufman J (2006) Methods in social epidemiology. Josey-Bass, San Francisco

Phelan JC, Link BG, Diez-Roux AV et al (2004) "Fundamental causes" of social inequalities in mortality: a test of the theory. J Health Social Behav 45:265–285

Putnam S, Galea S (2008) Epidemiology and the macrosocial determinants of health. J Public Health Policy 29:275–289

Rothman KJ, Adami HO, Ttichopoulos D (1998) Should the mission of epidemiology include the eradication of poverty? Lancet 352:810–813

Roy A (2010) Poverty capital: microfinance and the making of development. Routledge, New York

Ruffin J (2010) The science of eliminating health disparities: embracing a new paradigm. Am J Public Health 100:S8–9

Rychetnik L, Frommer M, Hawe P et al (2002) Criteria for evaluating evidence on public health interventions. J Epidemiol Community Health 56:119–127

San Sebastián M, Hurtig AK (2005) Oil development and health in the Amazon basin of Ecuador: the popular epidemiology process. Soc Sci Med 60:799–807

Sanson-Fisher RW, Bonevski B, Green LW et al (2007) Limitations of the RCT in evaluating population-based health interventions. Am J Prev Med 33:155–161

Savitz DA, Poole C, Miller WC (1999) Reassessing the role of epidemiology in public health. Am J Public Health 89:1158–1161

Schnarch B (2004) Ownership, Control, Access, and Possession (OCAP) or self-determination applied to research: a critical analysis of contemporary First Nations research and some options for First Nations communities. First Nations Centre, National Aboriginal Health Organization, Ottawa

Schwartz S, Carpenter KM (1999) The right answer for the wrong question: consequences of Type III error for public health research. Am J Public Health 89:1175–1180

Schwartz S, Susser E, Susser M (1999) A future for epidemiology. Ann Rev Public Health 20:15–33

Seabrook J (2007) The no-nonsense guide to world poverty, 2nd edn. New Internationalist Publications, Oxford

Smedslund G, Hagen KB, Steiro A, Johme T, Dalsbø TK, Rud MG (2006) Work programmes for welfare recipients. Rapport fra Kunnskapssenteret nr 20 - 2006. ISBN 82-8121-120-2 ISSN 1503-9544

Solar O, Irwin A (2007) A conceptual framework for action on the social determinants of health. Discussion paper for the Commission on Social Determinants of Health. World Health Organization, Geneva

Sorensen G, Barbeau E, Hunt MK et al (2004) Reducing social disparities in tobacco use: a social-contextual model for reducing tobacco use among blue-collar workers. Am J Public Health 94:230–239

Starfield B (2007) Pathways of influence on equity in health: a rejoinder to Braveman and Wilkinson. Soc Sci Med 64:1371–1372

Stuckler D (2008) Population causes and consequences of leading chronic diseases: a comparative analysis of prevailing explanations. Milbank Q 86:273–326

Syme SL (2008) Reducing racial and social-class inequalities in health: the need for a new approach. Health Aff (Milwood) 27:456–459

Thacker SB, Buffington J (2001) Applied epidemiology for the 21st century. Int J Epidemiol 30:320–325

Venkatapuram S, Marmot M (2009) Epidemiology and social justice in light of social determinants of health research. Bioethics 23:79–89

Walke HT, Simone PM (2009) Building capacity in field epidemiology: lessons learned from the experience in Europe. Euro Surveill 14:Pii = 19376

Wallace B (2008) Toward equity in health: a new global approach to health disparities. Springer, New York

Wallerstein N, Duran B (2010) Community-based participatory research contributions to intervention research: the intersection of science and practice to improve health equity. Am J Public Health 100:S40–46

Welsh BC, Farrington DP (2008) Effects of closed circuit television surveillance on crime. Campbell Systematic Reviews 17 http://www.campbellcollaboration.org/

Westley F, Zimmerman B, Patton MQ (2006) Getting to maybe: how the world is changed. Vintage Canada, Toronto

Whitehead M (2007) A typology of actions to tackle social inequalities in health. J Epidemiol Community Health 61:473–478

Wilkinson R (2007) The challenge of prevention: a response to Starfield's "Commentary: pathways of influence on equity in health". Soc Sci Med 64:1367–1370

Williams GH (2003) The determinants of health: structure, context and agency. Sociol Health Illn 25:131–154

Woodcock J, Aldred R (2008) Cars, corporations, and commodities: consequences for the social determinants of health. Emerg Themes Epidemiol 5:4

Yen IH (2005) Historical perspective: S. Leonard Syme's influence on the development of social epidemiology and where we go from there. Epidemiol Perspect Innov 2:3

Part I
Foundations

Chapter 2
"Explanation," Philosophy and Theory in Health Inequalities Research: Towards a Critical Realist Approach

James R. Dunn

Contents

2.1	Introduction	24
2.2	The Challenge	25
2.3	Philosophical Underpinnings of Social Epidemiology	26
2.4	Key Principles of Critical Realism	27
2.5	"Explanation": A Realist Approach	28
2.6	Causal Analysis	30
2.7	Types of Research	33
2.8	From Qualitative/Quantitative Research to Extensive/Intensive Research	34
2.9	Practical Adequacy	37
2.10	Implications for Social Epidemiology Research	39
References		40

Abstract The relative lack of attention to philosophy and theory in research on social inequalities in health and its consequences for explanation and methodology has been described in the social epidemiologic literature. Nevertheless, the field of social epidemiology, dominated as it is by the trappings of positivism, is arguably still in need of further development of epistemological frameworks that can adequately incorporate richer explanations of the phenomena we study. Some have advocated for the adoption of a critical realist perspective for the study of social inequalities in health in order to overcome some of the difficulties described above. This chapter uses critical realism as a means to identify some of the epistemological and methodological difficulties inherent in attempts to explain health inequalities (especially the connection between social and biological mechanisms) and offer an "affirmative" approach to health inequalities research based on the insights of critical realist philosophy. In both the physical and social sciences, concerns about

J.R. Dunn (✉)
Department of Health, Aging and Society, McMaster University, Kenneth Taylor Hall 226,
1280 Main Street West, Hamilton, ON L8S 4L8, Canada
e-mail: jim.dunn@mcmaster.ca

P. O'Campo and J.R. Dunn (eds.), *Rethinking Social Epidemiology:*
Towards a Science of Change, DOI 10.1007/978-94-007-2138-8_2,
© Springer Science+Business Media B.V. 2012

epistemology and philosophy are routinely left unexamined. This chapter argues that a more explicit engagement with such questions is an important next step in social epidemiology and health inequalities research. The chapter begins with a description of the explanatory problem faced by research on social inequalities in health. This explanatory task is difficult, but it is precisely that difficulty which cannot be adequately accommodated by the unacknowledged epistemological underpinnings of social epidemiology. The chapter highlights several key features of the critical realist approach and demonstrates how these can be usefully applied to health inequalities research to solve persistent problems of explanation and methodological pluralism. Specifically, the chapter argues that the complexity of the social phenomena implicated in this research demands a more detailed consideration of what is meant by causation, "explanation" and "theory," and of what the relationship of these concepts should be to empirical research.

2.1 Introduction

The relative lack of attention to philosophy and theory in research on social inequalities in health and its consequences for explanation and methodology have been the subject of several articles in the past several years (Forbes and Wainwright 2001; Wainwright and Forbes 2000; Krieger 1994, 1999, 2001; Muntaner 2004). The attention to theory, philosophy and explanation in such writings, however, has been dwarfed by the explosive growth of empirical research, which, it could be argued, has repeatedly generated highly similar findings regarding the differential distribution of health status by socioeconomic status, but produced far less "explanation." What little explanation has been produced has leaned heavily towards biological reductionism (Taylor et al. 1997), while relatively little has been accomplished in filling an obvious vacuum of *social* explanation.[1] This state of affairs, in turn, has prompted calls for more theory (Krieger 2001), but it is clear that the field of social epidemiology, dominated as it is by the trappings of positivism, is still in need of further development of epistemological frameworks that can adequately incorporate richer explanations of the phenomena we study.

Arguments similar to these are made very effectively by Forbes and Wainwright (2001) and Wainwright and Forbes (2000). They advocate the adoption of a critical realist perspective for the study of social inequalities in health in order to overcome some of the difficulties described above. I share Wainwright and Forbes' enthusiasm

---

[1] There are, of course, some examples of works that have been at least partly successful at mounting social explanations, including the work of Kawachi and others on social capital (Kawachi et al. 1997, 2004; Kawachi 1999), Wilkinson (1996) with regards to social capital and other psychosocial factors, Hertzman and Marmot's (1996) explanations of the health consequences of rapid economic change in central and eastern Europe, and the work of a number of authors offering sociopolitical explanations (e.g., Navarro et al. 2006; Bambra et al. 2009).

for the realist approach in general, but emphasize different components of that approach. Also, rather than using critical realism just to critique health inequalities research, as Forbes and Wainwright do, in this paper I also use it to identify some of the epistemological and methodological difficulties inherent in attempts to explain health inequalities (especially the connection between social and biological mechanisms), and I offer what I call an "affirmative" approach to health inequalities research based on the insights of critical realist philosophy. While I acknowledge the important role that philosophical approaches such as critical realism have to play in critiquing existing research, I believe that critical realism has more to offer the field than simply a critique. It can be a tool for mounting explanations of complex phenomena, drawing on knowledge from diverse disciplines, not unlike the idea of critical epidemiology described in Chap. 1. In both the physical and the social sciences, concerns about epistemology and philosophy are routinely left unexamined, but I argue that a more explicit engagement with such questions is an important next step in social epidemiology and health inequalities research.

I begin the paper by delimiting what I believe to be the explanatory problem faced by research on social inequalities in health. In so doing, I underscore the difficulty of the explanatory task, which a growing number of scholars have chosen to tackle. But it is precisely that difficulty which cannot be adequately accommodated by the unacknowledged epistemological underpinnings of social epidemiology. I then highlight several key features of the critical realist approach and demonstrate how these can be usefully applied to health inequalities research to solve persistent problems of explanation and methodological pluralism. Specifically, I argue that the complexity of the social phenomena implicated in this research demands a more detailed consideration of what is meant by causation, "explanation" and "theory," and of what the relationship of these concepts should be to empirical research. The discussion that follows is guided by philosophical investigations within scientific realism (Bhaskar 1975, 1979a, b, 1989; Pawson 1989), with particular emphasis on the work of Andrew Sayer, who provides an excellent translation of realist philosophy into practical terms for use in empirical social research (Sayer 1992, 1993, 1997).

2.2 The Challenge

Stated briefly, I take one of the main challenges of social epidemiology, and the focus of the remainder of this chapter, to be related to explaining the differential distribution of health status by socioeconomic position. This differential distribution is an enduring tendency that holds across a wide variety of health conditions and disease states, from accidents and injuries to mental illness to coronary heart disease, and for a variety of conceptions of socioeconomic position (e.g., social class, minority status, educational attainment) to different degrees at different stages of the life course, and the pattern is generally more pronounced for males than females. The explanatory task of social epidemiology, therefore, is to be able to combine both empirical and theoretical research that links: (1) "cell to society" (actually, sub-cellular as well) through some sort of "bio-psycho-social translation" or similar alternative (Tarlov 1996); (2) individuals to the experience of a quasi-nested, scaled and stratified social world ("neurons to neighbourhoods to nation-states") (Shonkoff and Phillips 2000); and (3) "cradle to grave" or, stated differently, research that can explain exposures, experiences and outcomes separated by differing, but often very long temporal scales (for example, from early childhood to late adulthood) through different possible modes, including latent, cumulative and pathways effects (Hertzman and Weins 1996). All of this, of course, must account for a complex background of both slowly evolving and punctuated historical changes and an increasingly complex set of geopolitical relations across the globe (Dunn 2006).

2.3 Philosophical Underpinnings of Social Epidemiology

Social epidemiology is a science that descends from the positivist tradition. The term positivism has its origins in French social theory. It is often attributed to Auguste Comte (1798–1857), but in fact Comte took the idea from enlightenment thinker Henri Saint-Simon (1760–1825) who was very concerned to establish a new order for society, one based upon the principles of science and industry, as opposed to traditional forms of social domination through nobility and the church.

As a philosophy to guide science, positivism is concerned with the development of knowledge in the form of general statements (ideally universal laws that apply across time and space) obtained through the application of accepted procedures about observable phenomena. Positivism asserts that the only authentic knowledge is that which is based on sense, experience and positive verification.

In its strongest formulation, positivism consists of a set of six principles (Halfpenny 1982; Keat 1981; Bryman 1988; Gartell and Gartell 1996; Ciaffa 1998):

1. The unity of science and its methods – i.e., belief that the methods of the natural sciences are appropriate to the social sciences and indeed, that the only legitimate knowledge of society can come from the application of such methods. Sometimes called methodological naturalism.
2. Knowledge can only be generated by empirical means, specifically, by observation with the senses. This excludes any phenomena that cannot be observed with the senses directly or indirectly with instruments (i.e., metaphysical notions like "social structure" or subjective experience). This principle is sometimes known as empiricism.
3. The objective of scientific research is to explain and predict, and these are symmetrical processes, achieved through the accumulation of empirically established regularities or laws. Most positivists would also say that the ultimate goal is to develop laws of general understanding by creating a model of the phenomenon in question that is simultaneously explanatory and predictive. This principle is often known as inductivism.
4. Scientific knowledge is testable. Research, according to this principle, should be mostly deductive. Scientific theories are seen as providing raw materials for hypotheses, which are developed so that they can be tested in empirical research.

5. Science must distance itself from common sense, which is seen as a source of bias in what is supposed to be an objective activity. Scientific procedures should be capable of generating knowledge that contradicts common sense.
6. Scientific knowledge must be value neutral. The goal of science, in fact, is to produce knowledge regardless of any values, morals or politics held by scientists. The quality of scientific research should be judged by logic, and it should, ideally, produce universal, generalized statements.

There are now numerous distinct versions of positivism, many of which do not subscribe to strong versions of all of these claims. For example, most contemporary social researchers do not believe in the existence of general social laws, and, increasingly, positivist research acknowledges the impossibility of value neutrality. Nevertheless, positivism still constitutes the philosophical basis for social epidemiology. This approach carries with it certain strengths, which are well documented, but also certain weaknesses. In this chapter, the underlying argument is that the realist approach could allow epidemiology's strengths to be maximized and its weaknesses to be minimized.

2.4 Key Principles of Critical Realism

Realist philosophy begins from several key propositions, a few of which are worth highlighting from the outset. The first is that the world exists independently of our knowledge of it; that is, there is a real world that exists whether we are aware of it or not (although our access to it is mediated by our senses and other factors) (Sayer 1992). This presupposition is in contradistinction to the viewpoint of idealist philosophy, which says that something only exists if it can be observed. Indeed, the term "realist" is meant to distinguish this school of thought from idealism.

The second key proposition is that all knowledge is fallible and theory laden. Indeed, realists are fond of saying that they are "inherent fallibilists," and that all knowledge is subject to review, change and correction. In this sense, the goal of science for realists is not to discover the truth or universal laws that apply in all times and all places, but rather to develop knowledge that is "practically adequate" but that is constantly subject to revision based on the fallibilist notion above. Practical adequacy will be discussed in more detail shortly. Indeed, as Sayer (1992) argues

> social science has been singularly unsuccessful in discovering law-like regularities. One of the main achievements of recent realist philosophy has been to show that this is an inevitable consequence of an erroneous view of causation. Realism replaces the regularity model with one in which objects and social relations have causal powers which may or may not produce regularities, and which can be explained independent of them.

Consequently, in realism, "less weight is put on quantitative methods for discovering and assessing regularities and more on methods of establishing the qualitative nature of social objects and relations on which causal mechanisms depend" (Sayer 1992).

As mentioned above, in addition to being fallible, all knowledge is theory laden. According to Sayer (1992), "concepts of truth and falsity fail to provide a coherent view of the relationship between knowledge and its object." But knowledge can be checked empirically, and its effectiveness in informing and explaining successful material practice is "not mere accident" (Sayer 1992). Indeed, this is what is intended by the term "practical adequacy."

A third proposition of realism that is important to the following discussion is that "there is necessity in the world; objects – whether natural or social – necessarily have particular causal powers or ways of acting and particular susceptibilities" (Sayer 1992). An important, but under-acknowledged goal of science is to distinguish between necessity (empirical events that occur because of the operation of internal causal mechanisms of objects) and contingency (empirical events that occur because of contingent factors that are unrelated to the operation of mechanisms). For example, it is because of necessary relations (the causal powers and liabilities of gunpowder, steel and human beings) that bullets fired from a gun can cause grave injuries or fatalities, but whether any particular gun is fired and wounds a particular person is a contingent matter.

A fourth proposition is that the "world is differentiated and stratified, consisting not only of events, but objects, including structures, which have powers and liabilities capable of generating events" (Sayer 1992). Most importantly, structures cannot be observed in the strict sense that positivism would insist (in other words, realism accepts metaphysics), and, like many things in the natural and social world, structures do not generate regular patterns of events.

Finally, realism argues that the social sciences, like epidemiology "must be critical of its object. In order to be able to explain and understand social phenomena we have to evaluate them critically." This concept is described more fully in a subsequent section. In the following section, the term "explanation" is recast from its positivist roots as a realist concept, with implications for rethinking social epidemiology.

2.5   "Explanation": A Realist Approach

Realism rejects the positivist assertion that prediction and explanation are symmetrical processes (i.e., that the ability of empirical models to predict events subsequently is a necessary condition for explaining the phenomena). Unlike positivism, from the realist perspective, identification of causal relationships *does not* depend on regularity of patterning of empirical events. The causes of World War I can be identified even though it only happened once and therefore does not constitute an empirical regularity. Indeed, in the social sciences regularities of patterning are rare because the objects of study in social science are typically open systems. Where regularities *are* observed in the social sciences, they "do not approach the universality and precision of those available to physicists and astronomers" (Sayer 1992). The reason for this is that in order for regularity of patterning to occur, the following two conditions must be met: first, "there must be no change or qualitative variation (e.g. impurities) in the object possessing the causal powers if mechanisms are to operate consistently. This is termed by Bhaskar the 'intrinsic condition for closure'" (Sayer 1992). Human beings have the capacity for learning, self-change and even resistance – to health promotion programs, for instance (see Chap. 12) – and therefore this condition is seldom met in the social sciences. The second condition that must be met for regularity of patterning to occur is that:

> the relationship between the causal mechanism and those of its external conditions which make some difference to its operation and effects must be constant if the outcome is to be regular (the extrinsic condition for closure). (Sayer 1992)

According to Sayer (1992), if *both* the intrinsic and extrinsic conditions are met, a *closed system* exists in which regularities may be produced, but, "most systems we encounter violate these conditions in some way and therefore any regularities they produce are at best approximate and short-lived; these are *open systems*" (Sayer 1992, emphasis in original; see also Bhaskar 1975, 1979a, b, 1989; Cloke et al. 1991; Pawson 1989). Now, the social gradient in health is a pattern that has been observed in hundreds of studies, but there is still a great deal of variance in health status that is not explained by socioeconomic position, strongly suggesting that the objects of study (societies) are open systems. It follows that close adherence to any form of positivism will be limited in terms of generating knowledge that can make a difference.

But not only is regularity of patterning of events rare in the social sciences, "patterns of events, be they regular or irregular, *are not self explanatory, but must be explained by reference to what produces them*" (Sayer 1992, emphasis added). This particular point is fundamental to moving forward in the field of social epidemiology. The observation of persistent inequalities in health status is the foundation of social epidemiology, and, to date, attempts to explain the pattern that do not take this observation as naively given are few in number compared to the number of publications that do little more than demonstrate the pattern empirically (Tarlov 1996; Wilkinson 1994, 1996 are exceptions[2]). Traditional approaches based on positivism (e.g., epidemiology) would suggest that more data is needed, with the expectation that eventually a regularity that better explains the phenomenon, or one that gives more certainty to an empirical relationship, will be found. According to the realist view, however, this relationship is not self-explanatory, but must be explained with reference to what produces it. Such an explanation would be expressed in terms of the mechanisms and structures thought to be responsible and, to use Sayer's (1992) terms, their "tendencies" to act in particular ways, their "ways of acting" or their "causal powers and liabilities." Human beings, for example, are vulnerable to suffocation or contagion of disease (a necessary relation), but who suffocates or contracts a contagious disease is a contingent matter.

---

[2] Link and Phelan's (1995) work on "fundamental causes" is a step in the right direction of deeper explanations, but I argue that the emphasis on social conditions and socioeconomic position is not fundamental enough, as its explanatory focus is situated primarily at the level of events (as opposed to mechanisms and structures – see Fig. 2.1) and it is not successful in distinguishing between necessary and contingent relations.

2.6   Causal Analysis

"To ask for the cause of something," argues Sayer, "is to ask what 'makes it happen', what 'produces', 'generates', 'creates', or 'determines' it, or, more weakly, what 'enables', or 'leads to' it" (1992). These common metaphors for describing causality are insufficient for scientific explanation, however, Sayer argues. According to the realist view, "causality concerns not a relationship between discrete events,… but the *'causal powers'* or *'liabilities'* of objects or relations, or more generally, their ways-of-acting or *'mechanisms'*" (Sayer 1992, emphasis in original). People have the causal powers of being able to work, speak, reason, walk, reproduce, learn, *et cetera*, and have causal liabilities such as susceptibility to persuasion, extremes of temperature, piercing by knives, *et cetera*. Causal powers often

> inhere not simply in single objects or individuals, but in the social relations and structures which they form. Thus the powers of a lecturer are not reducible to her characteristics as an individual but derive from her interdependent relations with students, colleagues, administrators, employer, spouse, etc. (Sayer 1992)

If causation is not a matter of linking discrete events, but rather a matter of causal powers and liabilities, it follows that "powers and liabilities can exist whether or not they are being exercised or suffered; unemployed workers have the power to work even though they are not doing so now" (Sayer 1992). It follows further – and this is a fundamental difference from positivistic methods and reasoning – that "a causal claim is not about regularity between separate things or events but about what an object is like and what it can do and only derivatively what it *will* do in any particular situation" (Sayer 1992).

Causal analysis, therefore, is about getting beyond the simple recognition that something produces some change, to understanding what it is about the object(s) that enables it (them) to do this. Often, however, relatively little is known about the mechanisms responsible for processes, for instance in the case of gravity, or the relationship between people's intentions and their actions (Sayer 1992). In the example of the electrical conductivity of copper, however, we do have knowledge of *how* the process works (presence of free ions in its structure) without reference to a "black box" – an actual causal mechanism has been postulated/identified, and it has been shown, at least to date, to be "practically adequate" for most purposes, scientific and otherwise (Sayer 1992). The "mode of inference" by which "events are explained by postulating (and identifying) mechanisms which are capable of producing them is called *'retroduction'*" (Sayer 1992, emphasis in original). Retroduction, it would seem, is crucial to the future of social epidemiologic research. Despite this, the depth with which epidemiological studies published in the top journals engage in retroduction is very shallow.

One final point on causation deserves attention before moving on to discuss types of research and the understanding of "explanation" from the realist perspective. Sayer (1992) reminds us that

> processes of change usually involve several causal mechanisms which may be only contingently related to one another. Not surprisingly then, depending on conditions, the operation

of the same mechanism can produce quite different results and, alternatively, different mechanisms may produce the same empirical result. At one level this seems unexceptional, although it does not rest easily with the orthodox view of causation in terms of regular associations.

As the analysis of the influences of social and economic factors upon health status at the individual and contextual levels involves a wide diversity of objects and relations stretched across time and space, it is going to be a complicated process that will belie orthodox conceptions of "proof" and certainty. Specifically, it demands identification of causal powers and liabilities of a diverse array of objects and relations and their conjunctures and will require different types of research and ways to integrate them.

But this raises an important question for the limits of epidemiology. As Sayer (1992) puts it, "can generalization and the search for regularities ever assist causal analysis?" He argues that in some cases "the discovery of empirical regularities may draw attention to objects whose causal powers might be responsible for the pattern and to conditions which are necessary for their existence and activation," providing an important role for standard epidemiologic methods. But, he argues, in order to confirm that such patterns point to the operation of causal mechanisms, "qualitative information is needed on the nature of the objects involved and not merely more quantitative data on empirical associations." In epidemiology, more data is routinely recommended in cases where uncertainty still exists, or, alternatively, an author may recommend improved measurement of "exposure" variables. However, more data without a better account of causal mechanisms is unlikely to reduce uncertainty and will do little to enhance explanation. As Sayer (1992) observes:

> So, for example, in epidemiology, ignorance of the causes and conditions of certain diseases may require a resort to mapping and charting quantitative data on a wide range of possible factors. It may seem reasonable to search for a factor which is common to all instances of the disease and hypothesize that this is the cause, or else a factor which is only present where the disease occurs. While they are worth trying, both methods fail to address the problem of finding a *mechanism* which *generates* the disease, as opposed to a factor which merely covaries with it. The weakness of the search for mere associations is illustrated in the well-known story of the drunk who tried to discover the causes of his drunkenness by using such methods: On Monday he had whisky and soda, and Tuesday gin and soda, on Wednesday vodka and soda and on other nights when he stayed sober, nothing; by looking for the common factor in the drinking pattern for the nights when he got drunk, he decides the soda water was the cause. Now the drunk might possibly have chosen alcohol as the common factor and hence as the cause. However, what gives such an inference credibility is not merely the knowledge that alcohol was a common factor, *but that it has a mechanism capable of inducing drunkenness.* (emphasis added)

Although this example may seem trivial, it is of critical importance to the future of social epidemiology. Given that one of the most common modes of analysis in social epidemiology is to identify common and distinguishing properties, it is essential to recognize the limitations of this approach. One obvious limitation is that it depends on the existence of counterfactuals, which might not always exist, and the search for which might miss important knowledge. There are two helpful examples of this. First is what Oakes (2004) calls "structural confounding," whereby in multilevel analysis there is not a full range of counterfactuals to test hypotheses about the relative influence of the neighbourhood or the individual on individual health (see also Chap. 7). In other words, it is often the case that there are too few poor people living in affluent neighbourhoods and *vice versa* to fully test the relative influence of individual versus neighbourhood income on health. The second example comes from the work of Geoffrey Rose (1985), who points out that typical, individual-based risk factor epidemiology, in its search for commonalities and differences among individuals, cannot account for risks to which whole populations are uniformly exposed.

This is not to say that epidemiology should stop doing such analysis, but as Sayer (1992) says, while many studies

> use available qualitative and causal knowledge to narrow down the list of possible factors to those which might have relevant powers and liabilities... *all too often the qualitative investigation is abandoned just at the point when it is most needed – for deciding the status and the causal (as opposed to statistical) significance of whatever patterns and associations are found.* When this happens, research may occlude rather than reveal causality. (Sayer 1992, emphasis added)

A good example of the kind of causal analysis that arguably needs to be encouraged in social epidemiology is illustrated by recent research by Mark Hunter. Working in South Africa, Hunter (2007) seeks to explain HIV infection rates in informal settlements in the early post-apartheid era via three interlinked dynamics critical to understanding the pandemic: (1) rising unemployment and social inequalities that leave some groups, especially poor women, extremely vulnerable; (2) greatly reduced marital rates and the subsequent increase of one-person households; and (3) rising levels of women's migration, especially through circular movements between rural areas and informal settlements in urban areas. He significantly improves upon previous explanations that lean on a specific culture of sex in South Africa and on the explanation of male migratory patterns and use of prostitutes. Specifically, Hunter identifies connections between poverty, the informal economy, money/sex exchanges and even the changing nature of love relationships in contemporary South African culture to explain HIV rates in these informal settlements where rates are said to be double the national average. To do this, he uses a combination of demographic, ethnographic and historical approaches to get beyond superficial explanations seen in strictly quantitative models focusing on strictly demographic factors. Although not explicitly approached from a realist perspective, Hunter's study illustrates a deeper notion of the term "explanation" than is typical in social epidemiology and reveals causal mechanisms with more detail and complexity, opening up more opportunities for intervention.

One of the vexing things about realist philosophy in science is that it is difficult, on the surface, to distinguish it from conventional social scientific research. It is rare that someone will say that they are doing a "realist analysis" of a phenomenon in the way that they would say they are practicing "realist synthesis" (see Chap. 11) or "realist evaluation" (see Chap. 12). In part this is because realism has penetrated into the core way of doing things for many social sciences,[3] and also because, unlike in systematic reviews or randomized trials, it is impossible to provide a standardized, formulaic way of doing realist-inspired science. Indeed, one of the challenges of adopting a realist approach is that it can look like it simply involves adopting "mixed methods." But realist science involves much more than that, as it is focused on identifying causal mechanisms and distinguishing between necessary and contingent relations. To learn to "do" realist social science, in other words, it is necessary to learn and apply its principles, as opposed to implementing some formulaic sequence of methods.

2.7 Types of Research

If explanation is not reducible to the establishment of statistical associations and predictive models, it follows that we must ask: what is the alternative? For Sayer (1992), "causal analysis is usually closely tied to abstraction and structural analysis and hence explanation to description" of the qualitative aspects of objects, relations, and processes. In some instances,

> the discovery of empirical regularities may draw attention to objects whose causal powers might be responsible for the pattern and to conditions which are necessary for their existence and activation. But in order to confirm these, qualitative information is needed on the nature of objects involved and not merely more quantitative data on empirical associations. (Sayer 1992)

Indeed, it is common in epidemiology to employ strategies to identify distinguishing or common factors in cases of diseases, and to conjecture causes from this information, but this fails to account for the mechanism that *generates* the disease and can lead to false and simplistic conclusions (for difficult and complex questions). One of the important activities of social science, therefore, is to identify those mechanisms, as discussed above, through retroduction. But the tools of retroduction, so to speak, are not obvious. According to the realist view, these tools are abstractions, and these are fundamental to explanation.

In common parlance, the adjective "abstract" often means vague, esoteric or removed from reality. The sense in which the term "abstraction" is used in research is different. According to Sayer (1992),

> an abstract concept, or an abstraction, isolates in thought a *one-sided* or partial aspect of an object. What we abstract *from* are the many other aspects which together constitute *concrete* objects such as people, economies, nations, institutions, activities and so on. (emphasis in original)

---

[3] Indeed, one of the criticisms of realism when people started writing about it in the social sciences is that many said "we're all realists now" (Cloke et al. 1991). Essentially, it codified the way many social scientists already worked. Even if this critique of unoriginality is valid, it is certainly advantageous that social scientists practice their craft in a way that is self-consciously aware of the philosophical underpinnings, and there is still plenty of relatively superficial analysis that could benefit from the insights of realist philosophy.

Abstract concepts need not be vague: abstractions such as temperature, gender, *et cetera*, are quite concrete and precise. Nor should the notion of abstract be equated with unreality or something residing only in thought – abstractions can and do refer to things that are real (Sayer 1992). "Class," "status," "identity," "neighbourhood," "context," "government" and even "society" are all abstractions that identify fundamental dimensions of human existence and have a certain degree of practical adequacy for explaining them.

On the other side of things, the concept of "concrete objects" "does not merely concern 'whatever exists' but draws attention to the fact that objects are usually constituted by a combination of diverse elements or forces" (Sayer 1992). A person, for instance, combines influences and properties from a wide range of sources (e.g., physique, personality, intelligence, attitudes, etc.), each of which "might be isolated in thought by means of abstraction, as a first step towards conceptualizing their combined effect" (Sayer 1992). As a consequence, understanding concrete events or objects involves a double movement:

> Concrete => abstract, abstract => concrete. At the outset our concepts of concrete objects are likely to be superficial or chaotic. In order to understand their diverse determinations we must first abstract them systematically. When each of the abstracted aspects has been examined, it is possible to combine the abstractions so as to form concepts which grasp the concreteness of their objects (Sayer 1992).

This activity forms the basis for research and, indeed, the relationship between empirical events, mechanisms and structures, on the one hand, and abstract and concrete research on the other, as shown in Fig. 2.1. The figure also shows different types of research and what sorts of activity they are concerned with. Orthodox empirical research operates only at the level of empirical events, seeking to make generalizations (extensive research). Abstract research "deals with the constitution and possible ways of acting of social objects" (Sayer 1992). Concrete research seeks to link abstractions and their concrete referents. Interpretive understanding is "presupposed in all of these types of research" (Sayer 1992), including the final type, synthesis research. Synthesis research seeks to combine all of these elements in a robust way (and is described more fully in Chap. 11).

2.8   From Qualitative/Quantitative Research to Extensive/Intensive Research

The previous section appears to advocate for qualitative research to inform quantitative research, or mixed methods. However, the distinction between qualitative and quantitative is of limited utility, as is the term "mixed methods." This distinction reflects an unfortunate tendency for people to acquire training and experience in either qualitative or quantitative methods, and then choose their research problems and questions on the basis of how amenable they are to study with the methods they know. Receptivity to mixed methods is a view that is often seen as progressive. This view is sometimes presented as if the mere mixing of methods *necessarily* produces

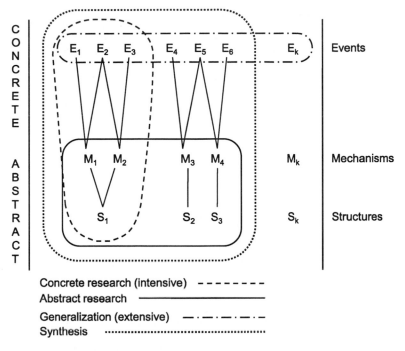

Fig. 2.1 Types of research (Reprinted from Sayer (1992). With permission from Taylor & Francis Books UK)

better research outcomes. Instead, the appropriateness of the method depends on the type of object and the question one is asking.

According to realism, it is preferable to distinguish between intensive and extensive research rather than qualitative and quantitative research, as intensive and extensive research designs are question driven (rather than method driven) (Sayer 1992; Harré 1979). Intensive research and extensive research differ in a number of their properties (Table 2.1). The chief difference is the kinds of questions that they allow researchers to ask about the phenomena under study. In extensive research, which often involves obtaining relatively superficial information on large numbers of people, questions relating to regularities, common patterns and distinguishing features of a population can be asked. It is also possible to ask how widely certain characteristics or processes are distributed or represented. Often this involves the use of surveys or other kinds of large, quantitative data sets. In extensive research, causal processes cannot be directly observed, as the only relations that can be observed are what Sayer (1992) calls "formal relations of similarity" among "taxonomic groups" (e.g., women under 45 years old). Intensive research, on the other hand, asks questions about how a process works in a small number of cases, often with identifiable people and/or institutions, by identifying substantial relations of connection between such factors as the reasons people give for their actions, their biographies and contingent factors.

Table 2.1 Intensive and extensive methods

	Intensive	Extensive
Research question	• How does the process work in a particular case or a small number of cases? • What did the agents actually do?	• What are the regularities, common patterns, distinguishing features of a population? • How widely are certain characteristics or processes distributed or represented?
Relations	• Substantial relations of connection	• Formal relations of similarity
Types of groups studied	• Causal groups	• Taxonomic groups
Type of account produced	• Causal explanation of the production of certain objects or events, though not necessarily representative ones	• Descriptive "representative" generalizations lacking in explanatory penetration
Typical methods	• Study of individual agents in their causal contexts, interactive interviews, ethnography • Qualitative analysis	• Large-scale survey of population or representative sample, formal questionnaires, standardized interviews. Statistical analysis
Limitations	• Actual concrete patterns and contingent relations are unlikely to be "representative," "average" or generalizable to other contexts, as they are necessary features of these objects	• Although representative of a whole population, they are unlikely to be generalizable to other populations at different times and places. Problems of ecological fallacy in making inferences about individuals. Limited explanatory power
Appropriate tests	• Corroboration	• Replication

Reprinted from Sayer (1992). With permission from Taylor & Francis Books UK

In intensive research, the groups studied are causal groups that may provide compelling accounts of causal mechanisms (or necessary relations) in real context. The generalizability of such mechanisms to other contexts, however, may be difficult to establish with certainty. This is not necessarily a weakness of intensive methods, as such mechanisms cannot be abstracted from extensive research. When the generalizability of a mechanism is in doubt, then further extensive research can be complementary. On the other side of the ledger, while extensive studies can give representative accounts of phenomena, these tend to lack explanatory penetration. Of course, different kinds of tests are appropriate for each kind of research as well. For intensive research, corroboration is the best way to establish rigour, while in extensive research it is replication (Sayer 1992).

Hunter's (2007) study of the social, economic, cultural and sexual factors that produced specific patterns of HIV transmission in South Africa in the early 2000s is an excellent example of the complementary use of both intensive and extensive methods (although primarily intensive). Hunter also successfully engages in retroduction by abstracting from events the mechanisms and structures that give rise to those events through a rich, complex but cogent account of an important phenomenon – more than would have been possible with extensive methods alone.

2.9 Practical Adequacy

One of the questions often raised when methods other than those with roots in positivism are suggested is: how will we know if the results of this research are valid if they are not conducted with objective, scientific methods? Realism offers a powerful and thoughtful perspective on this question through the notion of "practical adequacy," a substitute and, in many ways, a more powerful alternative to notions of truth. "[T]o be practically adequate," argues Sayer (1992), "knowledge must generate expectations about the world and about the results of our actions which are actually realized…" and it must be "…intersubjectively intelligible and acceptable in the case of linguistically expressed knowledge." Quite literally, according to this view, the adequacy of knowledge must be evaluated for its ability to guide practice (i.e., to accomplish some end) in a way that is sensitive to context. Moreover, to "acknowledge that a theory 'works' or has some practical adequacy in a particular context is not to suppose that every one of its constituent elements is 'true' or practically adequate" (Sayer 1992). This notion implies that because of the differentiated nature of the world, we can expect our knowledge of certain processes or phenomena can be unevenly developed yet practically adequate (Sayer 1992). The notion of practical adequacy steps outside conventional notions of truth and falsity, which is helpful partly because it avoids "giving the impression that to hold such false beliefs is necessarily to know nothing and hence to be able to do nothing" (Sayer 1992).

Indeed, the intention and ability to use knowledge to guide practice is an important aspect of the social role of social science. Sayer (1992) suggests that "social science must stand in a critical as well as an explanatory and interpretive relationship to its object and to common-sense knowledge." This implies that

> social science should not be seen as developing a stock of knowledge about an object which is external to us, but should develop a critical self-awareness in people as subjects and indeed assist in their emancipation. It does this first by remembering that its 'object' includes subjects, that the social world is socially produced and hence only one of many possible human constructions. It encourages emancipation and self-development by bringing to light formerly unrecognized constraints on human action. In capitalist societies, with their extraordinarily extended economic relations between anonymous people, the results of people's actions – their own products – take on 'nature-like' qualities in the sense that they react back on us as *blind forces* to which we must submit. (Sayer 1992, emphasis in original)

Taking the world as given, "nature like" or as if "what is, must be" is to naturalize social phenomena and to let common sense guide practice. This is highly problematic because, as Sayer (1992) suggests,

> [a] social science which builds uncritically on common sense, and reproduces these errors, may, at a superficial level, appear to produce correct results. On the other hand, from the standpoint of common sense, which takes its knowledge to be self-evident and beyond challenge, the knowledge produced by critical theories such as marxism will appear to be false because it *conflicts* with what it judges to be the case ("an affront to common sense!"). Yet such theories aim not just to present an alternative or to reduce the illusions inherent in social understanding, but to represent and explain what actually exists as authentically as possible. (emphasis in original)

Indeed, this passage points to the problem with many of the conclusions about health inequalities emerging from social epidemiology, some of which are strongly dependent on unexamined and unacknowledged common sense understandings of the nature of society. The possibilities for a richer theoretical treatment of health inequalities lie not just in the development of an alternative hypothesis, but also in the ability to represent and explain what actually exists in an authentic way that opens up some new possibility for intervention or change in the practices that create the differential distribution of health status. But even more boldly, a further possible outcome of a theoretically richer social epidemiology is a change in society's self-understanding about social inequality and the differential distribution of health status. This is not as outrageous as it may sound if it is recognized that

> part of "the facts" about human existence is that it depends considerably on societies' self-understanding, that it is socially produced, albeit only partly in intended ways, and that changes in this self-understanding are coupled with changes in society's objective form. (Sayer 1992, emphasis added)

According to this view, "it becomes possible to see how knowledge can simultaneously be not only explanatory and descriptive but also evaluative, critical and emancipatory" (Sayer 1992). That a society's objective form and its self-understanding are interdependent suggests the potential power and impact of theoretical research, if those insights can be successfully disseminated and translated into practice. These are important challenges for the future of social epidemiology. Social change as a result of the permeation of concepts from the social sciences into everyday knowledge is possible, owing to social science's unique relationship to its object of study – an internal one. Concepts from the social sciences differentially impact upon society's self-understanding and do so only in partly intended ways (allowing for the easy dodge of accusations of social engineering – a ridiculous concept on this view), but it is clear that they do have this impact, and often very quickly. Take, for example, Freudian psychology, which emerged in the late 1920s, only to permeate everyday understandings of internal family relations (Oedipus complex) and personality traits (ego) in the western world within a 40–50 year period.

Most individual papers or studies in social epidemiology are relatively limited in their scope with regards to providing a richly theoretically informed explanation of the phenomenon. In part this is because there are aspects of the phenomena that cannot be addressed by the data collected in any one study, so they must be supplemented by secondary reports of other studies and by retroduction – the abstraction of the causal powers and liabilities of the objects under study. To combine such knowledge is a challenging process requiring a careful assessment of the strength of evidence (in the strict empirical sense) and the cogency of theoretical perspectives on the structures and mechanisms that the empirical events are an expression of. And this is the critical point about developing an explanation of this type: the empirical events and data representing them, in addition to being scrutinized for their strength in the traditional positivist sense, must be understood as the concrete manifestation of a number of contingently-related and imperfectly-understood

structures and mechanisms whose causal powers and liabilities have been identified through abstract theoretical research. It is this kind of knowledge, not simply
evidence of empirical associations between explanatory and outcome variables
that will provide new openings and opportunities for social action to reduce
inequalities in health status.

2.10 Implications for Social Epidemiology Research

The scope and complexity of the realist perspective makes it difficult to explain in
anything less than a book-length project. Nevertheless, there are a few lessons for
social epidemiology that can be drawn from the foregoing. These, I would suggest,
provide a compelling direction for "rethinking social epidemiology."

The first implication is that the greatest challenge for social epidemiology is not
to achieve more accurate measurement of variables, nor is it a need for better or
more complete data, or more sophisticated statistical techniques. These kinds of
innovations are welcome, but greater precision will not lead to greater certainty,
better explanation or greater impact. The most important challenge for social epidemiology arising from the realist perspective is that more attention needs to be paid
to the theoretical accounts of causal mechanisms and the distinction between necessary and contingent relations. At some level, this rethinking is going to require more
comfort with uncertainty and a retreat from the standards imposed by such positivist
cornerstones as replication, hypothesis testing and generalizability. Indeed, if real
world impact is the aspiration of social epidemiologists, I would suggest that the
search for truth and certainty would be productively replaced by a concern for practical adequacy and the ongoing, reflexive search for fallibility in our knowledge so
that it can be refined. By no means does this imply a reduction in rigour, merely a
recasting of it.

If we are to provide richer explanations of the phenomena we study, then
social epidemiology needs to recognize that causality can never be decided by
empirical research alone. It must be expressed in terms of causal powers and
liabilities of objects, and in the description of necessary and contingent relations.
In order for more social epidemiologists to embrace the kind of research illustrated by Hunter's (2007) work, some institutional change is required. The careers
of social epidemiologists will have to be measured less on the number of publications they produce and the impact factor of the journals in which they appear, and
more on other factors, such as greater credit for writing books, that would allow
social epidemiologists to engage in more exploratory research that would provide richer explanations of social epidemiologic phenomena. Moreover, we need
publication outlets that accept longer articles that permit more in-depth exploration of the theoretical and conceptual bases of our work, as opposed to the few
paragraphs of speculative interpretation that we usually get at the end of articles
in typical epidemiological journals.

In order to aid investigations of richer accounts of causal mechanisms, a more nuanced understanding of the value of various kinds of methods is required. I strongly suggest that we eschew the distinction between qualitative and quantitative methods in favour of the distinction between intensive and extensive research. If more social epidemiologists and social scientists of health had a greater understanding of this distinction, then specialists in both qualitative and quantitative methods would have a better understanding of the relative strengths and weaknesses of their own approaches and also their complementarity.

This raises a critically important implication for training: learning how to execute the methods, the cornerstone of most graduate-level epidemiology programs, is simply inadequate. It is imperative that students understand where methods come from, both historically (i.e., positivism as part of the enlightenment era and as a reaction to the hegemony of the church) and in terms of their philosophical under-pinnings. Use of a realist perspective can be helpful in this regard, given how research decisions that need to be made must be made on an appeal to the key philosophical underpinnings.

To embrace a realist perspective and deeper inquiry into causal mechanisms and structures will require greater openness to experimentation with methodology, including natural experiments, ethnographic methods, *et cetera*, because these methods tell us how causal mechanisms work in context. Experimentation is espe-cially valuable because a system behaves differently when it is perturbed than when it is stable, and this perturbation can reveal dormant causal mechanisms in a system. Observational research, therefore, has critical limitations, so natural experiments are needed and welcomed. The non-random assignment of subjects and other messy aspects of such research, rather than things to be disdained, are useful, as they pro-vide learning opportunities. That said, social epidemiology has to embrace designs and methods that can capture much of the qualitative information about the messi-ness of the implementation of interventions and not the typically clean and sterile "did this intervention have an effect" research (see Chap. 12).

Social epidemiology is growing quickly and has never been more widely read by academics, practitioners and the general public. The realist perspective has a great deal to offer in transforming this popularity into impact. This theme is present in a number of the chapters that follow in this book, and hopefully it can be embraced.

References

Bambra C, Pope D, Swami V et al (2009) Gender, health inequalities and welfare state regimes: a cross-national study of thirteen European countries. J Epidemiol Community Health 63:38–44
Bhaskar R (1975) A realist theory of science. Leeds Books, Leeds
Bhaskar R (1979a) The possibility of naturalism. Harvester, Brighton
Bhaskar R (1979b) On the possibility of social scientific knowledge and the limits of naturalism. In: Mepham J, Ruben D-H (eds) Issues in Marxist philosophy, vol 3, Epistemology, science, ideology. Humanities Press, Atlantic Highlands

Bhaskar R (1989) Reclaiming reality. Verso, London

Bryman A (1988) Quantity and quality in social research. Routledge, London

Ciaffa JA (1998) Max Weber and the problems of value-free social science: a critical examination of the Werturteilsstreit. Bucknell University Press, Lewisburg

Cloke P, Philo C, Sadler D (1991) Approaching human geography: an introduction to contemporary theoretical debates. Guildford Press, New York

Dunn JR (2006) Speaking theoretically about population health: commentary on carpiano RM and daley DM "A guide and glossary on theory-building for population health". J Epidemiology & Community Health 60:572–573

Forbes A, Wainwright SP (2001) On the methodological, theoretical and philosophical context of health inequalities research: a critique. Soc Sci Med 53:801–816

Gartell CD, Gartell JW (1996) Positivism in sociological practice: 1967–1990. Can Rev Sociol 33:143–158

Halfpenny P (1982) Positivism and sociology: explaining social science. Allen and Unwin, London

Harré R (1979) Social being: a theory for social psychology. Blackwell, Oxford

Hertzman C, Marmot M (1996) The leading hypothesis and its discontents: a synthesis of evidence and outstanding issues regarding the east-west life expectancy gap. In: Hertzman C, Kelly S, Bobak M (eds) East-West life expectancy gap in Europe. Kluwer, Dordrecht

Hertzman C, Weins M (1996) Child development and long-term outcomes: a population health perspective and summary of successful interventions. Soc Sci Med 43:1083–1095

Hunter M (2007) The changing political economy of sex in South Africa: the significance of unemployment and inequalities to the scale of the AIDS pandemic. Soc Sci Med 64:689–700

Kawachi I (1999) Social capital and community effects on population and individual health. Ann NY Acad Sci 896:120–130

Kawachi I, Kennedy BP, Lochner K et al (1997) Social capital, income inequality, and mortality. Am J Public Health 87:1491–1498

Kawachi I, Kim D, Coutts A et al (2004) Commentary: reconciling the three accounts of social capital. Int J Epidemiol 33:682–690

Keat R (1981) The politics of social theory: Habermas, Freud, and the critique of positivism. University of Chicago Press, Chicago

Krieger N (1994) Epidemiology and the web of causation: has anyone seen the spider? Soc Sci Med 39:887–903

Krieger N (1999) Embodying inequality: a review of concepts, measures, and methods for studying health consequences of discrimination. Int J Health Serv 29:295–352

Krieger N (2001) Theories for social epidemiology in the 21st century: an ecosocial perspective. Int J Epidemiol 30:668–677

Link B, Phelan J (1995) Social conditions as fundamental causes of disease. J Health Soc Behav 35:80–94

Muntaner C (2004) Commentary: social capital, social class, and the slow progress of psychosocial epidemiology. Int J Epidemiol 33:674–680

Navarro V, Muntaner C, Borrell C et al (2006) Politics and health outcomes. Lancet 368:1033–1037

Oakes JM (2004) The (mis)estimation of neighborhood effects: causal inference for a practicable social epidemiology. Soc Sci Med 58:1929–1952

Pawson R (1989) A measure for measures: a manifesto for empirical sociology. Routledge, London

Rose G (1985) Sick individuals and sick populations. Int J Epidemiol 14:32–38

Sayer A (1992) Method in social science: a realist approach, 2nd edn. Routledge, London

Sayer A (1993) Postmodernist thought in geography: a realist view. Antipode 25:320–344

Sayer A (1997) Essentialism, social constructionism, and beyond. Sociol Rev 45:453–487

Shonkoff J, Phillips DA (eds) (2000) From neurons to neighbourhoods: the science of early child development. National Research Council and Institute of Medicine, Washington, DC

Tarlov AR (1996) Social determinants of health: the sociobiological translation. In: Blane D, Brunner E, Wilkinson R (eds) Health and social organization: towards a health policy for the 21st century. Routledge, London

Taylor SE, Repetti RL, Seeman T (1997) Health psychology: what is an unhealthy environment and how does it get under the skin? Annu Rev Psychol 48:411–47

Wainwright SP, Forbes A (2000) Philosophical problems with social research on health inequalities. Health Care Anal 8:259–277

Wilkinson RG (1994) The epidemiological transition: from material scarcity to social disadvantage? Daedalus 123:61–78

Wilkinson RG (1996) Unhealthy societies: the afflictions of inequality. Routledge, New York

Chapter 3
Values and Social Epidemiologic Research

Ahmed M. Bayoumi and Adrian Guta

Contents

3.1	Introduction	44
3.2	A Working Definition of Values	45
3.3	Epidemiology, Positivism and Values	47
3.4	Social Epidemiology as a Bridge Science	48
3.5	Social Justice	48
3.6	Two Examples	49
3.7	Theories of Ethics	50
	3.7.1 Deontological Ethics	51
	3.7.2 Consequentialist Ethics	51
	3.7.3 Rights Theory	52
	3.7.4 Virtue Ethics	52
	3.7.5 Communitarian Approaches	53
	3.7.6 The Capability Approach	53
3.8	Social Epidemiology Research, Values and Ethical Frameworks	54
	3.8.1 Harm Reduction Research and Values	54
	3.8.2 Obesity Research and Values	56
3.9	Values in Research Design	57
	3.9.1 Selecting and Framing a Research Question and Deciding on Data	57
	3.9.2 Analyzing Data	58
	3.9.3 Interpreting Results	59
	3.9.4 Knowledge Translation	59
3.10	Values, Objectivity and Rigour	60
3.11	Conclusion	62
References		63

A.M. Bayoumi (✉)
Centre for Research on Inner City Health, St. Michael's Hospital, 30 Bond Street,
Toronto, ON M5B 1W8, Canada
e-mail: ahmed.bayoumi@utoronto.ca

A. Guta
Dalla Lana School of Public Health, University of Toronto, 155 College Street, 6th floor,
Toronto, ON M5T 3M7, Canada
e-mail: adrian@guta.ca

P. O'Campo and J.R. Dunn (eds.), *Rethinking Social Epidemiology:
Towards a Science of Change*, DOI 10.1007/978-94-007-2138-8_3,
© Springer Science+Business Media B.V. 2012

Abstract Social epidemiology, although rooted in social justice and studies of health disparities, has not yet articulated a set of core values. We argue that recognizing such values is important when research is inherently value-laden and that, in such circumstances, establishing an evidence base for policy will be insufficient to bring about social change. Theories of ethics, including deontological ethics, consequentialism, rights theory, virtue ethics, communitarianism and the capability approach can inform how to consider valuation within research. We use two illustrative examples, from harm reduction and obesity research, to indicate how values underlie multiple aspects of the research process. Since a values-based approach requires moving beyond positivist conceptions of science, the social sciences, particularly critical theory and sociological models of public intellectuals, offer models for developing a value-based social epidemiology that is critical, engaged and relevant.

3.1 Introduction

One definition of social epidemiology distinguishes it from other frameworks by its focus on the social determinants of population health (Krieger 2001). While this approach might once have seemed revolutionary, it now has the status of an established mainstream framework. Yet studying the links between determinants and health does not seem to have influenced the prevalence of those determinants. From the mid-1990s to mid-2000s, the number of articles indexed annually in Medline that addressed poverty and health increased from 567 to 1,348. In the same time interval, the proportion of the population earning 50% or less of the median income after taxes and transfers increased from 9.5% to 12.0% in Canada and remained amongst the highest of all Organisation for Economic Cooperation and Development countries in the United States (18.1–17.1%) (Organisation for Economic Cooperation and Development 2010). Similar observations have led commentators to criticize social epidemiology for being "overly descriptive and analytical... [and] almost irrelevant to policy debates" (Muntaner et al. 2009). Heath (2010) has suggested that funding research into inequalities with no resultant improvement in the health of marginalized groups "seems to result in the paradox of the poor directly subsidising the more affluent."

Despite the advent of evidence-based decision making, the development of rigorous research methods and the amassing of a solid body of research findings, researchers regularly lament the lack of impact of this research on policy. This gap has sometimes been framed as a clash between evidence, on one hand, and ideology, entrenched interests, or the difficulty of social change on the other hand (Hemenway 2010; Godlee 2010). For instance, a discussion of the discrepancy between the evidence for harm reduction interventions and international drug policies called for greater advocacy for evidence-based approaches to counter "forces that seek to maintain the harmful status quo in the drug policy arena" and stated that "these forces would be overwhelmed if the medical, public health, and scientific communities stood together and called for evidence based approaches to tackle drug related harms" (Wood 2010). This chapter argues from a different approach. We believe that simply advocating for more evidence-based decision making is insufficient for policy-relevant research to make meaningful changes in people's lives. Plainly stated, there are no technical solutions to political problems. Muntaner et al. (2009) have characterized this distinction as one that pits "supposedly value-free public health policies vs policies rooted on a set of political views (e.g., egalitarianism)." Accordingly, health research that addresses social issues cannot escape a discussion of the values that underlie the frameworks and choices used by both researchers and decision makers. Jonathan Mann wrote, in 1997, that public health "is struggling to define and articulate its core values." Over a decade later, values in public health and epidemiologic research remain ill defined and discussion of the role of values in research remains controversial, even in disciplines such as social epidemiology that has a solid grounding in the study of inequities. Thus, establishing an evidence base for public health policy is necessary, but not sufficient, when the research itself is value laden.

Several authors, including authors of a chapter in this book (see Chap. 9), have called for a "political epidemiology" that moves beyond quantitative analyses of individual or group determinants of health to examine the political bases for health inequalities (Gil-González et al. 2009). A recent workshop in the United States similarly called for a "politicised orientation to analyzing and rectifying health problems" (Krieger et al. 2010). The study of how political processes determine health or the establishment of a politicized orientation to health research must start with the more rudimentary question of how to characterize values that are intrinsic to such discussions.

Consideration of values should not be seen as belonging solely to the "problem" of translating knowledge into practice. Burawoy (2004), when writing about sociology, distinguishes between research that focuses on developing instrumental knowledge, i.e. technical solutions to pre-defined problems, and research that focuses on reflexive knowledge, i.e. research that is explicitly concerned with how the results may be mobilized, and with the possible meanings of the "good society." The latter category, which is inextricably bound to consideration of values, is further divided into "critical" and "public" realms depending on whether the primary audience is academic or extra academic. We believe that adopting such a framework for social epidemiology will re-orient the field to being more critical, engaged and relevant.

3.2   A Working Definition of Values

Values imply the formation and ranking of preferences over some thing, usually with an ethical dimension attached to the valuation. Some definitions of value refer to behavioural norms; others focus on moral systems with classifications into "good" and "bad" categories. Similarly, many different *things* could be valued: an idea, a policy, an outcome, a behaviour, a person, wealth, material possessions, social interactions or many other things. Values guide decisions about morality, which refers to "norms about right and wrong human conduct" (Beauchamp and Childress 2001). Moral systems fully encompass principles, rules, rights and virtues. Values and morals relate more broadly to ethics, "a generic term for various ways of understanding and examining the moral life" (Beauchamp and Childress 2001).

We suspect that much of the reluctance to discuss values in scientific research relates to the concept of moral systems and the perceived inherent tendency of some moral systems to adopt normative frameworks. Such frameworks tend be universal and absolute in their judgments about those things that are least preferred. Such views may be seen as "subjective" and as inconsistent with good scientific practice. Furthermore, such perspectives might strike many (including us) as inconsistent with a pluralistic, non-judgmental attitude that emphasizes freedom of inquiry and expression. The critical point, however, is that rigid moral systems are only one of several ways to define values. As we discuss below, strict classification of acts into good and bad categories and a focus on moral rules is a deontological approach to values. That such a perspective on values is inconsistent with how social epidemiology research is conducted does not imply that the discussion of values should not occur. Rather, it mandates that researchers recognize how values are defined, which aspects of their work are value-laden and how differing concepts of values might lead to challenges or even conflicts when translating research into practice.

Values can also be difficult to define and are often not made explicit. We view values as being constructed and context-specific rather than fixed and universal. Dominelli (2002) states that "values develop over time, being modified through interaction, including conflicts about them… Moreover, values are subjective, although some of them may be presented as absolute because they are recognisable or persist over space and through time." In part because values may not be well formed, they are also frequently not explicit.

We are not, in this chapter, primarily concerned with individuals' values; rather, we are interested in values that are shared across groups, i.e. social or community values. Central to this approach is the recognition that social values are not the aggregation of individual values; rather, they are the values of the community *qua* community (Mooney 2009). A communitarian perspective locates individuals within communities and treats individuals as citizens who recognize obligations to others in the community rather than as consumers who seek only to maximize their own welfare. Accordingly, members of such communities define their values with regard to the community as a whole and not on the basis of their own self interest. This perspective also applies to the "community" of researchers who have their own set of shared values.

There are two related objectives in studying values in research. First, communities and scholars should be clear about what their values are. Indeed, the uncritical application of analytical tools or methods might result in scientists conducing research that is inconsistent with their own values. Accordingly, social epidemiologists can and should evaluate their research and that of their discipline not only relative to scientific standards but also relative to their own set of shared values. Institutional review boards, for example, provide a set of value standards based in individual ethics against which to evaluate research. An analogous set of standards (without the sanction of an official body) based in social values would allow for critical reflection and new research directions. Second, understanding values can provide a framework for understanding the role of research in guiding policy (or in failing to do so) and for developing interventions that might effect social change.

3.3   Epidemiology, Positivism and Values

Like quantitative sciences in general, epidemiology is firmly grounded in the positivist tradition that idealizes objectivity and seeks to separate facts from values (Krauss 2005). According to this perspective, clarifying the distinction between cognitive and social values helps in "relegating debates over social and emotional values to their proper sphere" (Machamer and Douglas 1999). In contrast, some disciplines within the social sciences have noted that facts and values are inextricable. Harrington (2005), echoing the Scottish philosopher David Hume, writes that the "difference between facts and values can be understood as the difference between the world as it is, or was, and the world as we would like it to be, or not to be." Many scholars have argued that to reject the role of values is a fruitless and, possibly, dangerous pursuit. Without defining values, science becomes reduced to being simply a technological or instrumental tool for analysis, open to manipulation (Maslow 2004). Furthermore, separating facts and values becomes particularly problematic when they are seen to be not just distinct but oppositional. As van Staveren (2007) notes: "The problem with a dichotomous positioning of fact and value…is that one excludes the other and is also favoured over the other, often without any ground other than that the favoured notion is not the unfavoured notion." For positivists, establishing facts is seen as a more important and legitimate research endeavour than studying values.

Within epidemiology there has been limited attention to defining values, but these have focused largely on extolling positivist values or values based in individualist research ethics. Coughlin (1998) writes that the core values of epidemiology are "fundamental ethical and scientific precepts (i.e., basic scientific values) that are consistent with and provide support for the mission and purpose of the profession." In this framework, explicit values include rigor in scientific research, the advancement of scientific knowledge, collegiality, general ethical principles and the importance of promoting population health. The guidelines for the American College of Epidemiology (2000) similarly state that epidemiologists "uphold values of free inquiry and the pursuit of knowledge" and "uphold the value of improving the public's health through the application of scientific knowledge." In a more limited way, there has been some recognition that epidemiology is concerned with providing service to communities, particularly ones that are disempowered, and that values may vary across cultures (Coughlin 1998). Of relevance for social epidemiology is that there has also been a recognition that epidemiologic specialities might develop their own "mission statements, statements of core values, and ethics guidelines" (Coughlin 1998).

3.4   Social Epidemiology as a Bridge Science

Some conceptions of social epidemiology view it as a critical engagement between the social sciences and epidemiology. Krieger (2000) has commented that "epidemiologic theory and methods overall will be invigorated and improved by acquiring a critical perspective that returns us to our roots, shared with social sciences, of finding meaning in and delineating accountability for the social patterning of human suffering." Spitzer (1986), writing in another context, described bridge sciences as those that join "two or more methods or fields" such as environmental toxicology or health economics. In this spirit, social epidemiology is accorded its "double designation" because it combines epidemiologic principles with social science research and methods. Furthermore, social epidemiology could also adopt critical theory frameworks from other social sciences that view health as a social institution imbued with power relations. A critical social science perspective defines a set of "reflexive" questions concerning the implicit assumptions and ideology underlying the research process and the role of power, contradiction and dialectical relationships in theory and research practice (Eakin et al. 1996).

Such considerations are important for a discussion of values because the array of theoretical perspectives within the critical tradition each explicitly endorse a set of values. To illustrate, social psychology has struggled with how anti-oppression research studies unjust social arrangements and explicitly advocates for resistance and social change. Similarly, feminist research, queer theory, anti-colonialist and indigenous studies as well as many other disciplines each have an established set of values as their starting point rather than a set of shared methods or populations of interest. Yet these disciplines have also struggled with how to balance an explicit statement of values alongside the concept of objectivity, a topic to which we return below.

3.5   Social Justice

The relationship between social justice and social epidemiologic research illustrates how one might start to consider values. We start by making three claims. First, the decision to study unjust health inequalities, or inequities, reflects not only the individual values of researchers but also a set of shared values among researchers. This point is important conceptually because it establishes a basis for how to think about social, as distinct from individual, values; it is important practically because it allows for a common starting point for discussion and critical analysis, even among differing ideologies. Second, this interest in social justice extends not just to the researcher's choice of a particular problem but also to how the problem is studied. Finally, as discussed above, we believe that making the social values of epidemiologic research explicit without asking researchers to apologize for holding such values is essential for informing and re-orienting the way epidemiologic research is conducted.

From the earliest emergence of social epidemiology as a distinct discipline, there has been a sustained focus on the examination of inequalities in health and health care delivery and on social determinants of health (Krieger and Birn 1998). Indeed, it is remarkable how frequently social justice has been identified as an underlying principle of social epidemiology or public health (Krieger et al. 2010; Peter 2001; Kirch and Vernon 2009; Venkatapuram and Marmot 2009; Sen 2002; Edwards 2009; Beauchamp 1976; Gostin 2007; Faden and Powers 2008). This emphasis is neither arbitrary nor accidental; rather, it reflects the implicit values of researchers working in the area. Stated boldly, if inequities are unjust then the goal of revealing and documenting social injustices must be to challenge them. A social justice perspective provides a framework for understanding who is harmed and who benefits from certain decisions (Krieger 2001). In adopting this framework, researchers reject others, in particular, those that are individualistic, atomistic or libertarian and that define justice solely based on the rights of individuals to maximize their own utility. Former British Prime Minister Margaret Thatcher famously remarked in 1987, that "there is no such thing as society. There are individual men and women, and there are families." Sometimes termed "market justice," perspectives such as these have been influential in health policy discussions in the United States and among proponents of neo-liberal social policies (Kirch and Vernon 2009; Beauchamp 1976).

While social justice stands in contrast to market justice (since the latter denies that individuals have social obligations), proponents of social justice do not share a single theory of justice, an ideological stance or even a complete set of shared values. Indeed, there are multiple theories of justice that disagree on key questions but that might all be consistent with a social justice orientation (Olsen 1997). Similarly, we anticipate significant disagreement among different ideological perspectives. For example, both a Marxist and a liberal researcher might value addressing social inequities, although we expect they might disagree both on how such inequities are defined and on the best method to address them. The approach to social justice consistently used in social epidemiologic research is one that is strongly egalitarian and focused on distributive justice, with particular attention to marginalized groups (Braveman 2006). We see these as some of the characteristics of shared values among social epidemiologic researchers, upon which we elaborate below.

3.6 Two Examples

Throughout this chapter, we will focus on two examples of issues that have been addressed by social epidemiologic research to demonstrate how research in these areas is value laden and how making such values explicit might advance research. Our goal is not to question the quality or integrity of research that has been done in these areas. Rather, we illustrate how thinking about these problems from different value frameworks yield distinct research questions and approaches as well as yielding different strategies for translating research into policy.

Our first example focuses on research on harm reduction interventions. Harm reduction refers to a policy and clinical approach to the use of psychoactive drugs that aims to minimize the associated health, social and economic harms. Examples of harm reduction interventions include disulfiram for alcohol addiction, methadone maintenance therapy for opioid addiction, needle exchange programs and supervised injection sites. Although a large body of work has demonstrated that harm reduction interventions improve health outcomes for drug users, they remain controversial in many jurisdictions.

Our second example is of obesity. Obesity research has become a major endeavour in North America with large investment contributions from national funding agencies. Researchers and policy makers have used the terminology of epidemiology, referencing the "epidemic of obesity," to justify the prioritization of this particular health issue. In contrast, some social theorists have been harshly critical of this approach arguing that it is victim blaming (Moffat 2010). Approaches to addressing obesity have included a range of interventions, including banning soft drink machines from schools, pharmacological therapy and calls for addressing features of the "built environment," such as locked stairways or urban sprawl, which discourage or deter physical activity (Booth et al. 2005).

We first consider how a "market justice" approach would address each of these research areas. A libertarian approach to drug use would hold that governments have no right to legislate or regulate what individuals choose to do with respect to drugs. A less extreme view, but still market driven, would hold that the state should not fund programs to address drug use or associated harms, except as they relate to harms that occur to others. Market justice would have a similar perspective regarding obesity, viewing individuals as consumers who choose to spend their money on foods that maximize their utility; that these choices result in some people being obese is seen as a particular, if perhaps unfortunate, preference. The problem in both cases, from a market justice perspective, is that some individuals make poorly informed choices. The solution, accordingly, is to give individuals better information with which to make decisions in the marketplace. Similar thinking underlies much of the health promotion literature. Missing is a perspective that focuses on the social determinants of the health behaviour, a conceptualization of the choice (to use drugs or overeat) as a consequence of social factors, or an examination of health interventions as elements of social institutions, whether these interventions are aimed at addressing the harms associated with drug use or decreasing excess weight (Dunn 2010).

3.7 Theories of Ethics

We have stated that the act of valuation often entails an ethical dimension and, further, that understanding differences in values is enhanced by understanding underlying theories. Accordingly, we now consider several such ethical theories and their application to the study of social epidemiology. These theories are normative in that they indicate how adherents should act when faced with questions in which value judgments are required. That is, they ask general questions but with "some relatively direct bearing on practice" (Reich 1995). Ethical theories provide ways of assessing moral reason and arguments and are used as frameworks for making judgments (Arras et al. 1999). For example, decision makers who adopt a particular ethical theory reveal something about what they value and how they rank those values. A detailed description of these theories is beyond the scope of this chapter; our goal is to provide an outline of some approaches and to relate these to issues in social epidemiology.

3.7.1   Deontological Ethics

Deontological (from *deon*, the Greek word for duty) ethics emphasize the moral nature of an action and whether it is morally permissible. Deontological ethics aims to both formulate and defend a particular set of moral rules and to develop and defend some method of determining what to do when the relevant moral rules come into conflict (Reich 1995). Immanuel Kant developed a form of deontological ethics that holds that the moral worth of an action should not be an outcome of its consequence but that the action itself must be grounded in reason and based on certain moral requirements. Deontological theories emphasize that human beings are considered equal and, accordingly, each individual's well-being is valued. Kant famously posited that humans "should never be turned into means for other people's ends," a recognition that sets limits on acceptable human behaviour (van Staveren 2007). Kantian ethics follows the "categorical imperative," which "commands unconditionally that I should act in some way...[and] apply to me no matter what my goals and desires may be" (Rohlf 2010).

Critics of deontological ethics point out that the approach is limited to situations in which individuals are able to make choices. Indeed, since it neglects the "vulnerabilities of human life that are outside the reach of the human will, such as scarcity of means and various contingencies to which social and economic life is so vulnerable," the approach may not offer insight into many epidemiologic problems (van Staveren 2007). Furthermore, deontological ethics are inherently rigid with no criteria for dealing with conflicting rules (or rights, see below) or allowances for exceptions to moral rules (van Staveren 2007).

3.7.2   Consequentialist Ethics

Deontological ethics contrasts with consequentialist (also teleological (from *telos*, the Greek word for end)) ethics, which emphasize the end consequence of an act to determine if it is good or bad. Consequentialist ethics aim to: (1) specify and defend some thing or list of things that are good in themselves; (2) provide some technique for measuring and comparing quantities of these intrinsically good things; and (3) to defend some practical policy for those cases where one is unable to determine which of a number of alternative actions will maximize the good thing or things (Reich 1995). Utilitarianism is a form of consequentialism that builds on the work of Jeremy Bentham and John Stuart Mill. Utilitarians hold that the most morally permissible action is one that will produce the most good. The utility of an action is the "total intrinsic value produced by an action" (Beauchamp and Steinbock 1999). Utilitarianism has the advantage of providing an impartial decision procedure, based on a single criterion of right action (happiness), which can be objectively and empirically measured and used to reach definitive conclusions about the best course of action to take (Arras et al. 1999). However, critics of utilitarianism object to the primary value placed on happiness, the difficulty of measuring the possible consequences of every action to calculate utility and the implied lack of responsibility associated with acts. Act-utilitarianism is a sub-stream of the theory, which focuses on the specific acts that will result in the greatest happiness. In contrast, rule-utilitarianism focuses on following rules that determine what is morally right and produce happiness.

3.7.3   Rights Theory

Most commonly espoused through the doctrine of liberal individualism, rights-based approaches have grown in popularity in philosophical, political and legal circles. Rights can be understood as "justified claims that individuals can make on other individuals or on society;" for each right there may be a complementary duty (Beauchamp and Childress 2001). Individuals have both positive (access to) and negative (freedom from) rights for which they may in turn have subsequent duties or obligations. Rights theories have challenged the supremacy of Kantian and utilitarian approaches through their broad appeal and seeming applicability to a range of contexts. However, conceptions of rights are varied and contested (Rainbolt 2006). Furthermore, this framework has been challenged by those who see conflicts between the notion of individual rights having primary moral ground when issues affect the common good.

3.7.4   Virtue Ethics

Theories of virtue ethics emphasize individual character with the aims of: (1) developing and defending some conception of the ideal person; (2) developing and defending some list of virtues necessary for being a person of that type; and (3) defending some view of how persons can come to possess the appropriate virtue (Reich 1995). A virtue is "a trait of character that is socially valuable, and a moral virtue is a trait of character that is morally valuable" (Beauchamp and Steinbock 1999). Accordingly, an act can be socially valued without necessarily having moral value; an example would be objectivity in epidemiologic research, which is highly valued within the research community but does not carry moral overtones. In a virtue ethics framework, both methods and ends can be defined as intrinsically "good" rather than as instrumental for other ends. Furthermore, emotions and intuitions are important for defining virtue ethics such that good motivations and good reasons combine to "produce moral goods like generosity, liberality, or kindness" (van Staveren 2007).

In contrast to other ethical frameworks, virtue ethics is contextual and pragmatic. Although this approach is personal (it defines someone who is good), it is not individualistic since "it regards people as social beings who can function only in relation to others" (van Staveren 2007). Virtue ethics is expressed in specific contexts and instances. In distinction to deontological approaches, which have rigid and universal rules, a virtue ethics approach is concerned with "concrete social life" (van Staveren 2007). Critics of virtue ethics point out that focusing on the "good person" makes it challenging to develop standards to judge situations or social institutions. Furthermore, critics emphasize that good intentions are no guarantee of good results.

3.7.5 Communitarian Approaches

Virtue ethics are central to communitarian approaches, which focus on finding common good and communal values through cooperation and deliberative dialogue (Mooney 2009; van Staveren 2007; Beauchamp and Steinbock 1999). Communitarian approaches are "guided by the values that are shared and contested in communities, supporting these values through a trial-and-error process, but recognizing that values are fallible" (van Staveren 2007). Communitarians reject liberalism's focus on individual rights as the starting point for establishing social order and instead consider other socially important interests in the establishment of polices to create livable communities (Arras et al. 1999). Critics of communitarianist approaches raise several concerns. First, individual or minority rights are not guaranteed of protection within a communitarian perspective. Second, since communitarian approaches (and virtue ethics more generally) are context-specific, they are by definition not generalizable. Thus, identifying the instrumental nature of an action to do good is severely constrained. Third, the relevance of communitarian approaches to larger communities remains uncertain.

3.7.6 The Capability Approach

A philosophical approach rooted in virtue ethics that has become increasingly popular is the capability approach (Sen 2002; Ruger 2004). Capabilities are defined as "the opportunity to achieve valuable combinations of human functionings – what a person is able to do or be" (Sen 2005). The approach emphasizes both the ability of a person to do those actions that they value and whether they have the necessary "means or instruments or permissions" to pursue their desires (Sen 2005). A disabled individual, for example, would not be assumed to have the same capabilities as non-disabled individuals even if they had similar means, since the disability might limit his or her ability to do those actions that he or she wants to do. Poverty, as well, is seen as denying individuals the ability to achieve their capabilities and, hence, their freedom. Ethical capabilities are an important virtue that act as moral guides for decision making and might include altruism, cooperation and trust. Sen (2005) declined to identify a list of capabilities and called instead for "open valuational scrutiny for making social judgements" (a perspective consistent with communitarian approaches). In contrast, Nussbaum's (2001) capability approach, based on a universalist concept of central human functions, lists central human capabilities (which she stresses is not a complete theory of justice). These capabilities (examples include life, bodily health, bodily integrity, emotions and control over one's environment) are akin to rights but focused on outcomes rather than on negative freedoms (Nussbaum 2001). Furthermore, Nussbaum incorporates the idea of a threshold level of each capability, which she argues should be the goal of public policy (Anand et al. 2009).

3.8 Social Epidemiology Research, Values and Ethical Frameworks

In the following section we examine how the values underlying harm reduction and obesity research and interventions might be viewed under these different ethical frameworks.

3.8.1 Harm Reduction Research and Values

Much of the opposition to harm reduction research and interventions is grounded in a deontological approach that views drug use as intrinsically wrong and, accordingly, any activity that facilitates drug use (such as a needle exchange program) is also wrong. Indeed, many of the public pronouncements against harm reduction interventions have an explicit deontological basis. In 2008, the Canadian federal Minister of Health, Tony Clement, in a speech to the Canadian Medical Association, commented on Vancouver's supervised injection site (which he opposed) by saying that: "This is a profound moral issue, and when Canadians are fully informed of it, I believe they will reject it on principle…The supervised injection site undercuts the ethic of medical practice and sets a debilitating example for all physicians and nurses, both present and future in Canada" (Clement 2008). Harm reduction research is intrinsically wrong under this approach, since it would seem to facilitate a bad behaviour. It is worth noting that these comments were criticized by both liberal and conservative medical practitioners.

Some have argued for harm reduction interventions as a means of protecting the rights of drug users, an approach that would situate harm reduction firmly in the deontological rights perspective (Keane 2003). Indeed, the Vancouver supervised injection site has remained open because the British Columbia supreme court has ruled that the right to health supersedes the right of the state to regulate drug use. In this formulation, the role of research is to generate the evidence that establishes the positive fact of improved health; decision makers (including elected officials and the judiciary) establish how the right to this improved health is weighed against other rights and social concerns. However, rights discussions invariably involve competing rights and contrasts between individual rights and social goods. Accordingly, there is no automatic policy direction that follows from a consideration of the evidence (Keane 2003). Social epidemiologic research, from a rights perspective, would thus constitute a relatively limited role in determining policy.

A seemingly common view among researchers and practitioners is that harm reduction is value-free or "amoral" when it comes to drug use (Keane 2003). Prominent proponents of harm reduction claim that the debate is the "age old battle between a deontological approach emphasizing righteousness, and a consequentialist approach emphasizing outcomes" (Wodak and McLeod 2008). However, a consequentialist approach to drug use requires a clear definition of what constitutes harm, which itself invokes value judgments. As Keane (2003) notes, "in a context where drugs are predominantly identified as bad (or even evil) and drug use as pathological, a view that drug use is neither right nor wrong is not neutral, but is itself a committed and critical standpoint." Furthermore, utilitarian frameworks within the consequentialist paradigm are notably neglectful of the distribution of harms and benefits. Thus, consequentialism offers no ethical basis for arguing against a heavy-handed law enforcement intervention, for example, if the end result is a net decrease in harm and an improvement in health even at the violation of individual freedoms.

An alternative approach to harm reduction "focuses attention on the effect of different programmes and campaigns on individuals' capacity for freedom and ethical self-formation, rather than promoting freedom as a moral principle or universal ideal" (Keane 2003). This approach is pragmatic and focuses on the generation and evaluation of the evidence base for decisions. This approach is most compatible with a virtue ethics framework. Like capability approaches, the emphasis is on promoting those interventions that enable substance users to achieve their full functioning that includes, but is not limited to, health. Like communitarian approaches, the ethical value of these interventions is determined in particular contexts of time and location. Social epidemiologic research in this perspective has a mandate to measure not only health outcomes but perhaps also other social outcomes or even to determine optimal methods for valuation of outcomes and processes for determining deliberation.

3.8.2   Obesity Research and Values

Although obesity research is perhaps less politically controversial than harm reduction research, we believe that values also determine how this research is conceptualized and conducted. Like addictions, obesity has frequently been cast as a problem of human will. The obese individual has chosen not to exercise sufficiently or has lost the ability to control his or her eating behaviour. Thus, an individuals' weight is not merely a positive fact, it also reflects a failing of the will and an indication of irrational behaviour. Deontological ethics would, therefore, endorse interventions that aim to correct this "aberrant" behaviour, such as imposition of taxes on sugary beverages. Overeating is conceptualized as analogous to cigarette smoking and public health interventions that focus on changing individual behaviour are endorsed in a similar manner as interventions that successfully reduced smoking. Similarly, being overweight, but not obese, is classified as a condition requiring intervention since it reflects the same failing of will, although to a lesser degree. The role of epidemiologic research from this value perspective is limited to establishing the evidence base for interventions that lead to weight loss.

To illustrate a consequentialist approach to obesity research, we focus on research design and analysis. A consequentialist approach might focus on weight reduction as the definition of a successful obesity intervention, as have several obesity intervention trials. This seemingly common-sense based approach neglects some aspects that might be important from other ethical frameworks. First, the mean weight loss between groups is an essentially utilitarian measure that neglects the distribution of weight loss. That is, interventions in which many people lose a little weight or a few people lose a great deal of weight are treated identically when the focus is solely on the mean effect. Second, it may be important to analyze which groups lose weight. The poor are disproportionately obese, indicating that the social determinants of obesity are significant (Braveman 2009). An equity perspective on obesity interventions might similarly focus on whether interventions to reduce obesity have similar effects among social groups, an approach that applies equally to individual- and group-level interventions. For example, an intervention that addresses changes to the built environment to reduce weight loss might neglect the association between neighbourhoods and poverty from a purely consequentialist perspective. Such "prioritarian" perspectives could be applied broadly to social conditions (such as giving priority to those living in poverty) or narrowly to health concerns (such as giving priority to the most unhealthy). Third, consequentialism mandates defining which consequences should be counted. Focusing only on health outcomes (such as weight, cholesterol, blood pressure and the adverse biological effects of medications) neglects how obesity is socially constructed and how weight gain, loss and re-gain influence both social well-being and interactions with others.

A virtue ethics approach to studying obesity might start from interrogating how the meaning and moral significance of obesity is socially constructed and how social forces (e.g., the built environment, food and agricultural policies, school-based policies) contribute to determining weight and how obesity and being overweight are viewed. As with research on harm reduction, the goal of such research is not the immediate short-term health goal (to reduce weight amongst obese individuals) but rather the larger aim of enabling individuals to attain their full capacity (Jan and Mooney 2006). A limitation of this approach is that this "full capacity" has no universal definition but rather must be interpreted in each time and context. Process also matters in this approach as does consideration of the distribution of benefits. Thus, the imposition of a tax on sugary beverages and reducing subsidies for the manufacturers of processed foods might have similar outcomes if overall sales are considered as an outcome but would need to be critically analyzed according to the perceived fairness of such policies and the differential impact on corporations, rich and poor consumers.

3.9 Values in Research Design

Values are explicitly or, more commonly, implicitly involved in each step of the research process including selecting and framing a research question and determining the data to be collected, selecting the analytical method, interpreting the findings and translating these findings into practice (Potts and Brown 2008). Choices at each step are usually framed as a meeting a desire for objective knowledge production. Yet these choices also reflect value structures beyond scientific rigor. Furthermore, these structures might not be the actual values of the researchers. We illustrate each step with representative examples; throughout, we adopt a value structure focused on advancing social justice.

3.9.1 Selecting and Framing a Research Question and Deciding on Data

Values rooted in social justice inarguably direct the choice of research themes and questions. The freedom of academics to ask the questions that interest them gives them considerable power, even as it is constrained by funding bodies, institutions and intellectual "chill." Asking a particular question can be a value-laden decision that has political implications. For example, framing questions of obesity in social contexts directly implies a rejection of a primary deontological approach. Furthermore, research grounded in the fight against oppression values dissent and anti-authoritarianism; that is, researchers that are dedicated to social change should reflect that spirit in their willingness to pose questions that challenge entrenched power. A critical social justice perspective would advocate that social epidemiology adopt a "Foucaultian hermeneutics of suspicion with respect to covert power, hidden ambitions, and cultural biases that infuse supposedly 'impartial' scientific research" (Wallwork 2008). Harm reduction research that challenges existing laws or the power of law enforcement is an example.

A commitment to community-based participatory action research similarly reflects a set of shared communitarian values, including a recognition that expertise is contextually specific and may be located outside of academia, a dedication to defining research goals from a set of shared communitarian values and an understanding that people are members of communities with claims and obligations defined relative to each other not just at the individual level (Guta et al. 2010). Thus, health research might focus on not only health outcomes but on all outcomes that are relevant to the community in which the research is being conducted (Mooney 2009). Such considerations might extend to social relations, privacy concerns, economic well-being, the impact of the research process and many more outcomes. More generally, social epidemiology is certainly interested in groups defined by social relations and in differences between such groups and not (only) disparities across individuals in an entire population. Such distinctions were at the heart of debates about World Health Organization measures of inequalities (Braveman et al. 2000). More generally, such deliberations might reflect not only value choices but also "program theories, which recognize the role of social determinants of health and the diverse actors involved in social change" (Potvin et al. 2005).

3.9.2 Analyzing Data

Harper and colleagues (2010) have demonstrated how various inequality measures contain implicit value judgments. For example, reporting differences between groups as relative differences values only the measure of equality between groups; in contrast, reporting differences as absolute places a value on the actual health of each group. Similarly, neglecting distributional concerns in health gains implies a set of implicit value judgments that might not be commensurate with the researchers' goals. As Harper et al. (2010) state: "choosing one or another measure to the exclusion of others may introduce normative criteria regarding the relative importance of inequality per se, whether individuals or groups count more, which groups (if any) should be prioritized and by how much, and what the appropriate target of inequality reduction should be."

Researchers must also make decisions about the appropriate unit of analysis. Fine (2006) writes that "research on the broad reach of injustice must account for all forms of social relations within…systems, not simply documenting the 'damage' or 'resilience' of the bodies or (un)consciousness of 'victims.'" This is not to say that social epidemiologic research can or should not collect data at the individual level, but it is to argue for also collecting and analyzing data at aggregate levels, since power relations at a societal level are expressed through such group relations as class and neighbourhood. This perspective resists the deontological approach of identifying ill health, or behaviours associated with ill health, as solely failings of individual will.

We also emphasize that analytical rigour and objectivity are also values of social epidemiologic research. Our emphasis on social justice and egalitarian values should not be read as a diminution of the importance of generating evidence that meets standards of scientific validity. We discuss the relationship between values, objectivity and reflexivity further below.

3.9.3   Interpreting Results

Just as the unit of analysis should recognize the social construction of health problems, so should the interpretation, an approach that necessitates theorization (Potvin et al. 2005). Fine (2006) writes that "the task of social researchers is to theorize across levels and resist the common sense explanations by which individuals are the site for analysis, blame, responsibility, and data collection." Such theorization is essential to both understand findings in context and to define those findings that are broadly generalizable. Krieger and colleagues (2010) note that "the point is not 'grand theory' that deterministically purports to explain 'everything', but rather critical uses of theoretical frameworks that can coherently orient inquiry and analysis within and across relevant levels and timeframes, situate different perspectives in relation to each other and make the invisible visible." Theorization is intrinsically linked to values, since the choice of theory and analytical framework directly reflects normative choices. For example, a review of 34 evaluation frameworks examining the gradient in health inequalities among families and children in Europe found considerable difference, notably among how outcomes were considered, including the role of health status measures and cultural aspects of community and individual well-being and the timeframe over which outcomes are measured. These studies differed not just in choice of outcome but also in which outcomes they considered to be both important and valid as a measure of health (Davies and Sherriff 2011).

3.9.4   Knowledge Translation

A particular challenge for social epidemiologic research comes at the point of translating the knowledge that has been produced into action. The predominant approach to knowledge translation presents the researcher as a value-free producer of technical information whose main role is to neutrally interpret the evidence for decision makers who will decide how to use this information. This approach recognizes that researchers might advocate for their findings when the researchers and decision makers have common values (such as approving pharmacological treatments for obesity). Advocacy is viewed much more suspiciously, however, when researchers' advocacy reflects values that conflict with those of decision makers.

Of course, we argue that avoiding a discussion of values is itself a political act of non-participation, a choice in direct conflict with social justice values. Yet engaging in political knowledge translation is not easy; particularly in the United States, where such engagement will often be in conflict with libertarian or other individualistic and market-oriented views. Thus, questions of power and conflict are unavoidable. Similar concerns are relevant when considering the openness of academic institutions, particularly as health research is increasingly tied to commercial interests.

Competing value frameworks can function as a seemingly impenetrable barrier to knowledge translation. Current knowledge translation paradigms, which fail to account for value clashes or to challenges to dominant power structures that might arise from policy-relevant research, are often of little help to understanding such value clashes. Yet such clashes provide a more coherent framework for understanding why decision makers might disregard the evidence for harm reduction interventions than analyses that simply decry the lack of due attention paid to evidence. Indeed, framing such discrepancies as value clashes offers some alternative approaches. First, as we noted above, many values are constructed and context-specific and, therefore, mutable. Engaging in public discussion about values (and not just evidence) is, therefore, essential. Second, researchers who are willing to acknowledge their values might usefully form collaborations with advocacy groups (or even advocate themselves) to influence political decision making.

Knowledge translation that takes politics seriously is discussed elsewhere in this volume (see Chap. 13). We concur that social epidemiology research is need of a model of the public intellectual. Burawoy (2005) has described public sociology as that which "brings sociology into a conversation with publics, understood as people who are themselves involved in conversation. It entails, therefore, a double conversation." This public engagement can take multiple forms and with many publics. Burawoy (2005) describes two complementary approaches of traditional and organic public sociology; the former entails engaging the public through popular media and instigating (though not necessarily participating in) debate, while the latter involves working with a "visible, thick, active, local and often counter-public." Fine (2006), citing Apfelbaum, similarly argues for the need to communicate findings to (organic) disadvantaged communities but also to (traditional) communities of privilege with the goal of awakening "a sense of injustice among those with material and cultural power; addressing the 'stubborn deafness' of the comfortable."

3.10 Values, Objectivity and Rigour

An undeniable benefit of a value-free approach to science is the ability to claim that the research is free of potential biases that might come with being explicit about values. However, acknowledging the value base of research does not make objectivity unobtainable. As Harrington (2005) notes, "if facts cannot be separated from values, it does not follow that evidence about social life cannot be collected, analysed in transparent and methodical ways." The key to objectivity lies not in negating an individual researcher's values but in having a system of checks and balances in place to prevent subsequent bias. As Parascandola (2003) has argued: "It is not the neutrality of individual investigators that keeps us honest, but the diversity of opinions and critical outlook of the scientific community as a whole. In fact, adversarial debate about methodology, and about values, drives advocates to marshal stronger evidence and clarify their reasoning." Fine (2006) evokes Harding who calls for "strong objectivity – achieved when researchers work aggressively through their own positionality, values and predispositions, gathering as much evidence as possible, from many distinct vantage points, all in an effort not to be guided, unwittingly, by predispositions and the pull of biography."

Reflexivity offers a useful approach to considering how to integrate values and maintain rigor that has been used extensively within the critical research tradition and among researchers who use qualitative methods. This approach involves taking a stance and "being able to locate oneself in the picture, appreciate how one's own self influences the research act" (Fook 2002). In qualitative research, "reflexivity implies the ability to reflect inward toward oneself as an inquirer; outward to the cultural, historical, linguistic, political, and other forces that shape everything about inquiry; and, in between researcher and participant to the social interaction they share" (Sandelowski and Barroso 2002). Critical theory, which rejects reductionism and the "forced choice between explanation and understanding" promoted by positivism (Bohman 2010), has its roots in the Frankfurt School of philosophy, which promoted analysis and discussion on the influence of late capitalism on social order (Daly 2006). Reflexivity was further developed in feminist theory to account for how research and theory are socially produced (Harding 1983).

From its theoretical roots, reflexivity has evolved into an important aspect of research and practice in health related disciplines (Lipp 2007). Reflexivity has been used to examine the role of the researcher, evaluate the research process and enable public scrutiny of the integrity of the research (Finlay 2002). Reflexivity has also been promoted to empower others by opening up a more radical consciousness; this concept is similar to the realist approach that views knowledge as simultaneously explanatory and descriptive yet also, through reflection, as evaluative, critical and emancipatory (Sayer 1992).

Pierre Bourdieu (2004) called for reflexivity in science (i.e., a science of science) to objectify scientific practice with the goal of improving it. Bourdieu and Wacquant (1992) differentiate their conceptions of reflexivity from others through three points: "First, its primary target is not the individual analyst but the social and intellectual unconscious embedded in analytic tools and operations; second, it must be a collective enterprise rather than the burden of the lone academic; and third, it seeks not to assault, but to buttress the epistemological security of sociology." When extended to the theory and practice of social epidemiology, Bourdieu's (2004) "reflexivity" challenges researchers to "objectify" their own practices and thereby use "its own weapons to understand and check itself." A reflexive social epidemiology researcher would not only analyze statistical data on differential health outcomes but also consider the categories of analysis used and the conditions of data gathering. The combination of these reflexive stances, one focused on the individual researcher and the other on a discipline, could help to explicate underlying value structures.

3.11   Conclusion

The adoption of a research perspective that recognizes the role of values would open new avenues for exploration for social epidemiology. Burawoy's (2004) division of sociology research into instrumental and reflexive categorizations has particular resonance for epidemiology, which has largely focused on the former type of knowledge. Whether intended for an academic audience or for a policy audience, this type of research is focused on answering specific questions and producing technically sound reports. Yet social epidemiology has the potential to do more than merely documenting disparities and should move to addressing systemic injustices. A willingness to incorporate a values framework would promote social epidemiologic research that is critical (whose primary audience is academic) or public (whose primary audience is the community). Both approaches would expand the realm of social epidemiology to develop new theories and frameworks and to engage more fully in politically controversial areas.

We foresee that "critical epidemiologists" would be explicit about their values in grant applications, presentations and publications and that these values would guide choices regarding theories, frameworks and methods. Such value statements already underlie much research that focuses on harm reduction or health disparities, although the theories underlying the frameworks are often not fully developed and the values are often implicit. We also foresee that "public epidemiologists" will not only engage in public discussion of epidemiologic findings but also advocate for the values that underlie this research, even at the risk of confrontation with those who hold opposite values.

We have not tried to catalogue all of the values that social epidemiologists might share. A non-exhaustive list, presented to illustrate our thoughts and provoke further discussion, might include: a commitment to social justice defined in egalitarian terms, at both the individual and group level; a corresponding focus on disadvantaged groups and distributive issues in health, its determinants and other outcomes; a recognition that health is only one of several outcomes that determine justice; avoidance of rigid judgments associated with deontological frameworks that lead, for example, to victim blaming; adoption of frameworks that consider health as socially constructed and health care as a social institution; a commitment to analyze findings at system levels; endorsing frameworks that value community opinions and expertise and that sees individuals as members of communities rather than as atomized entities; a commitment to free inquiry and a willingness to challenge authority; and dedication to rigorous research methods, self criticism and reflexivity.

We believe that a significant reason to define social epidemiology as a sub-discipline of epidemiology is not only to develop shared methods but also to focus on these shared values. Recognizing and endorsing these values leads to consideration of theories and frameworks that situate research in broader social contexts and provide frameworks for thinking about knowledge translation that move beyond blaming decision makers for failing to acknowledge evidence. Indeed, critical and public epidemiologists will have increased responsibility for defending and promoting their work. Social epidemiologists' values, however, might not be shared by other epidemiologists. Such conflicts might be unavoidable but could also be welcomed as a means to increase the scope of discussion about what is the role and relevance of social epidemiology.

Acknowledgements The authors thank Patricia O'Campo, James Dunn and Kelly Murphy for invaluable advice and reflection.

References

American College of Epidemiology Ethics Guidelines (2000) Ann Epidemiol 10:487–497

Anand P, Hunter G, Carter I et al (2009) The development of capability indicators. J Hum Dev Capab 10:125–152

Arras JD, Steinbock B, London AJ (1999) Moral reasoning in the medical context. In: Arras JD, Steinbock B (eds) Ethical issues in modern medicine, 5th edn. Mayfield Publishing, Mountain View

Beauchamp DE (1976) Public health as social justice. Inquiry 13:3–14

Beauchamp TL, Childress JF (2001) Principles of biomedical ethics. Oxford University Press, New York

Beauchamp DE, Steinbock B (1999) New ethics for the public's health. Oxford University Press, New York

Bohman J (2010) Critical theory. In: Zalta EN (ed) The Stanford encyclopedia of philosophy. http://plato.stanford.edu/archives/spr2010/entries/critical-theory/. Accessed 22 Feb 2011

Booth KM, Pinkston MM, Poston WS (2005) Obesity and the built environment. J Am Diet Assoc 105:S110–S117

Bourdieu P (2004) Science of science and reflexivity. University of Chicago/Polity Press, Chicago

Bourdieu P, Wacquant LJ (1992) An invitation to reflexive sociology. University of Chicago Press, Chicago

Braveman P (2006) Health disparities and health equity: concepts and measurement. Annu Rev Public Health 27:167–194

Braveman P (2009) A health disparities perspective on obesity research. Prev Chronic Dis 6:A91

Braveman P, Krieger N, Lynch J (2000) Health inequalities and social inequalities in health. Bull World Health Organ 78:232–234; discussion:234–235

Burawoy M (2004) Public sociologies: contradictions, dilemmas, and possibilities. Soc Forces 82:1603–1618

Burawoy M (2005) For public sociology. Am Sociol Rev 70:4–28

Clement T (2008) Speech by the Honourable Tony Clement Minister of Health Canadian Medical Association Annual Conference. http://www.hc-sc.gc.ca/ahc-asc/minist/speeches-discours/2008_08_18-eng.php. Accessed 22 Feb 2011

Coughlin SS (1998) Scientific paradigms in epidemiology and professional values. Epidemiology 9:578–580

Daly G (2006) Marxism. In: Wake P, Malpas S (eds) The Routledge companion to critical theory. Routledge, London

Davies JK, Sherriff N (2011) The gradient in health inequalities among families and children: a review of evaluation frameworks. Health Policy 101(1):1–10

Dominelli L (2002) Anti-oppressive social work theory and practice. Palgrave Macmillan, London

Dunn JR (2010) Health behavior vs the stress of low socioeconomic status and health outcomes. JAMA 303:1199–1200

Eakin J, Robertson A, Poland B et al (1996) Towards a critical social science perspective on health promotion research. Health Promot Int 11:157–165

Edwards NC (2009) Revisiting our social justice roots in population health intervention research. Can J Public Health 100:405–408

Faden RR, Powers M (2008) Health inequities and social justice. The moral foundations of public health. Bundesgesundheitsblatt Gesundheitsforschung Gesundheitsschutz [German] 51:151–157

Fine M (2006) Bearing witness: methods for researching oppression and resistance. A textbook for critical research. Soc Justice Res 19:83–108

Finlay L (2002) Negotiating the swamp: the opportunity and challenge of reflexivity in research practice. Qual Res 2:209–230

Fook J (2002) Social work: critical theory and practice. Sage Publications, Thousand Oaks

Gil-González D, Ruiz-Cantero MT, Alvarez-Dardet C (2009) How political epidemiology research can address why the millennium development goals have not been achieved: developing a research agenda. J Epidemiol Community Health 63:278–280

Godlee F (2010) Ideology in the ascendant. BMJ 341:c3802

Gostin LO (2007) Why should we care about social justice? Hastings Cent Rep 37:3

Guta A, Wilson MG, Flicker S et al (2010) Are we asking the right questions? A review of Canadian REB practices in relation to community-based participatory research. J Empir Res Hum Res Ethics 5:35–46

Harding S (1983) Common causes: toward a reflexive feminist theory. Women Polit 3:27–42

Harper S, King NB, Meersman SC (2010) Implicit value judgments in the measurement of health inequalities. Milbank Q 88:4–29

Harrington A (2005) Introduction. What is social theory? In: Modern social theory: an introduction. Oxford University Press, New York

Heath I (2010) Crocodile tears for health inequality. BMJ 340:c2970

Hemenway D (2010) Why we don't spend enough on public health. N Engl J Med 362:1657–1658

Jan S, Mooney GH (2006) Childhood obesity, values and the market. Int J Pediatr Obes 1:131–132

Keane H (2003) Critiques of harm reduction, morality and the promise of human rights. Int J Drug Policy 14:227–232

Kirch DG, Vernon DJ (2009) The ethical foundation of American medicine: in search of social justice. JAMA 301:1482–1484

Krauss SE (2005) Research paradigms and meaning making: a primer. Qual Rep 10:758–770

Krieger N (2000) Epidemiology and social sciences: towards a critical reengagement in the 21st century. Epidemiol Rev 22:155–163

Krieger N (2001) A glossary for social epidemiology. J Epidemiol Community Health 55:693–700

Krieger N, Birn AE (1998) A vision of social justice as the foundation of public health: commemorating 150 years of the spirit of 1848. Am J Public Health 88:1603–1606

Krieger N, Alegria M, Almeida-Filho N et al (2010) Who, and what, causes health inequities? Reflections on emerging debates from an exploratory Latin American/North American workshop. J Epidemiol Community Health 64:747–749

Lipp A (2007) Developing the reflexive dimension of reflection: a framework for debate. Int J Multiple Res Approaches 1:18–26

Machamer P, Douglas H (1999) Cognitive and social values. Sci Educ 8:45–54

Mann JM (1997) Medicine and public health, ethics and human rights. Hastings Cent Rep 27:6–13

Maslow AH (2004) The psychology of science: a reconnaissance. Henry Regnery, Chicago

Moffat T (2010) The "childhood obesity epidemic": health crisis or social construction? Med Anthropol Q 24:1–21

Mooney G (2009) Challenging health economics. Oxford University Press, New York

Muntaner C, Borrell C, Espelt A et al (2009) Politics or policies vs politics and policies: a comment on Lundberg. Int J Epidemiol 39:1396–1397

Nussbaum MC (2001) Women and human development: the capabilities approach. Cambridge University Press, New York

Olsen JA (1997) Theories of justice and their implications for priority setting in health care. J Health Econ 16:625–639

Organisation for Economic Cooperation and Development (2010) Income distribution: poverty 2010. http://stats.oecd.org/Index.aspx?DataSetCode=POVERTY. Accessed 8 Apr 2010

Parascandola M (2003) Objectivity and the neutral expert. J Epidemiol Community Health 57:3–4

Peter F (2001) Health equity and social justice. J Appl Philos 18:159–170

Potts K, Brown L (2008) Becoming an anti-oppressive researcher. In: Webber M, Bezanson P (eds) Rethinking society in the 21st century: critical readings in Sociology, 2nd edn. Canadian Scholars' Press, Toronto

Potvin L, Gendron S, Bilodeau A et al (2005) Integrating social theory into public health practice. Am J Public Health 95:591–595

Rainbolt GW (2006) Rights theory. Philosophy Compass 1:11–21

Reich WT (1995) Encyclopedia of bioethics. Simon & Schuster Macmillan, New York

Rohlf M (2010) Immanuel Kant. In: Zalta EN (ed) The Stanford encyclopedia of philosophy. http://plato.stanford.edu/archives/fall2010/entries/kant/. Accessed 26 June 2010

Ruger JP (2004) Health and social justice. Lancet 364:1075–1080

Sandelowski M, Barroso J (2002) Finding the findings in qualitative studies. J Nurs Scholarsh 34:213–219

Sayer RA (1992) Method in social science: a realist approach. Psychology Press, New York

Sen A (2002) Why health equity? Health Econ 11:659–666

Sen A (2005) Human rights and capabilities. J Human Dev Capab 6:151–166

Spitzer WO (1986) Clinical epidemiology. J Chronic Dis 39:411–415

van Staveren I (2007) Beyond utilitarianism and deontology: ethics in economics. Rev Political Econ 19:21–35

Venkatapuram S, Marmot M (2009) Epidemiology and social justice in light of social determinants of health research. Bioethics 23:79–89

Wallwork E (2008) Ethical analysis of research partnerships with communities. Kennedy Inst Ethics J 18:57–85

Wodak A, McLeod L (2008) The role of harm reduction in controlling HIV among injecting drug users. AIDS 22(Suppl 2):S81–S92

Wood E (2010) Evidence based policy for illicit drugs. BMJ 341:c3374

Chapter 4
Population-Based Data and Community Empowerment

Janet Smylie, Aisha Lofters, Michelle Firestone, and Patricia O'Campo

Contents

4.1	Introduction: Social Exclusion and Population Data Systems	68
4.2	Knowledge, Power and Data: A Post-colonial Approach	69
4.3	How Data Systems Can Undermine Communities and Perpetuate Health Inequities	70
	4.3.1 Data Processes That Exclude or Marginalize Communities	72
	4.3.2 Technical and Methodological Issues that Result in Inadequate Data	75
4.4	Transforming Health Data and Data Systems: Strategies for Change	77
	4.4.1 Re-envisioning Health Data and Social Data and Data Systems as Beneficial Tools to Advance Health and Social Equity	77
	4.4.2 Four Strategies for Change	81
4.5	Anticipating and Addressing Challenges	88
References		89

Abstract This chapter focuses on the transformation of population-based data and data systems into social resources that actively contribute to social, economic and political solutions to reduce health inequities. Our first underlying premise is that current systems of population health data collection, management, analysis and use are too often disconnected from the communities being described and whose data are being collected. Our second and related premise is that, in order for data to become a tool for social empowerment and social change, the social structuring of data governance and management must change from systems that reinforce social exclusion by marginalizing communities from their data to systems in which

J. Smylie (✉) • A. Lofters • M. Firestone • P. O'Campo
Centre for Research on Inner City Health, St. Michael's Hospital, 30 Bond Street, Toronto, M5B 1W8 ON, Canada
e-mail: SmylieJ@smh.ca; LoftersA@smh.ca; FirestoneF@smh.ca; O'CampoP@smh.ca

P. O'Campo and J.R. Dunn (eds.), *Rethinking Social Epidemiology: Towards a Science of Change*, DOI 10.1007/978-94-007-2138-8_4, © Springer Science+Business Media B.V. 2012

communities are fully and centrally involved in data decision making. The first part of this chapter rationalizes these premises by providing examples of the ways in which existing data systems undermine the broader mission of social epidemiology to identify effective interventions that alleviate conditions of social marginalization and poverty. The remainder of the chapter focuses on strategies for transformation in health and social data and data systems.

Abbreviations

RCT   Randomized controlled trial
PHAC   Public Health Agency of Canada
OCAP   Ownership, Control, Access and Possession
RHS   Regional Longitudinal Health Survey
DSM   Diagnostic and Statistical Manual of Mental Disorder
CCHN   Community Child Health Research Network
WHO   World Health Organization

4.1   Introduction: Social Exclusion and Population Data Systems

A key achievement of social epidemiology, to date, has been the expansion of our awareness of the need to link social, economic and political resources with health. Descriptive work has documented poorer health outcomes for social groups who have restricted access to employment, housing, health care, education and training as compared to social groups with unrestricted access (Marmot 2005; Commission on Social Determinants of Health 2008). Although this work has been important, social epidemiologists now need to go further. There is a need to uncover the mechanisms by which social exclusion affects the well-being of society and to apply these findings to the identification of effective strategies for social change. With these goals in mind, we have chosen a working definition of social exclusion that covers a broad range of resource domains (including but not limited to material needs) and that is explicitly linked to the social hierarchies in which social exclusion is rooted: "Social exclusion is the inability of certain groups to fully participate in society due to inequalities in access to social, economic, political and cultural resources, where these inequalities arise out of oppression related to race, class, gender, disability, sexual orientation, immigrant status and/or religion" (Public Health Agency of Canada 2004).

Earlier chapters have already identified that one of the major challenges facing social epidemiology is the movement from descriptive, problem-focused research to action-oriented, solution-focused research (see Chap. 1). This chapter will focus on the transformation of population-based data and data systems into social resources that actively contribute to social, economic and political solutions to reduce health inequities. Our first underlying premise is that current systems of population health data collection, management, analysis and use are too often disconnected from the communities being described and whose data are being collected. Our second and related premise is that, in order for data to become a tool for social empowerment and social change, the social structuring of data governance and management must change from systems that reinforce social exclusion by marginalizing communities from their data to systems in which communities are fully and centrally involved in data decision making. The first part of this chapter will rationalize these premises by providing examples of the ways in which existing data systems undermine the broader mission of social epidemiology to identify effective interventions that alleviate conditions of social marginalization and poverty. The remainder of the chapter will focus on strategies for transformation in health and social data and data systems.

For the purposes of this chapter, we define communities as any group of individuals sharing a common interest. This definition includes cultural, social, political, health and economic issues that may link together individuals who may or may not share a particular geographic association (North American Primary Care Research Group 1998). Within the context of social epidemiology, these communities would typically be the communities whose data is being collected, and the unifying issues would be the cultural, social, political, health and economic factors upon which social hierarchies and subsequent social privileging and social marginalization are based. We note that, while this chapter (and much of social epidemiology) primarily attends to social marginalization in the effort to enhance social well-being, there is a pressing need to concomitantly expand the examination of social privileging and recognize its fundamental importance as a driver of social conditions.

4.2 Knowledge, Power and Data: A Post-colonial Approach

Social epidemiology provides a unique opportunity to reconcile and enrich the rationalist scientific assumptions of conventional epidemiology with social theory. One of the limitations of conventional epidemiology is that there is a purposeful effort to acquire knowledge that is distanced from and even devoid of social context. This distancing is based on an assumption that there are "objective" and generalizable truths, the discovery of which will be "biased" if contextual factors contaminate data collection and analysis.

Critical social theory positions rationalist scientific inquiry into a larger epistemological framework in which knowledge and knowledge systems are woven into the architecture of social hierarchy. Foundational critical theorists such as Foucault (1977) asserted a vision of the collection of social data, or surveillance, as a form of externally controlled and pervasive social control that perpetuated oppressive societal power hierarchies. Foucault's work provides important insights into the intrinsic connections between knowledge, power, social hierarchies and data collection. However, it is less helpful with respect to the transformation of health and social data systems into tools that will alleviate oppression, since in Foucault's worldview there is a strong hegemony of oppressive state "knowledge:power" that leaves the oppressed at the margins with few explicit tools of resistance and very little discussion of alternate knowledge and power systems beyond the local level.

For an in-depth discussion of how to move forward with respect to knowledge and data systems that empower communities rather than perpetuate marginalization, one must turn to modern post-colonial theory and literature. Indigenous scholars such as Tuhawi Smith, Littlebear and Youngblood Henderson are particularly helpful in mapping out Indigenous knowledge systems including Indigenous sciences as sophisticated, diverse and epistemologically distinct entities from the Western European knowledge systems that were actively imposed on Indigenous peoples worldwide as part of colonization (Smith 1999; Little Bear 2000; Youngblood-Henderson 2000). Preserving, recovering and revitalizing Indigenous knowledge is critical to the dismantling of colonial processes and the re-empowerment of Indigenous people worldwide. In the words of Indigenous scholar Marlene Brant Castellano (2004): "Fundamental to the exercise of self-determination is the right of peoples to construct knowledge in accordance with self-determined definitions of what is real and what is valuable." Notably, in this effort to strengthen Indigenous knowledge systems, Indigenous scholars rarely repeat the colonialist approach of rejecting and/or subjugating outside scholarship, philosophy and ideas but rather adapt a pluralistic and practical approach in which knowledge and knowledge systems are understood to be complex and dynamic, and the ability to interface both locally and globally is critical to the attainment of thriving societies. Examples later on in this chapter will highlight how Indigenous communities have focused on taking ownership and control of data collection rather than rejecting surveillance because it can be a tool for oppression.

Health and social data and data systems provide a unique opportunity for all sectors of democratic societies to contribute to the exercise of the right to self-determination for Indigenous peoples and the rights to health equity for socially excluded groups more generally. Social epidemiologists can contribute to these efforts through technical and methodological expertise and, perhaps more importantly, by critically understanding the connections among data, knowledge and power to ensure that data systems are reducing rather than contributing to social exclusion.

4.3   How Data Systems Can Undermine Communities and Perpetuate Health Inequities

Individuals and systems external to communities are typically the gatekeepers who control access to data and data systems across the spectrum of research, dissemination and policy application processes (Fig. 4.1). Data processes and systems that

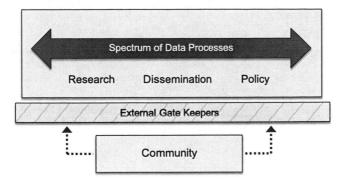

Fig. 4.1 Data and data systems that reinforce community marginalization

build on and perpetuate broader social exclusion by maintaining the barriers between communities and their data sets and/or contributing to the construction of inadequate data can be quite harmful to communities. For many communities, "data insults" resonate with historic human rights violations by health and social science researchers, such as the infamous Tuskegee experiments where syphilis treatment was purposely withheld from African American men without their knowledge to study the long-term effects of untreated syphilis; the immortalized HeLa human cell line, which was taken from a cancer-stricken African American woman, Henrietta Lacks, and used in decades of scientific research without her or her family's consent; or Dr. Richard Ward's unauthorized use of blood samples from members of the Nuu-chah-nulth First Nation in British Columbia, Canada for genetic studies that participants were never informed about (Randall 2006; Centers for Disease Control and Prevention 2008; Dalton 2002; Skloot 2010; Freimuth et al. 2001; Sateesh 2008). In recent decades, public privacy commissioners and health and social science research ethicists in democratic countries have challenged situations such as these where control lies outside the community as a violation of human rights, particularly in situations where the community of interest is already subject to one or more forms of social exclusion (Canadian Institutes of Health Research 2007; Battiste and Youngblood Henderson 2000; Battiste 2007; O'Neil et al. 1998; Israel et al. 2001; Minkler 2000). The underlying premise is that individuals and collectives should have access to information that is collected about them. However, with respect to health and social data, particularly for groups experiencing ongoing social exclusion, access itself is necessary but not sufficient. Ethicists and scientists agree that meaningful involvement throughout the data continuum is required, including involvement in data collection, data analysis, data management and governance and data dissemination and use (Royal Commission on Aboriginal Peoples 1993; Snarch 2004).

Unfortunately, there is a long list of ways in which health and social data and data systems can detrimentally impact communities whose data is being collected. For simplicity, we have identified two groupings of data system problems recognizing that there is, of course, overlap between groups and problems (Table 4.1).

Table 4.1 Ways in which health and social data and data systems can be detrimental to communities

Problem	References
Group A: exclusion or marginalization of community from data processes	
Absent, inadequate or late community engagement in data processes	Wenman et al. (2004) and Wallerstein (1999)
Indicators and/or measurement tools are in tension with community concepts of health and social well-being	Smylie and Anderson (2006), Smylie et al. (2006), and Altshuler and Schmautz (2006)
Euro-Western scientific analytical methods and assumptions are privileged over community epistemologies	Smith (1999) and Popay et al. (2008)
Data interpretation and dissemination perpetuate societal stereotypes and the marginalization of already marginalized groups	See Chap. 5
Community members are unable to access their community's data	Public Health Agency of Canada (2006)
Group B: technical and methodological issues that result in inadequate data	
Marginalized communities are excluded from, or are under-represented in, data collection	Statistics Canada (2000) and Canadian Hypertension Education Program (2010)
Data systems lack individual identifiers that enable for meaningful data disaggregation across strata of inequality	Health care utilization datasets in Canada (e.g., CIHI DAD) Anderson et al. (2006) and Rodney and Copeland (2009)
Uncoordinated health service performance measurement system and data sources	Anderson et al. (2006) and Anderson (1999)

Problems in Group A focus on the relationship between the data gatekeepers and the community. Problems in Group B highlight common technical and methodological issues that yield inadequate health and social data and data systems for marginalized groups. Cited references refer to either direct examples of detrimental data processes or additional information sources regarding the specific data problem. Problems and examples are further detailed in the text below.

4.3.1 Data Processes That Exclude or Marginalize Communities

4.3.1.1 Absent, Inadequate or Late Community Engagement in Data Processes

Data systems that exclude the communities whose data are being collected overwhelmingly predominate in current health and social sciences research and practice. Researchers and policy makers may not be aware of the importance of early and ongoing community engagement in health and social data work from either an ethical or a practical perspective. For example, when challenged on the absence of meaningful engagement of Aboriginal community stakeholders in a study of pregnancy risk factors and birth outcomes among Aboriginal women in Canada, Wenman et al. (2004) stated that this type of engagement was only required for studies using "participatory action research" methods and that, as a hospital based cohort, their study was excluded from the need to appropriately engage study subjects. Fortunately, there is a growing body of literature that clarifies the ethical requirements for and scientific merit of adequate community engagement in health and social research involving primary or secondary health and social data regardless of the subject or method (Canadian Institutes of Health Research 2007; Canadian Institutes of Health Research, Natural Sciences and Engineering Research Council of Canada, and Social Sciences and Humanities Research Council of Canada 2010; Israel et al. 2001; Wallerstein 1999).

A more insidious and increasingly common problem occurs when researchers, practitioners and policy makers are indeed aware of requirements to appropriately engage representatives of communities whose data are being collected and "learn the lingo" well enough to be successful in their acquisition of project funds, but upon project implementation do not have the commitment and/or skill set to adhere to existing standards. Wallerstein (1999) addresses this issue in her reflective examination of the New Mexico Partnership for Healthier Communities. The partnership was a community-based participatory research project with the goal of local communities creating collaborative planning and decision-making coalitions with the state to address community problems, such as domestic violence, and better meet community needs. Although the researchers and state agencies were committed to the study, several mistakes were made throughout the process. For example, state agencies did not provide communities with enough autonomy with regard to coalition development and organization, and the researchers did not seek out sufficient input from communities on the evaluation process, used language that distanced themselves from the community instead of using community definitions and did not openly acknowledge the power dynamics involved in the project. The non-community members of the study team did not have the skills to immediately recognize the inherent power imbalances in their project, which were expressed as communities being left out of the communication loop, not being consulted on key issues and having little or no decision-making authority (Wallerstein 1999). These power imbalances and lack of true collaboration led to tense relations between the researchers, state agencies and coalition members and to coalition members rejecting the negative aspects of the project evaluations as invalid and as "outsider" interpretations.

4.3.1.2 Indicators and/or Measurement Tools Are in Tension with Community Concepts of Health and Social Well-Being

When indicators and measurement tools are in tension with community concepts of health and social well-being, it is usually because they have been developed external to the community and are based on theories that are mismatched with community-based understandings and assumptions. For example, Indigenous communities internationally have articulated concerns that commonly used health indicators and health indicator systems marginalize Indigenous understandings of health and social well-being. In response, communities have responded by developing Indigenous-specific health indicator frameworks (Smylie et al. 2006).

A second example is found in the measurement of intelligence and academic ability through standardized tests. Although validated on mostly White, upper-middle class students and reflective of Euro-Western concepts of intelligence, these inherently biased tests continue to be used, which further perpetuate social marginalization and negatively affect self-perception as well as result in false assumptions about group cognitive ability (Altshuler and Schmautz 2006). The bestselling book *The Bell Curve* by Richard J. Herrnstein and Charles Murray (1994) argued that genes played a role in racial and class differences on IQ (intelligence quotient) tests and illustrated the significant and detrimental policy impacts such biased measurements can have (Muntaner et al. 1996). Subsequent reductions in welfare benefits in the United States have been linked to the policy recommendations of the authors of *The Bell Curve*, which included a call to end the subsidization of births among poor women in order to avoid an intellectually stratified society (O'Connor 2004).

4.3.1.3   Euro-Western Scientific Analytical Methods and Assumptions are Privileged over Community Epistemologies

In epidemiology (especially in clinical epidemiology) a hierarchy of evidence exists where randomized controlled trials (RCTs) are considered the strongest and most reliable form of evidence, and the opinions of respected authorities are considered the weakest. This hierarchy means that the knowledge of communities is automatically regulated to the weakest tier of evidence (assuming that community members are even viewed as respected authorities). Again, we see inherent power imbalances in the relationship between researcher and community. However, this community-based "lay" knowledge undoubtedly could provide critical information that is currently missing in epidemiologists' understanding of health inequalities (Popay et al. 2008; see also Burke et al. 2005 and O'Campo et al. 2009b for a discussion of concept mapping).

4.3.1.4   Data Interpretation and Dissemination Perpetuate Societal Stereotypes and the Marginalization of Already Marginalized Groups

Without awareness of its societal, political and economic context, research findings often lead to perpetuation of stereotypes and misguided interventions. For example, the higher prevalence of cigarette smoking among African Americans as compared to their White peers has been attributed to acculturation and to African Americans deeming themselves invulnerable to the harms of smoking due to "various culturally based, superstitious rituals" rather than to contextual factors such as targeted advertising, anti-smoking campaigns and coping mechanisms for chronic stress (Klonoff and Landrine 1996). Ethnicity or culture then becomes viewed as a risk factor when, in actuality, the problems that must be addressed are underlying inequities in the distribution of health and social resources. Chapters 1, 6, 8 and 10 in this book further discuss the importance of context in the interpretation of data.

4.3.1.5 Community Members Are Unable to Access Their Community's Data

When members of the community of interest, including practitioners and policy makers, are excluded from access to their own data, the obvious result is missed opportunities for individual- and community-level response, community empowerment and evidence-based advocacy. For example, Aboriginal groups in Canada have had extremely limited access to the Aboriginal data collected in the recent Maternity Experiences Survey, despite previous agreements with the Public Health Agency of Canada (PHAC) that they would be actively involved in the analysis and dissemination of this national dataset (Public Health Agency of Canada 2006). This exclusion has occurred despite longstanding expressed concerns by Aboriginal groups regarding their ability to access health and social survey data that has been collected in their communities by the federal government (Castellano 2004).

4.3.2 Technical and Methodological Issues that Result in Inadequate Data

4.3.2.1 Marginalized Communities Are Excluded from, or Are Under-Represented in, Data Collection

One sure way to mask health and social inequalities and, therefore, to further perpetuate them is to under-represent or even completely exclude marginalized populations from data systems. For example, First Nations people living on reserves are excluded from national health surveys in Canada and, therefore, are excluded from the statistics reported from these surveys and the benefits that are supposed to be gained (Smylie et al. 2006; First Nations Information Governance Committee 2007). Similarly, marginalized groups are frequently excluded from or are under-represented in clinical studies, and the results are often simply assumed to be applicable. For example, the Canadian hypertension guidelines make recommendations for the treatment of high blood pressure in Black Canadians based on the assumption that African American data are applicable, despite different histories, social circumstances and genetics between these two groups (Canadian Hypertension Education Program 2010; Campbell et al. 2010). Studies that do not recruit adequate subgroup samples may result in the combination of diverse populations into a single category for reasons of statistical power, which blurs important distinctions and limits the policy relevance of results. For example, the Canadian Community Health Survey (Statistics Canada 2000) and the Maternal Experiences Survey (Public Health Agency of Canada 2006) both had inadequate samples of First Nations, Inuit and Metis groups, therefore, requiring the collapsing of these three very distinct groups into one "Aboriginal" category in order to have statistically relevant results.

4.3.2.2   Data Systems Lack Individual Identifiers That Enable for Meaningful Data Disaggregation Across Strata of Inequality

Many vital registration data, health care utilization data and surveillance data sets in Canada lack consistent and meaningful ethnic identifiers. Even when racial or ethnic identifiers are present on vital records such as in the United States, it is not clear whether the identifiers used are sufficient to describe the populations of interest. Again, the result is the masking of health and social inequities, including the masking of inequitable access to health services. For those who may argue that there is no need to measure ethnicity in Canada or who argue that inequities do not exist, Rodney and Copeland (2009) have shown that whenever data are disaggregated in Canada, based on racial and ethnic categories, disparities are observed among Black Canadians. The systematic underestimation of disparities among marginalized populations is a direct result of this lack of consistent identifiers. For example, if one is trying to use rates to identify health status disparities for ethnic minority groups compared to White populations in North America, the tendency will be to miss events among individuals belonging to ethnic minority groups since they may be more likely to be misclassified as White than vice versa. This scenario is encouraged by the lack of systematic, effective methods for data collection and is exemplified by the underestimation of First Nations infant mortality rate in Canada (Smylie et al. 2006).

4.3.2.3   Uncoordinated Health Service Performance Measurement System and Data Sources

Perplexingly, current data sources are not yet well coordinated into integrated health performance measurement systems. In fact, the expression "water, water, everywhere, nor any drop to drink" from Samuel Taylor Coleridge's 1798 poem *Rime of the Ancient Mariner* (which describes the plight of sailors stranded at sea with no freshwater to drink) could aptly be applied to the availability of useful and relevant social and health equity data (Coleridge 1965). For example, Indigenous groups worldwide have complained that they are being "researched to death." Yet the large majority of Indigenous health and social research has been non-systematically driven by the interests of the academic researchers, and entire populations and subject areas have been overlooked (Young 2003). The resulting research data is a non-integrated "patchwork" of information characterized by large "holes," which are for the most part of little use to Indigenous health and social policy makers, particularly at the community level (Smylie and Anderson 2006; Smylie et al. 2006; Anderson and Smylie 2009; Anderson et al. 2008).

It is clear that solutions to the many harms that data and data systems have on marginalized communities need to be found. In the next section, we will outline four strategies for change that address the challenges that we have just detailed. Addressing the problems and power imbalances, which characterize the relationship between data gatherer and data owner, is of paramount importance. We will describe how addressing these challenges can lead naturally and directly to solutions for the technical and methodological problems described above.

4.4 Transforming Health Data and Data Systems: Strategies for Change

The focus of the remainder of this chapter will be to answer the following two questions: (1) What do data and measurement systems that are actively contributing to social, economic and political processes, which are in turn reducing health inequities, look like? and (2) What types of change strategies will help us get there?

4.4.1 Re-envisioning Health Data and Social Data and Data Systems as Beneficial Tools to Advance Health and Social Equity

Up to this point, we have emphasized the ethical, scientific and practical problems that result from the disconnection of data systems from the communities whose data is being collected. Figure 4.1 illustrates how this disconnection is often formalized with external gatekeepers controlling community access to their data. Our re-visioning of health and social data systems shown in Fig. 4.2 builds on clearly articulated aspirations from diverse communities across equity strata. Despite varied contexts, communities experiencing a wide range of social inequities have clearly indicated a desire to move from a marginal to a central role in the processing and management of their health and social data (Pivik and Goelman 2011; Kobeissi et al. 2011; Shalowitz et al. 2009).

Health and social data systems need to be re-conceptualized as a resource designed to serve communities that is located within communities and managed and governed in partnership with the appropriate community authorities. It is these authorities, rather than external stakeholders, who need to be the gatekeepers for managing the interface among researchers, policy makers and practitioners.

Researchers and policy makers external to a particular community may find it challenging to identify the appropriate community representatives with whom to

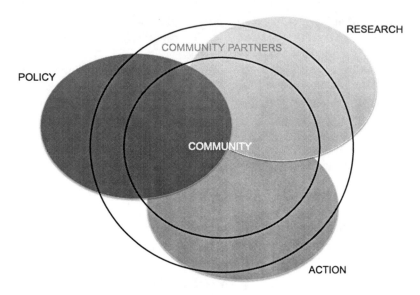

Fig. 4.2 Data and data systems that support community self determination

engage and/or partner. There is also the issue of understanding whether or not the identified community representatives have the relevant delegated authority and community-based legitimacy to hold this role. Familiarity with specific community contexts will greatly assist in addressing these challenges. In general, most communities of shared interest – no matter how small – have existing protocols and processes to identify leaders or representatives. While not always perfect, these existing protocols and processes can be a good place for the external researcher or policy maker to start. Another useful approach is to look for leaders or representatives who hold authority at a level of jurisdiction that matches the level of aggregation of data held in the data system of interest (e.g., a national-level data system link with national-level representatives).

It is not only the relationships upon which data systems are structured that need to change but also the content of what is being measured. The facilitation of social, economic and political processes that result in the reduction of health inequities requires data that enables social explanations of health problems. The processes that drive social exclusion clearly occur at the collective rather than the individual level. Therefore, it is at this collective, community level that they need to be studied, challenged and reversed. This approach will require a radical shift away from the over-reliance on individual-level data and the ongoing development of analytic methods that will facilitate community-level understandings of the social phenomena that drive health inequity. In our experience, community partnerships can naturally inform this process, since community stakeholders are acutely aware of the day-to-day collective social, economic and political constraints that impact community health and well-being.

Table 4.2 Ways in which health data and social data and data systems can be beneficial to communities

Benefit	Examples
Informing community planning, including identification of gaps in services and barriers in access to care	First Nations Regional Longitudinal Health Survey (First Nations Information Governance Committee 2007); South Asian Health Equity Report (Council of Agencies Serving South Asians 2010)
Highlighting disparities and unmet needs to external community funders and policy makers	Street Health Report (Khandor and Mason 2007); First Nations Regional Longitudinal Health Survey (First Nations Information Governance Committee 2007); South Asian Health Equity Report (Council of Agencies Serving South Asians 2010)
Identification and/or affirmation of community strengths that contribute to positive community self-image and challenge negative stereotypes	Community Child Health Research Network (CCHN) (National Institute of Child Health and Human Development 2002)
Demonstrating effectiveness of community-based programs, services and policies	Partnered realist review on concurrent mental health and substance use disorders (O'Campo et al. 2009a); Baltimore City Healthy Start program (Boroff and O'Campo 1996); Kanawahke Schools Diabetes Project (Kahnawake Educations System 1998; Macaulay et al. 2006; Paradis et al. 2005)
Identification of programs and service areas in need of improvement	Realist review on concurrent disorders (O'Campo et al. 2009a)

Community partnerships facilitate the dissemination of data into readily useful formats, since community policy makers are well aware of their own data needs. In the community-centric model, the translation of data into policy and practice is intrinsically "built-in." With respect to external community dissemination, community policy makers are already interfaced with external policy makers, research and practitioners and are seasoned in their ability to appropriately package information for these diverse audiences. Table 4.2 provides a list of ways in which communities can benefit from social data and health data and data systems when they are active data partners, along with examples of research that exemplify these benefits. In most cases, the benefits to communities are multiple and overlapping.

Box 4.1 presents a vision of perinatal surveillance that was developed by a joint working group of national Indigenous health stakeholders in Canada. This group included four national Indigenous organizations representing the interests of different Indigenous groups as well as representatives from Health Canada and PHAC. This statement exemplifies the transformation of health and social data systems that we have described above. The leadership role of Aboriginal organizations in all data processes is clearly articulated. This data system is about serving community interests – so much so that a more general vision of family and community wellness precedes the description of the ideal perinatal surveillance system.

Box 4.1 A Vision of Aboriginal Family and Community Well-Being Supported by Perinatal Surveillance

The arrival of infants is celebrated by their families and communities. Infants, children and their families are 100% healthy, happy and safe. Mothers, fathers and their families are supported before, during and after childbearing. Primary health care, including access to traditional healing and traditional midwifery, is universally accessible to all individuals and communities regardless of geographic location. Meaningful, relevant and tailored prevention and education programs are in place for all Aboriginal peoples. Through this nurturance and protection of our infants and children our communities are strengthened and renewed.

Infant mortality rates in Canada are available for all Aboriginal peoples (First Nation and Status Indians living on reserve, Status Indians living off-reserve, Non-status Indians, Inuit and Métis). The method of data collection and calculation of infant mortality rates is standardized across provinces and territories. Aboriginal organizations are active and full partners in the governance and management of the data. The methods of data collection, analysis and reporting are appropriate for all Aboriginal people. Aboriginal organizations are recognized as the owners of the data, and with their approval, data is publicly available. Flexibility and adaptability are built into the data system. The accuracy and reliability of the data is internationally recognized.

Birth outcomes data are linked to a longitudinal, comprehensive and inclusive Aboriginal health information system that includes data regarding the social and environmental determinants of health such as income, housing, family size, family and community environment, including culture-based nurturance and parenting, geographic location and environmental issues. This system is also linked to health and social services and their data. This system allows us to track how each infant blossoms. It creates a picture of what each child is arriving into and flags adversity as required. This information is then communicated to local health and social service providers and policy makers and is used to empower infants, children and their families. Drawing on this information, providers and policy makers can then identify the best strategies for further assessment and community-based assistance in the form of a "hand up" versus a "hand out."

The disparities and gaps between the health of Aboriginal people and other Canadians no longer exist. Canada has surpassed the commitments of international conventions, declarations and agreements regarding the rights of children and Aboriginal people.

4.4.2   Four Strategies for Change

In this section, we outline four strategies to facilitate the transformation of health and social data and data systems into tools that support community empowerment. We will illustrate each strategy using specific examples, with the provision that the complexity and diversity of processes that contribute to inequity in different settings and in different communities preclude highly prescriptive approaches. Our intention is that community leaders and researchers interested in change may be able to draw both principles and practical ideas from the discussion that can then be adapted to the specific community contexts.

4.4.2.1   Strategy One: Community-Centric Approach

The first strategy for change involves the shift from a researcher- or policy maker-focused method to a community-centric approach, where the community is truly at the centre of the data system (Fig. 4.2). This shift in focus and approach requires the development of a meaningful and truly collaborative partnership with the community where the community is the initiator of data processes or engaged in the very first stages of data work. In a community-centric model, the community is the centrepiece of the governance, management, dissemination and application of their data sets, measurement tools and measurement systems. With such an approach, the Ownership, Control, Access and Possession (OCAP) of information lies within the community, necessitating meaningful community involvement throughout each of the data production, analysis, dissemination and use processes.

Researchers should not assume that they have the skills or knowledge to implement this strategy if they have limited prior experience or training in community partnership work. The implementation of this strategy requires on the part of researchers the ability to collaborate with community partners, which to some might be a newer skill set. Specific elements of this collaborative skill set include but are not limited to: the ability to communicate effectively within the community context; the ability to appropriately demonstrate respect for the community; the ability to earn community trust and respect; and the ability to foster mutual understanding. Even the skilled and experienced collaborative researcher cannot expect these elements to occur without a considerable investment of time and energy. Another critical reflection for the researcher wanting to implement this strategy involves his or her internal comfort level and ability to adapt to a paradigm where the community, rather than the researcher, controls the data.

Despite these challenges, the benefits of acquiring this skill set and approach are clear. When properly and appropriately applied, data and data systems instantly become more relevant and useful, and community participation in the provision of data can markedly improve. Two examples illustrate this point. The first example is a community-based project focused on African Americans and the second is a national survey for First Nations populations. Through a true community-based participatory research framework, the African American Health Initiative Planning Project was able to actively engage a population considered "hard to reach" in planning of research and prevention activities (Woods 2009). In this project, the community was at the centre of deciding what information needed to be collected, how to collect it, what instruments to use and how to analyze and interpret data. Community participation was high, and after the release of the study report, the community selected a steering committee to ensure recommendations would be translated into practical solutions. The authors postulated that the traditional "hard to reach" moniker placed on African Americans was erroneous and was in fact rooted in the disconnection between the perceived versus real needs of this community. Of note is the fact that the community members in this initiative found it insulting that they could not be considered the lead agency for the associated grant, emphasizing the point that research ethics boards and funding agencies need to be vigilant on the true meaning of community involvement and engagement (Woods 2009).

The second example of a community-centric approach to using data as a tool of empowerment is the relatively new First Nations Regional Longitudinal Health Survey (RHS), the only First Nations-governed national health survey in Canada and the only national survey for the First Nations on-reserve populations (First Nations Information Governance Committee 2007). The purpose of the survey was to fill the void left by previous national surveys on the collection of relevant data for Aboriginal populations. In the past, other national surveys either completely excluded First Nations people living on reserve or were not able to reach enough on-reserve communities. The RHS serves to obtain data that is centred around First Nations conceptualizations of health, is controlled by First Nations, reflects the priorities of First Nations communities and uses both Western and First Nations traditional understandings of health and well-being. A community health governance policy framework called the OCAP (Ownership, Control, Access and Possession) of Data has been developed and successfully by the RHS governing committee. In RHS Phase I (2002–2003), the adult, youth and children surveys were collected from 22,602 individuals in 238 First Nations communities. RHS Phase II (2008–2009) covered a wide range of priorities, including health conditions and services, language, culture, education, housing, employment, sexuality, water quality, traditional medicine, mental health and disabilities.

These two examples demonstrate that, by putting the community at the centre of data processes and systems, we can ensure that they will feel a true sense of benefit from the collection of data and, therefore, will be willing participants in the process. The shift from externally- to community-controlled data and data systems can be challenging for researchers and policy makers who may fear that by giving up control of data sets means that their research findings will be tampered with or suppressed. It can also put pressure on community stakeholders who may not have the same infrastructure and/or human resources to govern and manage data. However, we would contend that there are far more examples of data suppression by researchers and policy makers than by community-governed data banks. Furthermore, the rebalancing of the distribution of data resources and building community-level data capacities not only will contribute to higher quality data that is more relevant and policy ready, it is also the only way to ensure that data work reduces rather than perpetuates social exclusions.

4.4.2.2 Strategy Two: Changing What We Measure

Secondly, we must change what we measure. We need to change both the focus of *what* we measure (i.e., data that can enable social solutions as opposed to just point out social gaps) and the tools that are developed for *how* to measure (i.e., match community perspectives, concepts and knowledge systems). As noted earlier, the processes that drive social exclusion and health inequities clearly occur at the collective rather than the individual level. Therefore, it is at this collective, community level that they need to be studied, challenged and reversed.

This change requires an emphasis on developing and assessing interventions designed to impact social and economic processes at a systems level in ways that decrease health inequities. Examples of these types of interventions include wage supplementation programs, accessible housing programs, affirmative hiring programs and health insurance programs. Clearly this kind of research is closely tied to policy and subsequently requires a high level of policy awareness and good working relationships with policy makers. One of the benefits of community-centric research approaches, as described above in Strategy One, is that this type of close interaction with policy and policy makers is typically built-in, since it will be community policy makers who are leading the research process.

Poverty research provides a good case study regarding the need to shift from descriptive research that documents social phenomena at the individual level to the evaluation of interventions that address social determinants of health at the systems level. Decades of poverty research in the United States have failed to create new knowledge on the modifiable societal-level causes of poverty because the focus of the research has been on individual characteristics of poverty such as dependency or employment history. The results of this individually-focused poverty research have thus informed interventions that address the causes of "dependency" in the United States versus interventions that focus on societal-level processes linked to poverty. This research has subsequently led to the dismantling of the "welfare" program and active maintenance (rather than reduction) of health inequities (O'Connor 2001). In contrast, the Mincome guaranteed income experiment that took place in the 1970's in three areas of Manitoba and the Self-Sufficiency Project in British Columbia and New Brunswick, which was designed to evaluate the impact of an income supplement for lone working parents, are both examples of intervention research aimed at addressing lack of money as an underlying and modifiable system-level cause of poverty. The Mincome experiment, although it was prematurely terminated due to changes in policy priorities, suggests that income assistance does not lead to significant decreases in labour force participation (Hum and Simpson 2001). The Self-Sufficiency Project demonstrated that income supplementation for full-time lone working parents led to wage progression over time (Zabel et al. 2006).

This example illustrates the need to strategically focus on the societal-level processes that maintain inequities, rather than the individual-level determinants of disparity, if the desire is to empower the communities experiencing the inequities. The data that we produce must provide the basis for convincing arguments to make social, economic and political changes – not for the perpetuation of marginalization and stereotypes. Furthermore, community representatives who have expertise in policy need to be active participants in the elucidation of meaningful causal models and mechanisms for change.

Community input is also essential in the development of relevant measurement tools or the identification and adaptation of existing ones. In order to avoid the imposition of indicators and measurement tools that are mismatched with community concepts of health and social well-being, there also needs to be a careful and thorough dialogue among community representatives and researchers who will be supporting measurement tool development. Concept mapping is one research tool that has been helpful in supporting communities in the process of articulating and documenting their understandings of health and social well-being and their measurement of priorities (Burke et al. 2005; O'Campo et al. 2009b). This type of baseline work is critical to ensuring that measures and measurement tools fit with community priorities and contexts. It is important to note that simple validity testing of an existing tool within the community setting does not ensure community relevance. For example, one could test the reliability and face validity of a psychometric scale designed to detect psychosis according to the Diagnostic and Statistical Manual of Mental Disorder (DSM) cross-culturally in an Indigenous population and arrive at the conclusion that the scale was reliable and valid. However, this approach would completely miss the profound issue of content validity that is created by differences in the ways in which the authors of the DSM and members of Indigenous communities might conceptualize mental health. The disciplines of psychiatry and psychology almost always consider visual and auditory hallucinations pathological, while in Indigenous contexts, it is relatively common for hallucinations to be sought out and those who have them may be considered gifted.

A final consideration with respect to changing what we measure is the importance of working in partnership with community and organizational representatives to ensure that appropriate identifiers are in place in all data systems and that sampling of each group is adequate to ensure that data can be disaggregated across equity strata. Carefully articulated agreements that mandate the active involvement of community representatives in the governance and management of these disaggregated data sets and appropriate and respectful protocols for the collection of equity information (e.g., ethnicity, race, income) are necessary prerequisites for this type of work. Studies must be designed so that samples across ethnicity strata are adequate in size to ensure "equal explanatory power" for each subgroup.

Box 4.2 illustrates how this partnership has been achieved with respect to the measurement of ethnicity in New Zealand (Curtis et al. 2005; Te Rōpū Rangahau Hauora a Eru Pōmare 2002). We note that when making efforts to include marginalized groups in research studies, researchers need to be mindful of the skills required for effective community engagement, which we have detailed in the preceding section on community-centric approach (Hasnain-Wynia 2005; Baker et al. 2006, 2007; Kandula et al. 2009).

Box 4.2 Equal Explanatory Power in New Zealand

There has been recent debate around the sampling frame for the New Zealand Health Survey and its inability to generate productive health information for Mäori development. Furthermore, there is a growing body of literature that describes disparities in Mäori and non-Mäori health, yet very few efforts have been made to provide explanations for these inequalities, thereby allowing the gap to widen further. With a legislative imperative, the New Zealand Ministry of Health currently has a mandate to reduce health disparities by improving the health outcomes of Mäori and other population groups.

The principle of equal explanatory power "recognizes Mäori statistical needs as having equal status with those of the total New Zealand population… Including equal numbers of Mäori and non-Mäori in survey samples allows data to be analyzed to equal depth and breadth for each population" (Te Rōpū Rangahau Hauora a Eru Pōmare 2002). It is this principle that will support the government's goals to reduce inequities in New Zealand.

In order to understand the implications of this principle, we can look at the age-mortality structure of the New Zealand population as an example. The Mäori population has a an age-mortality pattern with most deaths occurring around 10 years earlier than the non-Mäori population, resulting in higher rates of co-morbidity, disability and more severe health needs at earlier ages. The funding of health services, however, are structured around mortality patterns of the total New Zealand (or non-Mäori) population, which has obvious negative impacts on the health care needs of the Mäori. Sample sizes will, therefore, need to be large enough to produce adequate age-specific data for the Mäori, which is a critical component of ethnic data analysis, policy and intervention development.

Using data obtained from the New Zealand Health Information Service for 1996–2000, Curtis et al. (2005) applied the principle of equal explanatory power in the first New Zealand study to conduct an analysis of age-specific breast cancer incidence and mortality, adjusting for ethnicity misclassification. Specifically, the analysis found that, despite similar age-specific breast cancer incidence rates, Mäori women had higher age-specific mortality rates from breast cancer than non-Mäori women, particularly below the age of 60 years. These results have important implications for the delivery of accessible and culturally appropriate breast cancer screening services to Mäori women.

4.4.2.3   Strategy Three: Cross-Community, Cross-Sector Partnerships and Alliances

Cross-community, cross-sector partnerships and alliances are an additional strategy for optimizing the effectiveness of health and social data systems as tools to address inequities. Partnerships and alliances across communities and across equity strata can optimize political leverage and prevent a "divide and conquer" resistance to change both within and across groups experiencing social exclusion. Practically, these partnerships and alliances require an investment of time, energy and open dialogue among community representatives to ensure that every communities' interests are fully represented by the collective. This investment is beneficial because leaders working together across jurisdictions are usually better able to advocate for change and can maximize the perceived credibility of data sets. Box 4.3 illustrates a multisite project concerned with documenting the social determinants of infants', young children's and families' well-being. It is one of the first community and university partnerships funded by the United States' National Institute of Child Health and Human Development (2002).

Box 4.3 Community Child Health Research Network: Five Communities Across the United States

The Community Child Health Research Network (CCHN) was established in 2003 in response to a call for community-academic partnerships across the United States. Five sites were selected and represented urban, suburban and rural environments and communities that were predominately African American or Latina. The network has been collaborating for 8 years, and for several of those early years the division between community priorities and academic or funder priorities was apparent. Examples of challenges included timelines for deliverables (e.g., research questions, study design details, research proposal), balance at the initiation of the project between community desires and academic foci and the development of a common "culture" of collaboration. From the start, the community sought to implement an intervention or provide services to the communities being researched, but funders made it clear that the original call for proposals was for a longitudinal study. Hard work, common vision and growth in trust on all sides (including funder, community and university partners) led to strong working relationships after several years.

All stages of the research project from conceptualization of the research foci to the design of surveys and to the prioritization of papers and analyses of the data have been enriched by the community-university partnerships. University partners have deepened their understanding of the issues facing residents of high risk communities and been challenged to operationalize such understandings in the research being undertaken. Communities learned a great deal about how research is conducted and how it can be used to improve the community even if it is not an intervention. The processes developed to enhance multisite collaboration have, over time, evolved to be respectful of differences in priorities of the partners.

(continued)

Box 4.3 (continued)

The existence of multiple sites has meant multiple challenges as well as multiple benefits. Systematic differences between the partner priorities were more easily understood to be due to the nature of the collaboration when observed to be true across sites (e.g., when communities needed more time to sign off on deliverables) and were less likely to be interpreted as personality or personal flaws. Given the power differentials due to academic institutions holding the purse strings and university partners having more research experience, communities could draw from the strength of multiple sites to bring forth their issues and be heard more easily than they would have had only one site been involved. Finally, the funder has grown from being concerned with internal deadlines early on in the project to understanding the unique needs of a community-partnered project.

4.4.2.4 Strategy Four: Integration of Data Systems with Social, Economic and Political Levers for Change

Our final strategy for change involves working toward the integration of health system performance measures – with each other, with mainstream data and with services, policies and programs. We need integrated health and social data systems that can monitor and compare resource utilization. Such systems could highlight both over- and under-access to resources for various communities and confront the underlying causes for social gaps and gradients. They would also directly and effectively track the impacts of health assessments on the reduction of health inequities. As described in Box 4.1, these systems would be governed by communities and operate for communities.

This final tactic is perhaps the most complex, and we do not have any examples of an operational integrated health and social data system that is directly and effectively monitoring the impacts of policies, programs and services on the distribution of social resources and linking these impacts to a reduction in health inequities. In fact, it appears that this type of work is just beginning. For example, some researchers have now begun to investigate the contribution of Cochrane-type reviews to the reductions of health inequities (Welch et al. 2009; Ogilvie and Petticrew 2004; Tsikata et al. 2003). We believe that the effective implementation of this strategy is closely linked to the earlier three strategies such that if there is a community-centric approach to data (i.e., where communities have control over linked data and thus are supportive of integrated data systems; where the data collected are meaningful to the community with opportunities to incite social change; and where partnerships are in place across communities, jurisdictions and domains) then an integrated data system could be a crucial step toward meaningful and lasting change for many communities.

4.5   Anticipating and Addressing Challenges

We would be remiss to not explicitly state that the adoption of the aforementioned or similar strategies will not be without its challenges. Tensions between community groups and researchers are longstanding and rooted in differences that need to be understood and negotiated. These differences include but are not limited to: differences in needs; differing capacities; differences in the desired outcomes from the use of data; differences in expectations about data ownership and control; and differing ways of valuing expertise.

Researchers and community representatives do not necessarily have the required skills to effectively interface these differences. Furthermore, the systems that they are working within are usually structured in ways that amplify rather than bridge differences. For example, research funding structures (with few exceptions) are set up to be accessible only to "eligible institutions" such as universities, colleges and hospitals, and it can be very difficult for other, community-based agencies to access these funds directly. This undermines attempts at a "community-centric" partnership, as it is usually the academic researcher who has initial access to and control of the research funds. The existing protocols of research administration at universities, colleges and hospitals have been set up for researcher-controlled and -initiated projects, usually from the basic science and clinical or pharmaceutical domains. Research agreement templates, for example, are usually focused on ensuring that the commercial and liability interests of the institution and the researcher are protected, and they are not set up to deal with issues of community ownership, control and access to data.

Finally, with respect to challenges it is important to remember that research institutions and community agencies do not operate in a vacuum. Rather, their day-to-day reality is heavily influenced by the larger political, economic and social policy context. It is this context that controls the large majority of funding for both groups in Western democracies. It is also this context that can impose policy decisions that can negate decades of work with a single policy decision. For example, in Canada the federal cabinet recently imposed a decision on the national statistics agency (Statistics Canada) to cancel its mandatory long-form census and replace it with a voluntary household survey. Since Canada does not ask questions about race or ethnicity on the short-form census questionnaire or in the large majority of its health care utilization and vital surveillance databases, this decision, if implemented, will severely undermine the already compromised ability of researchers and communities to document and address health and social inequities across ethnic groups.

All of these challenges will not easily be overcome. However, as illustrated in Sects. 4.1 and 4.2 of this chapter, community sentiments are not born out of irrational paranoia but are instead the creation of many years of policies that produce ongoing social exclusion, whether deliberate or unintended. Therefore, it is crucial that external stakeholders see community involvement in the research, provider and policy arenas as enhancing rather than undermining the credibility and capabilities of the data system.

The current global context provides a rich opportunity for change. The World Health Organization (WHO) released its report on social determinants of health in 2008, and subsequently in May 2009 the World Health Assembly passed Resolution 62.14. This resolution calls upon the international community to consider health equity when working toward the achievement of the core global development goals, including developing indicators to monitor progress and strengthening international collaboration (Commission on Social Determinants of Health 2008; World Health Organization 2009). New measurement tools and processes will be critical to ensuring that measurement systems that result from this policy empower communities to address the social, economic and political processes that drive social exclusion rather than reiterate the harms described in Sect. 4.2.

In closing, it is our belief and experience that population-based data can be a tool for community empowerment. In this chapter, we have provided evidence regarding the need for a transformation of social epidemiology into a discipline that is focused on the development of community-owned and -driven health and social data systems. This work needs to be done in partnership with community representatives. A key role for social epidemiologists will be the bridging of differences between researchers and the community at the individual, collective and systems levels.

References

Altshuler SJ, Schmautz T (2006) No Hispanic student left behind: the consequences of "high stakes" testing. Child Sch 28:5–14

Anderson I (1999) Performance indicators in Aboriginal health services. In: Handock L (ed) Health policy in the market state. Allen and Unwin, Sydney

Anderson M, Smylie J (2009) Health systems performance measurement systems in Canada: how well do they perform in First Nations, Inuit, and Métis Contexts. Pimatisiwin 7:99–115

Anderson M, Smylie J, Anderson I et al (2006) First Nations, Métis, and Inuit health indicators in Canada. A background paper for the project: action oriented indicators of health and health systems development for Indigenous peoples in Canada, Australia, and New Zealand, Indigenous Peoples' Health Research Centre, Saskatoon

Anderson I, Anderson M, Smylie J (2008) The national Indigenous health performance measurement system. Aust Health Rev 32:626–638

Baker DW, Cameron K, Feinglass J et al (2006) Development and testing of a system to rapidly and accurately collect patients' race and ethnicity. Am J Public Health 96:532–537

Baker DW, Hasnain-Wynia R, Kandula NR (2007) Attitudes toward health care providers collecting information about patients' race, ethnicity and language. Med Care 45:1034–1042

Battiste M (2007) Research ethics for protecting Indigenous knowledge and heritage: institutional and researcher responsibilities. In: Denzin N, Giardina M (eds) Ethical futures of qualitative research: decolonizing the politics of knowledge. Left Coast Press, Walnut Creek

Battiste M, Youngblood Henderson J (2000) Protecting Indigenous knowledge and heritage. Purich Publishing, Saskatoon

Boroff M, O'Campo P (1996) Baltimore City Healthy Start Medical Reform for reducing infant mortality. Patient Educ Couns 27:41–52

Burke JG, O'Campo P, Peak GL et al (2005) An introduction to concept mapping as a participatory public health research method. Qual Health Res 15:1392–1410

Campbell N, Kaczorowski J, Lewanczuk RZ et al (2010) Canadian Hypertension Education Program recommendations: scientific summary. University of Calgary, Calgary

Canadian Hypertension Education Program (2010) CHEP recommendations for the management of hypertension. http://hypertension.ca/chep/wp-content/uploads/2010/04/FullRecommendations2010. pdf. Accessed 4 Aug 2010

Canadian Institutes of Health Research (2007) CIHR guidelines for health research involving Aboriginal peoples. http://www.cihr-srsc.gc.ca/e/documents/ethics_aboriginal_guidelines_e. pdf. Accessed 26 Apr 2010

Canadian Institutes of Health Research, Natural Sciences and Engineering Research Council of Canada, Social Sciences and Humanities Research Council of Canada (2010) Tri-council policy statement: ethical conduct for research involving humans, The Agencies, Ottawa

Castellano MB (2004) Ethics of aboriginal research. J Aborig Health 1:98–114

Centers for Disease Control and Prevention (2008) Tuskegee study timeline. http://www.cdc.gov/ tuskegee/timeline.htm. Accessed 2 Aug 2010

Coleridge ST (1965) The rime of the ancient mariner. In: Gardner M (ed) The annotated ancient mariner. Clarkson Potter, New York

Commission on Social Determinants of Health (2008) Closing the gap in a generation: health equity through action on the social determinants of health. Final report of the Commission on Social Determinants of Health, World Health Organization, Geneva

Council of Agencies Serving South Asians (CASSA) (2010) A diagnosis for equity: an initial analysis of South Asian health inequities in Ontario. http://www.cassaonline.com/index3/ downloads/Front/DiagnosisforEquity_May14_report.pdf. Accessed 12 Apr 2011

Curtis E, Wright C, Wall M (2005) The epidemiology of breast cancer in Maori women in Aotearoa New Zealand: implications for ethnicity data analysis. J N Z Med Assoc 118:U1298

Dalton R (2002) Tribe blasts "exploitation" of blood samples. Nature 420:111

First Nations Information Governance Committee (2007) First Nations Regional Longitudinal Health Survey (RHS) 2002/03: results for adults, youth and children living in First Nations communities, 2nd edn. Assembly of First Nations, Ottawa. http://www.rhs-ers.ca/english/pdf/ rhs2002-03reports/rhs2002-03-technicalreport-afn.pdf. Accessed 28 Feb 2009

Foucault M (1977) Discipline and punishment. Tavistock, London

Freimuth VS, Quinn SC, Thomas SB et al (2001) African Americans' views on research and the Tuskegee Syphilis Study. Soc Sci Med 52:797–808

Hasnain-Wynia R (2005) Patients' attitudes toward health care providers collecting information about their race and ethnicity. J Gen Intern Med 20:895–900

Herrnstein RJ, Murray C (1994) The Bell curve: intelligence and class structure in American life. Free Press Paperbacks, New York

Hum D, Simpson W (2001) A guaranteed annual income? From Mincome to the millennium. Policy Options Jan/Feb:78–82

Israel BA, Schulz AJ, Parker E et al (2001) Community-based participatory research: policy recommendations for promoting a partnership approach in health research. Educ Health (Abingdon) 14:182–197

Kahnawake Education System (1998) Kahnawake schools diabetes prevention project code of research ethics. Kahnawake Education System, Kahnawake

Kandula NR, Hasnain-Wynia R, Thompson JA et al (2009) Association between prior experiences of discrimination and patients' attitudes towards health care providers collecting information about race and ethnicity. J Gen Intern Med 24:789–794

Khandor E, Mason K (2007) The street health report. Street Health/The Wellesley Institute, Toronto

Klonoff EA, Landrine H (1996) Acculturation and cigarette smoking among African American adults. J Behav Med 19:501–514

Kobeissi L, Nakkash R, Ghantous Z et al (2011) Evaluating a community based participatory approach to research with disadvantaged women in the Southern suburbs of Beirut. J Community Health. 11 Feb 2011 [Epub ahead of print]

Little Bear L (2000) Jagged worldviews colliding. In: Battiste M (ed) Reclaiming indigenous voice and vision. University of British Columbia Press, Vancouver

Macaulay AC, Cargo M, Bisset S et al (2006) Community empowerment for the primary prevention of type 2 diabetes: Kanien'keha:ka (Mohawk) ways for the Kahnawake Schools Diabetes Prevention Project. In: Ferreira ML, Lang GC (eds) Indigenous peoples and diabetes: community empowerment and wellness. Carolina Academic Press, Durham

Marmot M (2005) Social determinants of health inequalities. Lancet 365:99–104

Minkler M (2000) Using participatory action research to build healthy communities. Public Health Rep 115:191–198

Muntaner C, Nieto FJ, O'Campo P (1996) The bell curve: on race, social class, and epidemiologic research. Am J Epidemiol 144:531–536

National Institute of Child Health and Human Development (NICHD) (2002) Development of community child health research. RFA: HD-02-008, National Institutes of Health, Rockville

North American Primary Care Research Group (1998) Responsible research with communities: participatory research in primary care. A policy statement. http://www.napcrg.org/resources-responsible.cfm. Accessed 10 Apr 2011

O'Campo P, Kirst M, Schaefer-McDaniel N et al (2009a) Community-based services for homeless adults experiencing concurrent mental health and substance use disorders: a realist approach to synthesizing evidence. J Urban Health 86:965–989

O'Campo P, Salmon C, Burke J (2009b) Neighbourhoods and mental well-being: what are the pathways? Health Place 15:56–68

O'Connor A (2001) Poverty knowledge: social science, social policy, and the poor in twentieth-century U.S. History. Princeton University Press, Princeton

O'Connor B (2004) A political history of the American welfare system: when ideas have consequences. Roman and Littlefield, New York

O'Neil JD, Reading JR, Leader A (1998) Changing the relations of surveillance: the development of a discourse of resistance in aboriginal epidemiology. Hum Organ 57:230–237

Ogilvie D, Petticrew M (2004) Reducing social inequalities in smoking: can evidence inform policy? A pilot study. Tob Control 13:129–131

Paradis G, Levesque L, Macaulay AC et al (2005) Impact of a diabetes prevention program on body size, physical activity, and diet among Kanien'keha:ka (Mohawk) children 6 to 11 years old: 8-year results from the Kahnawake Schools Diabetes Prevention Project. Pediatrics 115:333–339

Pivik JR, Goelman H (2011) Evaluation of a community-based participatory research consortium from the perspective of academics and community service providers focused on child health and well-being. Health Educ Behav 38(3):271–281

Popay J, Williams G, Thomas C et al (2008) Theorising inequalities in health: the place of lay knowledge. In: Bartley M, Blane D, Smith GD (eds) The sociology of health inequalities. Blackwell Publishers, Oxford

Public Health Agency of Canada (2004) Social inclusion as a determinant of health. http://www.phac-aspc.gc.ca/ph-sp/oiar/03_inclusion-eng.php. Accessed 10 Apr 2011

Public Health Agency of Canada (2006) The Canadian maternity experiences survey. Public Health Agency of Canada, Ottawa

Randall V (2006) Dying while Black: an indepth look at a crisis the American healthcare system. Seven Principles Press, Dayton

Rodney P, Copeland E (2009) The health status of Black Canadians: do aggregated racial and ethnic variables hide health disparities? J Health Care Poor Underserved 20:817–823

Royal Commission on Aboriginal Peoples (1993) Royal commission on Aboriginal peoples. Appendix B: ethical guidelines for research, Royal Commission on Aboriginal Peoples, Ottawa

Sateesh MK (2008) Bioethics and biosafety. IK International Publishing House, New Delhi

Shalowitz MU, Isacco A, Barquin N et al (2009) Community-based participatory research: a review of the literature with strategies for community engagement. J Dev Behav Pediatr 30: 350–361

Skloot R (2010) The immortal life of Henrietta Lacks. Crown Publishers, New York

Smith LT (1999) Decolonizing methodologies: research and Indigenous peoples. Zed Books Ltd., London/New York

Smylie J, Anderson M (2006) Understanding the health of Indigenous peoples in Canada: key methodological and conceptual challenges. CMAJ 175:602–605

Smylie J, Anderson I, Ratima M et al (2006) Indigenous health performance measurement systems in Canada, Australia, and New Zealand. Lancet 367:2029–2031

Snarch B (2004) Ownership, control, access, and possession (OCAP) or self-determination applied to research: a critical analysis of contemporary First Nations research and some options for First Nations communities. J Aborig Health 1:80–95

Statistics Canada (2000) Canadian Community Health Survey (CCHS), cycle 1.1. http://www. statcan.gc.ca/imdb-bmdi/instrument/3226_Q1_V1-eng.pdf. Accessed 21 July 2010

Te Rōpū Rangahau Hauora a Eru Pōmare (2002) Mana Whakamarama – Equal explanatory power: Maori and non-Maori sample size in national surveys, Ministry of Health, Wellington

Tsikata S, Robinson V, Petticrew M et al (2003) Is health equity considered in systematic reviews of the Cochrane Collaboration? Cochrane Systematic Reviews, 11th Cochrane Colloquium, Barcelona

Wallerstein N (1999) Power between evaluator and community: research relationships within New Mexico's healthier communities. Soc Sci Med 49:39–53

Welch V, Tugwell P, Wells GA et al (2009) How effects on health equity are assessed in systematic reviews of interventions (Protocol). Cochrane Database Syst Rev (3):MR000028

Wenman WM, Joffres MJ, Tataryn IV (2004) The Edmonton perinatal infections group: a prospective cohort study of pregnancy risk factors and birth outcomes in Aboriginal women. CMAJ 171:585–589

Woods V (2009) African American health initiative planning project: a social ecological approach utilizing community-based participatory research methods. J Black Psychol 35:247–270

World Health Organization (2009) Sixty-second World Health Assembly. Geneva, 18–22 May 2009, resolutions and decision, annexes, World Health Organisation, Geneva. WHA62/2009/REC/1. http://apps.who.int/gb/ebwha/pdf_files/WHA62-REC1/WHA62_REC1-en.pdf. Accessed 31 Aug 2010

Young TK (2003) Review of research on aboriginal populations in Canada: relevance to their health needs. BMJ 327:419–422

Youngblood-Henderson J (2000) Ayupackhi: empowering Aboriginal thought. In: Battiste M (ed) Reclaiming Indigenous voice and vision. University of British Columbia Press, Vancouver

Zabel J, Schwartz S, Donald S (2006) Analysis of the impact of SSP on wages, Human Resources and Skills Development Canada, Ottawa. http://www.srdc.org/uploads/zabel_et_al-wages.pdf. Accessed 7 Mar 2011

Chapter 5
Differences That Matter

Aisha Lofters and Patricia O'Campo

Contents

5.1   Introduction 94
5.2   The Need for Theory 96
5.3   The Risks of Essentialism 97
5.4   The Importance of Context 98
    5.4.1   The Misguided Focus on Individual-Level Factors 98
    5.4.2   The Role of Power Relations 99
    5.4.3   Measures Reflective of Context 100
5.5   Heterogeneity 102
    5.5.1   Heterogeneity Within Common Socially Defined Groups 103
    5.5.2   Heterogeneity Through a Realist Lens 105
5.6   Conclusion 106
References 106

Abstract The practice of stratification based on variables or indicators such as race, ethnicity, gender and socioeconomic position has been integral in the development of a substantial body of the social epidemiologic literature demonstrating significant and persistent inequalities in health outcomes. However, it is time for social epidemiologists to recognize that mere demonstration of gradients is no longer enough. The identification of gaps and gradients based on these variables flags the presence of a potential problem but does not explain the underlying mechanisms. Yet these proxies are often treated as if they *are* the exposures responsible for the gaps in outcomes. In this chapter, we will explore how the practice of stratification in epidemiologic research can evolve to identify the real causes of the gaps and to

A. Lofters (✉) • P. O'Campo
Centre for Research on Inner City Health, St. Michael's Hospital, 30 Bond Street,
Toronto M5B 1W8 , ON, Canada
e-mail: loftersa@smh.ca; O'CampoP@smh.ca

P. O'Campo and J.R. Dunn (eds.), *Rethinking Social Epidemiology:*
Towards a Science of Change, DOI 10.1007/978-94-007-2138-8_5,
© Springer Science+Business Media B.V. 2012

inform interventions and evaluations of interventions that target identified health inequities. The key recommendations of this chapter are to:

1. Draw from strong theories about causal mechanisms, which must take into consideration the relational aspects of the groups we are comparing;
2. Undertake measurement of, and stratification by, the modifiable societal and contextual factors that lead to hierarchical power relations between socially defined groups; and
3. Undertake measurement of variables that accurately explain the heterogeneity of experiences within socially defined groups to ensure that groups or individuals are not essentialized, with a particular focus on the solution-linked variables responsible for the heterogeneity.

5.1 Introduction

A fundamental strategy employed in epidemiology is to stratify study populations to investigate differences between groups such as those distinguished by age, sex or gender and race or ethnic group (Shim 2002). With a growing interest in social and health inequities and the emergence of the sub-discipline of social epidemiology, many epidemiologists have focussed in on the differential impact of social, economic and demographic variables on health-related processes and outcomes (Berkman 2009; Putnam and Galea 2008). This practice of stratification has been integral in the development of a substantial body of international literature that has demonstrated significant and persistent inequalities in health outcomes based on variables such as race, ethnicity, gender and socioeconomic position (e.g. income and education) (Berkman 2009; Hofrichter 2006; Shim 2002).

However, social epidemiology is becoming increasingly at risk of stagnation unless researchers acknowledge that the demonstration of gaps and gradients is no longer enough, in part, because they only flag the presence of a potential problem and do not explain why a problem exists or how to address that problem. For example, knowing that infant mortality is two times higher among African Americans compared to Whites does not yield information about which interventions should be implemented to reduce the gap. As has been argued throughout this book, social epidemiologists need to move the emphasis of the field away from problem description and toward identifying actionable mechanisms and the generation of evidence to inform the development of viable interventions (see Chap. 1). Although it is commonplace to see a discussion on action that could be taken to reduce the identified inequity in many social epidemiologic papers, these discussions are often speculative and not based in strong theory or direct evidence regarding the causes or contributors of the gaps. In order to determine the best actions to take to reduce inequities, one requires a firm basis in the underlying and modifiable mechanisms that lead to these same inequities, and this foundation is often where social epidemiology is still lacking (Engel 2002; Krieger 2001; Krieger et al. 1993, 1997; Randall 2006; Syme 2008).

The increased level of distress experienced by many homosexuals upon coming to terms with their own sexuality when compared to heterosexuals realizing their sexuality provides one example. This marked distress was at one time viewed as a mental disorder (listed as "ego dystonic homosexuality" in *The Diagnostic and Statistical Manual of Mental Disorders*, 3rd edition), instead of as a fairly predictable result of the prospect of having to deal with both internalized and societal homophobia (Zucker and Spitzer 2005). One can imagine two markedly different paths towards ameliorating this mental distress based on these two explanations, one focussed on changing the individual, e.g. the use of fluoxetine to suppress sexual activity (Elmore 2002), the other focussed on changing societal biases and/or helping those affected with coping mechanisms and de-stigmatization strategies (Lamont 2009). Clearly, it is only through direct exploration of causes of distress level gaps (i.e., societal-level discrimination toward homosexuals) that we arrive at feasible ways to begin to close the gaps (i.e., *not* to feel the need to fix the individual).

In this chapter, we seek to view stratification through a realist lens (see Chap. 2). We aim to encourage social epidemiologists to rethink the current reflexive practice of stratification based on variables or indicators such as race or income, as it does little to explain why gaps exist or shed light on achievable solutions to the gaps observed. As they are currently conceptualized and operationalized, some of these stratification variables are often uninformative, serving as poor proxies for the true mechanisms that underlie health inequities (Coburn 2004; Gravlee 2009; Manly 2006; Sayer 1992). Yet we regularly treat these poor proxies as if they *are* the exposures responsible for the gaps in outcomes. "Race" itself is almost never the reason a gap exists; instead it is the exposure to interpersonal racism or being subjected to institutional racial discrimination, the intergenerational transmission of its effects or particular experiences that are associated with race that lead to inequities. Indicators, in other words, are proxies *of something*, and it is imperative that social epidemiology have a clear explanation of what that something is (see Chap. 2). Moreover, when such proxies are used, the reader can insert their own interpretation as to whether it is a cultural, genetic (e.g., Muntaner et al. 1996), economic or discriminatory practice that has lead to the observed gaps, resulting in confusion as to the real causes of the inequities. Further evidence of the weakness of these proxies is apparent when we consider that many are measured cross-sectionally; yet, the life course and legacy effect literature tell us that the cumulative and intergenerational effects of social deprivation could be much more revealing (David and Collins 2007; Love et al. 2010; Singh-Manoux et al. 2004; Smith et al. 1997).

In this chapter, we will explore how, using new and complementary indicators and methods, stratification can evolve to inform interventions and evaluations of interventions that target identified health inequities. We aim to move social epidemiology from only examining the *who* of health inequities to a focus on *how to change* health inequities. In particular, our recommendations are threefold: (1) draw from strong theories about causal mechanisms, which must take into consideration the relational aspects of the groups we are comparing; (2) undertake measurement of, and stratification by, the modifiable societal and contextual factors that lead to hierarchical power relations between socially defined groups; and (3) undertake measurement of variables that accurately explain the heterogeneity of experiences within socially defined groups to ensure that groups or individuals are not essentialized, with a particular focus on solution-focused variables responsible for the heterogeneity.

We begin the chapter with a discussion of the need for supporting theories. Such information is currently sparse in the literature but is essential to inform attainable solutions to the problems identified when we demonstrate gaps by race, gender or class.

5.2 The Need for Theory

Epidemiology and public health, as applied fields, have tended to de-emphasize theory or relied on implicit biomedical and biological-based theories that predominate within the field to explain health and health inequities. Yet all research, and especially all causal claims, including those concerned with social, economic, racial and gender inequities, are based upon explicit or implicit theory. Epidemiology and public health in the twentieth century have relied heavily on biomedical theories to explain the occurrence of and inequities in health and well-being (Engel 2002; Krieger 2001; Stallones 1980; Susser 1985). Thus, despite much research challenging the scientific validity of the categories of "race" or "ethnicity" as they are typically used in public health studies (American Anthropological Association 1998; Gunaratnam 2003; Stanfield and Dennis 1993) and ample evidence dispelling the myth that racial groups reflect inherent biological or genetic homogeneity (American Anthropological Association 1998; U.S. Department of Energy Office of Science 2003), we still encounter studies that invoke such explanations for demonstrated racial or ethnic gaps (Cooper et al. 2003).

At the other end of the spectrum, there are those who argue that race and ethnicity are socially determined categories shaped by societal processes like slavery, colonization, discrimination and/or privilege (Fujishiro 2009; Muntaner et al. 1996; Randall 2006). Thus, examination of racial differences should be explained by historical, materialist or cultural processes (Gunaratnam 2003). There is even the suggestion that the categories of race be abandoned in favour of the study of the processes that contribute to so-called racial gaps (Stanfield and Dennis 1993).

While we focus on "race" here as an example, it is important to note that stratification by race is primarily an American practice. Race, and in particular African American race, is a proxy for the history of slavery and continuous discrimination unique to this population and is not applicable in other settings such as neighbouring Canada. Historical differences between the United States and Canada means that references to Black race would represent an entirely different set of circumstances and is very rarely used in Canadian epidemiologic research. Because of the history of immigration in Canada, the term "visible minority" has been used instead by federal agencies to represent "persons, other than Aboriginal people, who are non-Caucasian in race or non-white in colour" (Statistics Canada 2009). Visible minority status was developed to study labour market disadvantages of this group (Statistics Canada 2009). Thus, the evolution of these variables used for stratification often reflects a historical context that is rarely made explicit.

5.3 The Risks of Essentialism

To progress in our understanding of why inequalities by race or ethnicity exist and, therefore, to reduce the gaps, we must avoid essentializing categories such as race, ethnicity, sex or gender and even poverty. When we *essentialize* we "impute a fundamental, basic, absolutely necessary constitutive quality to a person, social category, ethnic group, religious community, or nation" (Werbner 2003). At the same time, we are not likely to discard the use of race, ethnicity or the other categories in our research as they reflect socially relevant groupings of populations (more so in some countries, such as the United States, than others). Moreover, even when using variables such as "racial identity," or discrimination, epidemiologists seek to simplify their categories, thus contributing to continued essentialism.

If we accept that the theories of inherent biological or genetic differences by race are invalid and that using race or ethnicity as a proxy for social explanations is too limiting in its ability to explain complex gaps, then how should epidemiologists approach the examination of inequities by race or ethnicity? To avoid essentialism, Gunaratnam (2003) recommends that our research: (1) take into account the relational nature of the categories being compared; (2) connect the categories to their context; and (3) focus on heterogeneity within categories of difference to ensure that groups or individuals are not defined by a single category.

Our theories of inequities must take into consideration the relational aspects of the groups we are comparing. Thus, rather than categorizing or stratifying groups into, for example, low or high income, we must articulate *how* wealth matters to health and also investigate the ways in which individual and institutional practices, through power, status, resources and connections, serve to maintain the wealth gap and maintain poverty (Wright 2008). Although individuals on both ends of the spectrum may not be aware of these institutionalized practices, competition and control for scarce resources where the wealthy consume more than their fair share, exploitation of those with less power by the wealthy, such that those in power benefit while the powerless suffer, and the ability of the wealthy to utilize power and connections to maintain their wealth at the expense of those with less wealth, are meaningful relations that should be incorporated into our research to explain why the gaps exist. Currently, strata or categories of income are devoid of such acknowledgements. Class-based measures (O'Campo and Burke 2004; Wright 2008) incorporate the relations between classes or potential "warfare" between the class strata and provide a theoretical explanation for why gaps exist. Measures on inequities by gender in the workplace, as reported in a study illustrating unique indicators of employment-based gender discrimination for income, job strain, job demands and control that were informed by strong theories, suggests that these factors illustrate large disparities in these areas even when controlling for occupation and are important predictors of health (O'Campo and Burke 2004).

The idea that we must connect the categories to the larger contexts is the second recommendation of Gunaratnam. The larger contexts that have contributed to the differences observed between groups will be discussed at length in the following section. Focussing on heterogeneity within groups being compared is a third strategy. This, too, will be discussed in the section on heterogeneity below. This acknowledgement of heterogeneity not only prevents groups from being reduced to simple homogeneous categories but also ensures that research reflects the multiple identities and experiences that can simultaneously shape risks and determine health. Thus, using strong theory to inform the key stratification variables and measuring indicators that avoid essentializing these groups will lead to progress in ensuring that epidemiologic evidence begins to point to appropriate interventions that move beyond the simple demonstration of disparities.

5.4   The Importance of Context

5.4.1   The Misguided Focus on Individual-Level Factors

Our second key recommendation for stratification in social epidemiology is to measure modifiable contextual factors that underlie the gradients and gaps we frequently observe. Too often within social epidemiology research, the analyses of the determinants of inequalities have focussed at the level of the individual. Consequences of this misguided focus have included epidemiology's long history of reductionist genetic and biological explanations for racial and ethnic health inequities (although it must be noted that a misconstruction of race as a biological classification has also strongly contributed to these misguided explanations) as well as suppositions such as "downward drift" (the hypothesis that mental disorders are more represented in lower social classes because individual weaknesses in mental functioning lead to low social class attainment (Perry 1996)) and similar individually focussed explanations for socioeconomic health inequities. While more recently there has been a growth in the inclusion of societal-level factors in research concerning health inequities, determinants are still primarily focussed on an individual's lifestyle and perceived choices without the requisite examination of the context of how power is embedded in the society around that individual (Krieger 2000; Muntaner et al. (2011); Putnam and Galea 2008; Shankardass et al. 2010a; Syme 2008). The subsequent explanations and range of interventions emerging from this evidence are therefore targeted at changing the behaviours of the individual, not at changing the contextual problems that shape and determine behaviours and the health of the individual.

For example, a major risk factor for the leading cause of mortality, cardiovascular disease, is physical activity. As physical activity rates have been suggested by some authors to be lower among people of lower income compared to their more well-to-do counterparts, proposed solutions are often focussed around ways to increase motivation of disadvantaged individuals to exercise more often (Hallal et al. 2005; McMurray et al. 2000). Factors such as accessibility of opportunities to exercise (e.g., time, cost, geographic proximity) are often ignored. Similarly, many of the discussions about poverty and low income frequently focus on individual-level characteristics such as employment readiness or educational attainment, which are modeled as determinants of low-income status. Factors such as labour markets, state or federal employment and minimum wage policies or business practices of cutting wages to increase profits, to name a few examples, are rarely considered in the examination of health inequities despite being the drivers of income levels. Similarly, more immediately actionable contextual factors such as the local availability of employment, employment training programs or traditional and alternative educational opportunities are rarely considered. Tellingly, in a review of how health inequities are addressed in the American media, Kim et al. (2010) found that behavioural explanations dominated the discourse.

The choice to frame health inequities as individual-level issues and to explain them with individual-level behaviours can be a counterproductive one. This choice often encourages, whether intended or not, the practice of "blaming the victim" (Green and Darity 2010; Wallace 2008) and encourages the erroneous use of resources on inappropriate interventions. In the case of physical activity, if the appropriate action is believed to be to encourage the individual to exercise, then the implicit (or even explicit) suggestion is that the individual has chosen to be lazy or does not have the knowledge or intelligence to recognize that they are lazy. If we focus on the demographic characteristics of low-income individuals, then we are choosing to not focus on the larger economic and political context that exclude them from obtaining quality education and employment training. This example illustrates how the wrong solutions, or solutions that will do little to ameliorate the true causes, will be implemented if contextual factors are not taken into consideration.

5.4.2 The Role of Power Relations

As social epidemiologists we can no longer afford to ignore that, on a global level, the wealthy or those of the lightest shade of skin color consistently have access to both micro- and macro-level privileges that have been determined by social, historical and economic societal-level contexts. Correspondingly, the poor and those of darker shades of skin color are consistently and actively excluded from receiving these same privileges (O'Campo 2007; Wallace 2008). In fact, many of the determinants of health and social inequalities observed the world over emanate from the societal processes of White privilege or privilege of the majority group, inequitable access to quality education, unjust labour markets, unjust financial policies and neo-liberalist economies and/ or political systems. Researchers need to examine these processes, especially those that are more readily actionable with community-based interventions (Green and Darity 2010; James 2009; Krieger 2003; Manly 2006; Wallace 2008).

The magnitude of the effects of the unequal distribution of power was captured in words by the African American physician, Charles Roman, in 1917 and still hold truth over 90 years later, once we interpret "strength of the white man" to represent the political power of the dominant social class: "The greatest difficulties confronting us from a sanitary and hygienic standpoint arise not from the physiological weakness of the colored man but from the psychological strength of the white man" (Roman 2010). Yet the aforementioned article by Kim et al. (2010) tells us that less than 5% of media articles on health inequities invoked a social justice explanation. To truly advance the field of social epidemiology, researchers need to constantly challenge the implicit idea that particular socially defined groups do not do well because they are not allowing themselves to integrate into the mainstream and instead develop explanations that incorporate the role that institutionalized power relations created by larger society play in actively perpetuating health inequities (Muntaner et al. 2011; Putnam and Galea 2008; Shankardass et al. 2010a; Syme 2008). These power relations are manifested not only at the larger level (national, state, provincial) but also at the more local level (neighbourhood, district), suggesting that the route to change will not only require widespread political upheaval but also community-based interventions that researchers can undertake immediately.

To unearth the true mechanisms generating inequities and to develop effective interventions, the contexts that generate the social inequalities must be measured and incorporated into our research. In essence, instead of comparing the number of calories that an individual from an empowered group is burning versus the number of calories an individual from a disempowered group is burning, we need to compare: the walkability of their neighbourhoods; whether each feels safe walking or cycling in their neighbourhood; the ability of their local schools to incorporate physical education into their curriculums based on their resources; and the availability of local community recreation centres with free activities, while explicitly acknowledging that a difference in political and societal empowerment exists. We need to recognize that if race is a socially defined construct, then racial inequities must be socially defined as well and are, consequently, socially actionable.

5.4.3   Measures Reflective of Context

So if current stratification variables do not represent the all-important societal context, what are examples of variables that could? Income level, possibly the single most commonly used stratification variable in social epidemiology in one form or another, does not accurately capture the underlying causes of health inequities by social class, in part because income levels themselves are the end result, not the cause, of larger societal processes that also contribute to health inequities. However, depending on the research question and specific context, there are many other variables that are directly reflective of underlying processes that researchers could consider. If the association between income and detrimental dietary practices are being questioned, exploration of access (both geographical and financial) to healthy and high-quality foods and the processes by which there might be systematic exclusion or diminished access to such health promoting resources becomes necessary. It is well documented that many foods available in high-income neighbourhoods tend to be of better quality, healthier and cheaper (Cummins and Macintyre 2002; Glazier et al. 2007; James 2009; Krieger et al. 1997). If the relationship between socioeconomic status and chronic stress is being studied, the ability to participate in the same recreational and family activities to which those of higher socioeconomic position are privy to becomes an important factor to measure (Krieger et al. 1997).

Race and ethnicity are also commonly used stratification variables in the social epidemiology literature, and many large and persistent health inequities based on race and/or ethnicity have been unearthed as a result. However, in addition to measuring race or ethnicity, at a minimum, epidemiologists should measure experiences of discrimination. As we have discussed above, the use of race/ethnicity in epidemiologic studies can be problematic, in part because it is routinely the inequitable race relations to which one is subjected to due to race that are the cause of inequalities and not one's race itself (Krieger 2003; Krieger et al. 1993; Wright 2008). For example, high blood pressure has been found to be associated with one's perceived and culturally ascribed color but not with one's measured skin pigmentation (Gravlee 2009), suggesting that it is one's place in the social hierarchy, as determined by the dominant group, that matters and not the geographic location from which one's ancestors originate. Although both attitudinal and institutionalized discrimination are important to acknowledge and measure, and although most people think first of attitudinal discrimination when they think of racism, discrimination and prejudice, we recommend a particular emphasis on the latter.

In the section above, we discussed the importance of power relations, many of which negatively impact racialized groups. The concept of institutionalized or structural discrimination is closely related and consists of systems in which public policies, institutional practices and/or societal norms interact to actively maintain inequities (Putnam and Galea 2008; Randall 2006). Instances of institutionalized discrimination are numerous, some of which have been mentioned before, and include: the under-representation of minorities in the health professions; the disproportionate marketing of tobacco and alcohol to racial minorities; name-based discrimination in the workforce; active maintenance of segregation from education and employment opportunities and from safe, healthy environments; and health care systems that are structured to disadvantage particular marginalized groups (O'Campo 2007; Randall 2006). This discrimination has far-reaching repercussions. For instance, discrimination in housing and lending markets leads to segregated neighbourhoods (Farley et al. 1993). These neighbourhoods, specifically those neighbourhoods in which disempowered groups live, are often subject to under-resourced schools and an inability to provide an adequate education to their students, limited employment opportunities, particularly for males, and a subsequent shift to illicit forms of earning money as other viable options rapidly disappear (Krieger 2000; Putnam and Galea 2008). Similarly, inability to access high quality, culturally competent medical care because of structural discrimination within the health care system can lead to a long-term deterioration in health for socially excluded groups (James 2009). The concept of cultural safety in health care, which recognizes that it is a group's position within society that is most relevant as opposed to the specific things members think or do, and that every health care interaction is influenced both by the cultural mindset of the provider and by the cultural context in which it occurs, is a direct response to this discrimination within the health system (Polaschek 1998).

We have emphasized the measurement of institutionalized discrimination because it has implications over and above any particular individual (Gravlee 2009; Krieger 2003) and, inevitably, also involves recognizing the contextual factors that actively maintain oppression based on race and/or ethnicity. As a result, it has the potential to lend itself more easily to movement into solution-focused research than does exclusively focusing on attitudinal discrimination; the former means acknowledging that we are all either active or passive participants, and the latter suggests that some mysterious and distant "they" are racists (Randall 2006). Therefore, we re-emphasize that the focus of social epidemiologists should be on measures of institutionalized discrimination that more readily lend themselves to action and toward targeted interventions. For example, as a direct result of a research report by Germany's Institute for the Study of Labor, which found that otherwise equivalent applications with German-sounding names had a 14% greater chance of landing an interview than those with foreign-sounding names, five major corporations agreed in 2010 to participate in a 1-year pilot project where personal information is removed before job applications are processed (Donath 2010). By using an actionable measure of institutionalized discrimination, instead of simply measuring employment based on ethnicity, the authors were able to directly affect an intervention targeted at some of the processes that underlie differences in employment based on ethnicity.

Importantly, whereas attitudinal prejudices are usually relatively easy to discern, institutionalized discrimination may not always be perceived by those toward whom it is targeted or, indeed, by those who are perpetuating it (Green and Darity 2010; Krieger 2003; Randall 2006). For instance, employers may not be aware of their name-based biases, and potential employees may not be aware that they are being passed over for interviews because of their perceived ethnicity. However, the effects are just as damaging, regardless of perception. Therefore, in studies where perceived discrimination has not been found to have a significant effect on health outcomes, but where health inequities still remain partially unexplained (Albert et al. 2010; Barnes et al. 2008), actionable processes of institutionalized discrimination should be strongly considered.

5.5   Heterogeneity

Our third and final recommendation is for researchers to address meaningful sources of heterogeneity within socially defined groups as a further method to elucidate underlying mechanisms of health inequalities. Socially defined groups,

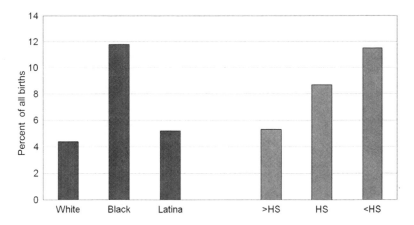

Fig. 5.1 Low birthweight by race and education separately, based on vital records data for a U.S. state

although so categorized because of some common characteristic, are not homogeneous and consist of many subpopulations with differing cultural, historical and societal experiences (Ruffin 2010). The sources of this experiential heterogeneity within any particular marginalized population become crucial to explore in a researcher's quest for moving toward solution-focused research. By investigating heterogeneity, we may discover important but more subtle inequities that can further hone in on whom action and intervention are most needed, help to further demystify the root causes of the inequities and subsequently facilitate the movement toward action (Kramer and Hogue 2009; Krieger 1992; Krieger et al. 1993, 1997; O'Campo et al. 2004; Wallace 2008).

5.5.1 Heterogeneity Within Common Socially Defined Groups

Two examples illustrate the importance of exploring heterogeneity within socially defined groups as well as of defining a meaningful referent group. A routine practice in epidemiology is to examine health outcomes by race or socioeconomic position such as those presented for low birthweight by race and education in Fig. 5.1. When examined separately, we see a familiar pattern of non-White and less educated individuals having the worst outcomes. Yet, when we combine race and education, as is shown in Fig. 5.2, we see the heterogeneity within and between races more clearly. We see just how much improvement is required across all races in order to bring all groups up to the standard of health experienced by the most privileged subgroup, namely White women with more than a high school education.

As a second example, Bleich et al. (2010) found that the well-known racial disparities in obesity among women in the United States, where African American

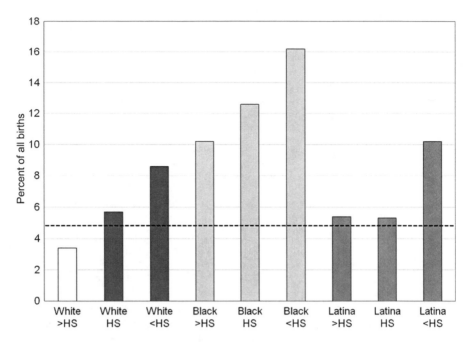

Fig. 5.2 Low birthweight by race and education together

women are significantly more likely to be obese, do not exist among poor, urban women subject to the same social context. Among these women, race had no significant bearing on obesity rates. These findings suggest that policies to target the obesity disparity should focus on social aspects of the environment around a woman, such as availability of healthy yet affordable foods and availability of an environment that promotes safe and regular physical activity as mentioned above, instead of focus on trying to change the cultural dietary choices of that woman. They also suggest that policies to fight obesity should not exclude non-African American women. However, without examining both race and social class and without identifying a meaningful referent group, the researchers would likely have produced misguided and erroneous recommendations for addressing the obesity problem.

These examples demonstrate an important point to remember. Variables that lead to heterogeneity within marginalized groups may not only act independently, they may also be variables that act synergistically. There are individuals who are simultaneously members of several marginalized groups, and the oppression that they experience as a result is more than additive (Krieger 2000; Krieger et al. 1993; Randall 2006). Author Vernellia Randall (2006) has described the impact of the intersection of race and gender in the United States with the phrase "all women are white, all blacks are men" to illustrate how African American women are often excluded from both gender and racial issues. Neglecting the potential synergistic effects of socially defined characteristics for an individual or group is unacceptable when we are concerned with targeting the social determinants of health. Therefore, social epidemiologists must not only simultaneously examine the effects of multiple variables in their analyses but must also examine their interactions (Wallace 2008). Through an exploration of heterogeneity and use of an appropriate referent group, and bearing in mind the possibility of synergistic effects, we can highlight the most vulnerable subgroups where action is most urgently needed and ensure the best use of resources for ameliorating inequities.

5.5.2 Heterogeneity Through a Realist Lens

However, it must be stressed that researchers need to be thoughtful on the sources of heterogeneity that they choose to investigate. Again, we need to ensure that we approach heterogeneity with a realist lens. Acknowledgement of heterogeneity within strata is not a new concept, but studies usually focus on individual-level factors that may serve as a source of distraction if used in isolation and rarely concurrently investigate the solution-focused variables responsible for the heterogeneity. When we explore the heterogeneity within disadvantaged groups, we must continue to address the contextual and societal factors that could be the basis of action to reduce inequities. For example, differential access to, eligibility for and participation in the financial arena (e.g., home ownership, ability to get credit) and various social services may explain differences in health or well-being among low-income populations in a more meaningful way than only sub-categorizing by race or ethnicity and in a way that guides us toward underlying mechanisms for hetero-geneity within groups (Krieger 2000; Krieger et al. 1997; Manly 2006). Gender differences within an income stratum might be better explained by also exploring differences based on childcare responsibilities and age and number of family members in the household (Krieger et al. 1993, 1997). Underlying mechanisms such as unequal access to political power, lack of accommodation for child-rearing responsibilities within the work force and the need to distribute the same amount of income over multiple household members need to be addressed (O'Campo et al. 2004). Within any particular racialized or ethnic group, important differences in experiences may exist based on level of acceptance by the privileged group, per-ceived threat by the privileged group, exposure to segregation, exposure to quality education and employment opportunities (Krieger 2003; Manly 2006). For exam-ple, babies born to African-born Black women have been found to have identical distributions of birth weight as babies born to American-born White women and higher than that of babies born to American-born Black women. Within one genera-tion, this advantage disappears (Gravlee 2009). If we want to explore the underlying causes for these differences, is birthplace the only appropriate source of heterogene-ity to target? Or should we also consider potential underlying mechanisms such as social supports, feelings around sense of self, sense of empowerment and chronic exposure to discrimination, segregation and stress? Tellingly, African American neonatal mortality has been independently associated with less relative political power (Krieger 2000).

A related example illustrates how the investigation of heterogeneity can directly inform evidence-based intervention. With the knowledge that infant mortality and low birth weight are more common in non-White ethnic groups, Norbeck et al. (1996) examined the effects of high stress, low social supports and high anxiety as sources of heterogeneity on pregnancy outcomes for African American, Hispanic and White women. The authors found that low social support from the woman's partner or mother was of especial importance for birth complications for African American women only. As a result of their findings, the authors created a social support intervention aimed at preventing low birth weight among African American women with known low social support. The intervention was designed to provide the support usually provided by mothers or partners and was effective in reducing the rate of low birth weight. By exploring actionable sources of heterogeneity within racial groups and not stopping at simply describing the differences in pregnancy outcomes by racial group, the authors were able to create an effective intervention targeted at an underlying mechanism for an observed inequity.

5.6 Conclusion

Epidemiologists may be hesitant to approach stratification in the way we have suggested for fear of appearing as advocates instead of scientists or for fear of appearing to lack subjectivity (Krieger 2003). Yet, it is advocacy groups, not academics, who have traditionally been most likely to propose solutions to health inequities (Kim et al. 2010). As well, the changes we propose to the approach to stratification may be difficult for peer reviewers and editors to accept (Syme 2008). However, the development of strong theoretical frameworks to guide the research may help to assuage some of these fears. Researchers should also consider, however, that a conscious choice to not acknowledge the underlying mechanisms that lead to health inequities is in itself a political decision based on implicit assumptions about the root cause of inequities (see Chap. 3). Finally, though reviewers and editors may be reticent to accept these changes, we suspect that interested policy makers will appreciate the advent of measures that will be directly transferable to action.

References

Albert MA, Cozier Y, Ridker PM et al (2010) Perceptions of race/ethnic discrimination in relation to mortality among Black women: results from the Black Women's Health Study. Arch Intern Med 170:896–904

American Anthropological Association (1998) Statement on "race". http://www.aaanet.org/stmts/racepp.htm. Accessed 25 Mar 2011

Barnes LL, de Leon CF, Lewis TT et al (2008) Perceived discrimination and mortality in a population-based study of older adults. Am J Public Health 98:1241–1247

Berkman LF (2009) Social epidemiology: Social determinants of health in the United States: are we losing ground? Annu Rev Public Health 30:27–41

Bleich SN, Thorpe RJ, Sharif-Harris H et al (2010) Social context explains race disparities in obesity among women. J Epidemiol Community Health 64:465–469

Coburn D (2004) Beyond the income inequality hypothesis: class, neo-liberalism, and health inequalities. Soc Sci Med 58:41–56

Cooper R, Kaufman J, Ward R (2003) Race and genomics. N Engl J Med 348:1166–1170

Cummins S, Macintyre S (2002) A systematic study of an urban foodscape: the price and availability of food in greater Glasgow. J Urban Stud 39:2115–2130

David R, Collins J (2007) Disparities in infant mortality: what's genetics got to do with it? Am J Public Health 97:1191 1197

Donath J (2010) Anonymous job applications: German pilot project aims to reduce discrimination. Spiegel Online International. http://www.spiegel.de/international/business/0,1518,713711,00. html. Accessed 30 Dec 2010

Elmore JL (2002) Fluoxetine-association remission of ego-dystonic male homosexuality. Sex Disabil 20:149–151

Engel G (2002) The need for a new medical model – a challenge for biomedicine. In: Marks D (ed) The health psychology reader. Sage, London

Farley R, Steeh C, Jackson T et al (1993) Continued racial residential segregation in Detroit: "Chocolate city, vanilla suburbs" revisited. J Hous Res 4:1–38

Fujishiro K (2009) Is perceived racial privilege associated with health? Findings from the Behavioral Risk Factor Surveillance System. Soc Sci Med 68:840–844

Glazier R, Booth G, Gozdyra P et al (2007) Neighbourhood environments and resources for healthy living – a focus on diabetes in Toronto: ICES Atlas. Institute for Clinical Evaluative Sciences, Toronto

Gravlee CC (2009) How race becomes biology: embodiment of social inequality. Am J Phys Anthropol 139:47–57

Green TL, Darity WA Jr (2010) Under the skin: using theories from biology and the social sciences to explore the mechanisms behind the black-white health gap. Am J Public Health 100: S36–S40

Gunaratnam Y (2003) Researching race and ethnicity: methods, knowledge and power. Sage, London

Hallal PC, Azevedo MR, Reichert FF et al (2005) Who, when, and how much? Epidemiology of walking in a middle-income country. Am J Prev Med 28:156–161

Hofrichter R (2006) Tackling health inequities through public health practice: a handbook for action. The National Association of County and City Health Officials, Washington, DC

James SA (2009) Epidemiologic research on health disparities: some thoughts on history and current developments. Epidemiol Rev 31:1–6

Kim AE, Kumanyika S, Shive D et al (2010) Coverage and framing of racial and ethnic health disparities in US newspapers, 1996–2005. Am J Public Health 100:S224–S231

Kramer MR, Hogue CR (2009) Is segregation bad for your health? Epidemiol Rev 31:178–194

Krieger N (1992) The making of public health data: paradigms, politics, and policy. J Public Health Policy 13:412–427

Krieger N (2000) Discrimination and health. In: Berkman LF, Kawachi I (eds) Social epidemiology. Oxford University Press, Oxford

Krieger N (2001) Theories for social epidemiology in the 21st century: an ecosocial perspective. Int J Epidemiol 30:668–677

Krieger N (2003) Does racism harm health? Did child abuse exist before 1962? On explicit questions, critical science, and current controversies: an ecosocial perspective. Am J Public Health 93:194–199

Krieger N, Rowley DL, Herman AA et al (1993) Racism, sexism, and social class: implications for studies of health, disease, and well-being. Am J Prev Med 9:82–122

Krieger N, Williams DR, Moss NE (1997) Measuring social class in US public health research: concepts, methodologies, and guidelines. Annu Rev Public Health 18:341–378

Lamont M (2009) Responses to racism, health, and social inclusion as a dimension of successful societies. In: Hall PA, Lamont M (eds) Successful societies: how institutions and culture affect health. Cambridge University Press, New York

Love C, David RJ, Rankin KM et al (2010) Exploring weathering: effects of lifelong economic environment and maternal age on low birth weight, small for gestational age, and pre-term birth in African-American and white women. Am J Epidemiol 172:127–134

Manly JJ (2006) Deconstructing race and ethnicity: implications for measurement of health outcomes. Med Care 44:S10–S16

McMurray RG, Harrell JS, Deng S et al (2000) The influence of physical activity, socioeconomic status, and ethnicity on the weight status of adolescents. Obes Res 8:130–139

Muntaner C, Nieto J, O'Campo P (1996) The bell curve: on race, social class, and epidemiologic research. Am J Epidemiol 144:531–536

Muntaner C, Borell C, Ng E et al (2011) Politics, welfare regimes, and population health: controversies and evidence. Sociology of Health & Illness 33(6):946–964

Norbeck JS, DeJoseph JF, Smith RT (1996) A randomized trial of an empirically-derived social support intervention to prevent low birthweight among African American women. Soc Sci Med 43:947–954

O'Campo P (2007) Equity and Distributive Justice. Background paper prepared for the 10th International Medical Workforce Conference, Vancouver, Canada 2006

O'Campo P, Burke J (2004) Recommendations on the use of socioeconomic position indicators to better understand racial inequalities in health. In: Ver Ploeg M, Perrin E (eds) Eliminating health disparities: measurement and data needs. National Academies Press, Washington, DC

O'Campo P, Eaton W, Muntaner C (2004) Labor market experience, work organization, gender inequalities and health status: results from a prospective analysis of US employed women. Soc Sci Med 58:585–594

Perry M (1996) The relationship between social class and mental disorder. J Prim Prev 17:17–30

Polaschek NR (1998) Cultural safety: a new concept in nursing people of different ethnicities. J Adv Nurs 27:452–457

Putnam S, Galea S (2008) Epidemiology and the macrosocial determinants of health. J Public Health Policy 29:275–289

Randall V (2006) Dying while Black: an indepth look at a crisis the American healthcare system. Seven Principles Press, Dayton

Roman CV (2010) Fifty years' progress of the American Negro in health and sanitation. Am J Public Health 100:S66–S68

Ruffin J (2010) The science of eliminating health disparities: embracing a new paradigm. Am J Public Health 100:S8–S9

Sayer A (1992) Method in social science: a realist approach, 2nd edn. Routledge, London

Shankardass K, Solar O, Murphy K et al (2010a) Health in all policies: a snapshot for Ontario. Results of a realist-informed scoping review of the literature. In: Getting started with Health in All Policies: a resource pack. Report to the Ministry of Health and Long-Term Care (Ontario). Centre for Research on Inner City Health, St. Michael's Hospital, Toronto. http://www.stmichaelshospital.com/knowledgeinstitute/search/details.php?id=18218&page=1. Accessed 12 May 2011

Shim J (2002) Understanding the routinised inclusion of race, socioeconomic status and sex in epidemiology: the utility of concepts from technosicence studies. Sociol Health Illn 24:129–150

Singh-Manoux A, Ferrie J, Chandola T et al (2004) Socioeconomic trajectories across the life course and health outcomes in midlife: evidence for the accumulation hypothesis? Int J Epidemiol 33:1072–1079

Smith GD, Hart C, Blane D et al (1997) Lifetime socioeconomic position and mortality: prospective observational study. Br Med J 314:547–552

Stallones R (1980) To advance epidemiology. Ann Rev Public Health 1:69–82

Stanfield J, Dennis R (1993) Race and ethnicity in research methods. Sage, Newbury Park

Statistics Canada (2009) Visible minority population and population group reference guide, 2006 Census. Catalogue no. 97-562-GWE2006003. http://www12.statcan.gc.ca/census-recensement/2006/ref/rp-guides/visible_minority-minorites_visibles-eng.cfm. Accessed 25 Mar 2011

Susser M (1985) Epidemiology in the United States after World War II: the evolution of technique. Epidemiol Rev 7:147–177

Syme L (2008) Reducing racial and social-class inequalities in health: the need for a new approach. Heal Aff 27:456–459

U.S. Department of Energy, Office of Science (2003) Exploring genetics issues relevant to minority communities. http://www.ornl.gov/hgmis/elsi/minorities.html. Accessed 25 Mar 2011

Wallace B (2008) Toward equity in health: a new global approach to health disparities. Springer, New York

Werbner P (2003) A "treacherous bind": working with and against racial categories. In: Gunaratnam Y (ed) Researching race and ethnicity: methods, knowledge and power. Sage, London

Wright E (2008) Logics of class analysis. In: Lareau A, Conley D (eds) Social class: how does it work? Russell Sage, New York

Zucker KJ, Spitzer RL (2005) Was the gender identity disorder of childhood diagnosis introduced into DSM-III as a backdoor maneuver to replace homosexuality? A historical note. J Sex Marital Ther 31:31–42

Part II
Context

Chapter 6
Place-Based Stress and Chronic Disease: A Systems View of Environmental Determinants

Ketan Shankardass

Contents

6.1	Stress as a Mediator of Sociospatial Disparities in Chronic Diseases	114
6.2	The Need for Cross-Disciplinary Synthesis on Place-Based Stress and Chronic Diseases	115
6.3	The Experience of Stress	117
	6.3.1 Sources of Stress	117
	6.3.2 Mediators of Stress	118
	6.3.3 Manifestations of Acute Stress	118
	6.3.4 Manifestations of Chronic Stress	119
6.4	Place-Based Stress	120
6.5	Environmental Stressors and Resources	122
6.6	A Systems View	125
6.7	Implications for Social Epidemiology	127
References		130

Abstract The global burden of chronic diseases (CD) has resulted in significant negative societal impacts, such as long-term disability, premature death and costs to health care systems (Cohen et al. 2007; Daar et al. 2007); a recent estimate suggests that such diseases account for approximately 60% of all deaths worldwide (Daar et al. 2007). As social epidemiologists begin to more closely investigate how environmental circumstances contribute to social disparities in CD, such as cardiovascular disease, diabetes, obesity and asthma, there has been growing interest in the mediating role of chronic stress. To date, many studies have speculated about the relevance of this pathway. However, stress-related mediation is rarely examined directly in epidemiologic research; and when it has been, it has often not been rigorously conceptualized and a biomedical focus has been predominant. As a

K. Shankardass (✉)
Department of Psychology, Wilfrid Laurier University, 75 University Avenue West,
N2L 3C5, Waterloo, ON, Canada
e-mail: KShankardass@wlu.ca

P. O'Campo and J.R. Dunn (eds.), *Rethinking Social Epidemiology:
Towards a Science of Change*, DOI 10.1007/978-94-007-2138-8_6,
© Springer Science+Business Media B.V. 2012

result, the potential mediating role of stress in CD disparities has been vaguely described and, arguably, over-simplified in epidemiology. In this chapter, a multi-disciplinary narrative review of the stress discourse is presented to facilitate a deeper understanding of inter-relationships among these factors, including how social and physical attributes of the environment can shape the experience of stress and how physiological and behavioural responses that characterize chronic stress can directly and indirectly foster chronic disease via multiple, overlapping pathways over time. In particular, the experience of stress is described in terms of sources, mediators and manifestations based on work from the disciplines of sociology, psychology and psychoneuroimmunology, and then integrated with notions of place from geography in order to facilitate a complex understanding of sociospatial disparities in CD. A conceptual framework is also presented that articulates a systems view of two key general pathways describing environmental determinants of chronic stress and CD. This tool can be used to support the development of elaborate hypotheses and study designs on this topic in social epidemiology and to support translational work related to chronic disease prevention.

Abbreviations

CD   Chronic diseases
GIS   Geographic Information Systems

...each exposure leaves an indelible scar...

–Hans Selye (1956)

6.1 Stress as a Mediator of Sociospatial Disparities in Chronic Diseases

Many studies describe small-area spatial disparities in CD (e.g., differences between residential neighbourhoods) that often indicate clustering in places characterized by low socioeconomic status (e.g., Creatore et al. 2007; Diez-Roux et al. 1997; Matheson et al. 2008). These differences often persist even after comprehensively accounting for individual-level risk factors (i.e., using multilevel models) (e.g., Shankardass et al. 2010). Such unexplained disparities suggest the importance of explanations that are not purely *compositional* (Diez-Roux and Mair 2010; Macintyre et al. 2002) – that is, there is increasing recognition that the context of places matters for health, well-being and aging, including a "mutually reinforcing and reciprocal relationship" between people and their context (Cummins et al. 2007). Moreover, there may be multiple healthy and harmful attributes that comprise the context of a specific place, with multiple implications for the onset of CD

(Aneshensel 2005; Auchincloss and Diez-Roux 2008; Buzzelli and Jerrett 2007; Curtis 2004; Evans and English 2002; Jerrett and Finkelstein 2005; Morello-Frosch and Shenassa 2006).

Sociospatial patterns in CD may partly reflect an oft-hypothesized but rarely studied (in epidemiology) mediating role of psychosocial processes. In particular, pathways involving chronic stress are often posited to explain why people in lower socioeconomic status places are less healthy (Adler and Stewart 2010; Thoits 2010; Chen et al. 2006; Clougherty and Kubzansky 2009; Hayward and Colman 2003; Morello-Frosch and Lopez 2006; Taylor et al. 1997; Wright 2006). Growing evidence suggests the plausibility of direct and indirect relationships between chronic stress and the onset of a range of CD, including (but not limited to) obesity, cardiovascular disease, chronic respiratory disease and diabetes (Adam et al. 2010; Wright et al. 2005; Baum et al. 1999; Bruce et al. 2009; Chen et al. 2006; Dave et al. 2011; de Vriendt et al. 2009; Holmes et al. 2009; McEwen 1998; McEwen and Gianaros 2010; Orpana et al. 2009; Shankardass et al. 2009; Steinberger et al. 2009; Steptoe 2006; Wright 2006; Turner 2010; Tsiotra and Tsigos 2006).[1] Many authors have noted also inter-relationships between the experience of chronic stress and other risk factors for various CD. For example, stress has been linked to increased cigarette smoking (Weaver et al. 2008); increased blood pressure (Steptoe and Willemsen 2004); weight gain (Chandola et al. 2008; Kivimaki et al. 2006); low physical activity (Chandola et al. 2008); and poor diet (Chandola et al. 2008).

6.2 The Need for Cross-Disciplinary Synthesis on Place-Based Stress and Chronic Diseases

While epidemiology (at large) has contributed to a better understanding of disease-specific aetiology and individual-level risk factors, and facilitated clinical treatment of and health promotion targeted at individuals to reduce disparities in the incidence and burden of CD, much remains to be understood about how and why

---

[1] There is also a substantial discourse on the relationship between chronic stress and mental health outcomes that are often chronic, particularly in sociology. This includes much work based on the stress process paradigm utilized in this chapter (e.g., Avison et al. 2010); in fact, the stress process paradigm was originally created in order to understand the onset of depression (Pearlin et al. 1981). There is also growing interest in incorporating broader social contexts in the use of the stress process to study mental health outcomes (e.g., Aneshensel 2010). Although the conceptual framework outlined in this chapter may be relevant to mental health researchers in terms of how environmental attributes can shape the experience of chronic stress, implications for sociospatial disparities in chronic mental health conditions may be fundamentally different in comparison to other chronic diseases. For example, addictions are commonly studied as a chronic mental health outcome having some antecedent role for chronic stress; whereas in this chapter, we consider the healthy and unhealthy habits reflected by addictive behaviour as manifestations of chronic stress that ought to be considered as on the pathway to the onset of other chronic diseases.

environments – including places of residence, work, play and study – shape our health and well-being. In particular, there has been less evidence (i.e., fewer studies) to support *specific* types of interventions that address the environmental attributes of *specific* places. Importantly, there has also been little theoretical discussion about generalizable mechanisms to understand why certain *types* of people in certain *types* of places may be at higher risk for both chronic stress and CD (Diez-Roux and Mair 2010; Evans and English 2002), although growing evidence suggests the relevance of explanations at the mesosocial- and microsocial-level that involve both psychological and physiological pathways.

For example, a recent study in *The Lancet* shows that the health gap between people of high and low social class in all-cause and circulatory disease mortality is diminished in places in England with more green space. The authors suggest that social disparities in mortality may be reduced in places with more green space, in part, because of the restorative effects of natural spaces that may ameliorate stress and also because of increased physical activity in greener places, which may have both psychological (read: stress buffering) and physiological health benefits (Mitchell and Popham 2008). While these types of studies support the notion of "environmental determinants of stress" that can be modified to address problems of chronic stress and chronic disease, they do not explicitly demonstrate the multiple specific and inter-related pathways from environment to stress to disease (or social disparity in disease, for that matter) to facilitate interventions. In turn, they also do not illuminate the extent to which such complex observations may be generalizable to other places.

Given the multifactorial nature of this problem, this may partly reflect the lack of cross-disciplinary synthesis that speaks to these pathways (Adler and Stewart 2010; Dankwa-Mullan et al. 2010; Krieger et al. 2010). In outlining the ways that *stressful* and *resourceful* (i.e., amenable to coping with stress) aspects of place can influence risk for CD, this chapter presents: (1) a narrative review of place-based stress (cf. Morello-Frosch and Shenassa 2006) and CD using Pearlin et al.'s (1981) notion of a *stress process* as a heuristic model (also see Pearlin 1999); and (2) a conceptual framework that offers a systems view of these complex relationships. In particular, the conceptual framework represents a "practically adequate" synthesis of various fields of research (cf. Sayer 1992), including several perspectives that may be less familiar to epidemiologists, while outlining two key etiologic pathways.

Although there may be controversies about these perspectives within specific disciplines – or in the proposed synthesis of knowledge from these disciplines – the framework identifies parts of the system that need to be clearly understood in order to have a more comprehensive understanding of how stress mediates sociospatial disparities in CD. In this spirit, it is also worth noting that other authors have offered valuable conceptual models of stress as a driver or mediator of social and sociospatial health disparities (e.g., Clougherty and Kubzansky 2009; Elliott 2000; Gee and Payne-Sturges 2004; Morello-Frosch and Shenassa 2006; Stockdale et al. 2007; Turner 2010; Wright 2006), although this framework is the first that uses a place-based notion of stress to focus on multiple chronic disease outcomes.

The proposed framework highlights the potential for multiple and inter-related effects of environmental attributes that characterize places and chronic stress on CD via psychological and physiological mechanisms. As further elaborated in the following discussion, a systems view particularly contributes to the practice of applied social epidemiology (e.g., public health) by facilitating the clarification and quantification of the health costs and benefits to developing "stress-sensitive" policies (Juster et al. 2009) and urban development strategies oriented toward healthier environments (see Chap. 15).

6.3   The Experience of Stress

Stress has been alternately defined across several seminal papers (e.g., Evans and English 2002; McEwen and Gianaros 2010; Pearlin et al. 1981; Selye 1936; Cohen et al. 1995). Rather than implying tremendous conflict over what stress *is*, these differences more likely reflect the fact that the experience of stress is multifaceted and can be associated with several negative (and positive) impacts on the human body. Moreover, our understanding of stress continues to grow more complex as a result of it being examined closely and simultaneously from several disciplinary perspectives (namely psychology, sociology, psychoneuroimmunology). Adapting Cohen et al.'s (1995) definition, this chapter considers stress as a process in which demands strain on an individual's ability to adapt – physiologically and emotionally – with implications for physiological and behavioural pathways that may compound over time and foster CD pathology. The discussion of the inter-relationship of place, stress and CD later in this chapter can be further clarified by first reflecting on the *stress process* paradigm (as discussed by Pearlin et al. 1981), which is a "general orienting framework" for the interlinked domains that comprise the experience of stress: sources, mediators and manifestations.[2]

6.3.1   Sources of Stress

The sources of stress are typically referred to as "stressors," and include major life events (e.g., moving to a new home); ambient strains (e.g., concern for safety in a particular neighbourhood); role strains (e.g., those related to workplace hierarchy); and those of a quotidian nature (e.g., a difficult or tiring commute) (Almeida et al. 2005). Stressors, in general, may contribute immediate and extended adaptive demands on individuals that may manifest as emotional, behavioural and

---

[2] Wheaton (1994) further examines the meaning and inter-relationships of similar domains of "stressors, stress, and distress."

physiological responses and the dysfunction of these systems in the long term (McEwen 2008).[3] However, as outlined below, all stressors should not be assumed to affect all individuals in the same way.

6.3.2 Mediators of Stress

To the extent that the sources of stress are external to the individual (i.e., they are objective), the manifestation of stressors on the individual is mediated by several internal factors.[4] In addition to genetic features (e.g., Iqbal Kring et al. 2011), this includes some processes that require the interpretation of stressors and other features of the environment vis-à-vis how to *perceive of* and *respond to* stressors (i.e., a subjective response). Importantly, a stressor must be perceived for it to elicit a response; but this need not be a *deliberate* process of recognizing and assessing potential threats, as changes in key stress hormones have been observed in response to noise disruption during sleep (Evans and English 2002; Maschke and Hecht 2004). An individual's perception of potential stressors may also be conditioned by early life circumstances that shape cognitive and socioemotional development (Maccari et al. 2003; Weinstock 2001), as well as prior experiences with specific types of stressors (Dave et al. 2011; Hertzman and Wiens 1996; McEwen 2008). In response to perceived stress, the assessment of social and material resources can be viewed as a precursor to the process of dealing with (or "coping with") stress (as described below), which may in turn be shaped by one's personality (e.g., positive affect, self-esteem) (McEwen 2008; Mällo et al. 2009) and by personal resources that may have been developed earlier in life (e.g., self regulation and executive function) (Karoly 1993; Riggs et al. 2007; Farah et al. 2006; Dunn 2010).

6.3.3 Manifestations of Acute Stress

The manifestations of *acute* stress events can be described in terms of physiological, emotional and behavioural sequelae. Acute stress events (both positive and negative) are normally met with an excited physiological response (often referred to as the "fight or flight" response; Cannon 1915) followed by a return to normal functioning, but there are also coping responses that involve "thoughts and behaviours" (Folkman et al. 1986) to deal with emotions and problems brought on by demands (Lazarus and

---

[3] It is also important to note that stressors can be positive in nature such that the emotional rush of participating in (or watching) a thrilling sporting event can also elicit stress responses. Selye (1975) referred to this type of stress as eustress. It is less clear to what extent positive stressors can be damaging in the long-term.

[4] Mediation in how the sources of stress are manifested is not to be confused with the role of chronic stress as a mediator of sociospatial disparities in CD.

Folkman 1984). The process of coping may involve the use of social support (e.g., friends, family, neighbours) and behavioural responses (e.g., drug use, sleeping, eating, exercising) (Umberson et al. 2008).

6.3.4 Manifestations of Chronic Stress

Where perceived stressors are particularly demanding or recurrent over time, longer-term (i.e., *chronic*) stress may result. A popular – and evolving – heuristic for understanding the manifestations of chronic stress is allostatic load (Korte et al. 2005; McEwen 2008; Morello-Frosch and Shenassa 2006). Allostasis denotes the capacity of the human body to adapt to stressors that bring the body out of the normal range of functioning (homeostasis, which is broken by the aforementioned "fight or flight" response). Allostatic load describes the "wear and tear" on the body in maintaining homeostasis in response to repeated stress challenge, leading to inter-related emotional, behavioural and physiological changes directly or indirectly related to dysregulation of brain function at some point of "allostatic overload" (Juster et al. 2009; McEwen 2008). Impacts on neuroendocrine, immune, metabolic, and cardiovascular system function related to dysfunction of the hypothalamic-pituitary-adrenal axis and the sympathetic-adrenal-meduallary system have been demonstrated and implications for multiple chronic disease pathologies are evident (McEwen 2008; Wright et al. 2005). In this way, the multimodal allostatic load model is largely compatible with Selye's (1936) original notion of stress as a General Adaptation Syndrome and shares many similarities with other recent perspectives on this topic (e.g., Adler and Stewart; Carlson and Chamberlain 2005; Chrousos and Gold 1992; Hayward and Colman 2003).

While the manifestations of chronic stress have often been described in terms of physiology, the aforementioned "thoughts and behaviours" (Folkman et al. 1986) that naturally accompany stress events, such as coping, should also be considered as *stress-related* determinants of CD (Laugero et al. 2011; McEwen 2008; Umberson et al. 2008). Over the long term, the resources that one has available to cope with stress also appear to be related to CD (House et al. 1988; Kawachi et al. 1999), and effective coping appears to buffer the negative impacts of chronic stress (McEwen and Gianaros 2010; Thoits 2010). For example, social support has been negatively associated with risk for CD and premature mortality (Hayward and Colman 2003), while healthy and unhealthy behavioural habits that may reflect more long-term, habitual coping responses (e.g., diet, exercise and smoking) more clearly determine CD pathology directly (Adler and Stewart 2010; Dunn 2010; Hayward and Colman 2003; Hughes et al. 2010; Lynch et al. 1997; Rod et al. 2009; Umberson et al. 2008; Tsatsoulis and Fountoulakis 2006; Epel et al. 2001) and indirectly, by increasing exposure and susceptibility to other risk factors (e.g., drug use leading to HIV infection (Larrat and Zierler 1993)).

In summary, long-term exposure to perceived stressors stimulates individuals acutely, while culminating in emotional, behavioural and physiological dysfunction over the long term that may contribute to the onset of CD. Individual variation in the extent to which such dysfunction occurs may be conditioned early in life, but also according to social and behavioural coping responses that occur over the life course and in relation to available resources.

6.4   Place-Based Stress

Previous work suggests that the environment plays a key role in both our experience of stress (Evans and English 2002) and our risk for CD (e.g., Aneshensel 2005; Elliott 2000; Hill et al. 2005; Juster et al. 2009). While the last section described the experience of stress and implications for CD using the stress process and allostatic load concepts, this section expands on how a complex notion of place can facilitate a clearer understanding of environmental determinants of stress and CD, including how experiences with stressors and the accessibility of resources over the life course can condition one's responses to stress (Marmot and Singh-Manoux 2005; Singh-Manoux et al. 2004).

The stress process – an individual-level construct – has been previously embed-ded within a broader context not only in terms of environmental attributes that may reflect potential stressors (Aneshensel 2010; Pearlin 1999), but also in terms of how consciously perceived stressors are appraised and coped with (Folkman et al. 1986; Lazarus and Folkman 1984; Pearlin 1989), as described by the *transactional model*. Here, people are viewed as being "in a dynamic mutually reciprocal, bidi-rectional relationship" with their context and stressors are comprised of "a specific set of environmental characteristics" being appraised by "a particular person with particular psychological characteristics" (Folkman et al. 1986). More broadly, Pearlin (1989) suggested that stressful experiences do not exist in a vacuum, but can be traced to "social structures" and the "location" of individuals within these structures. In this way, individual variation in one's response to stress – in both behavioural and physiological terms – may be determined in complex ways by one's perception of their surroundings as well as their socioeconomic position (interpreted broadly).

The social structures and location of individuals that Pearlin refers to, as well as the complex relationship described by the transactional model, share great similar-ity with geographic perspectives on place and health. For example, Cummins et al. (2007) recently proposed a "relational" approach to understanding place in health research that challenges us to account for not only the "processes and interactions occurring between people and places and over time," but also the "dynamic and changing characteristics of places and the place-to-place mobility of populations on a daily basis, and over the life course." In turn, this and other geographic approaches to place and health (see Cutchin 2007) have implications for how social epidemio-logists gauge whether individuals may be more or less susceptible to stressors according to how they perceive their surroundings and how they access local resources for coping. For example, Luginaah et al. (2002) describe a process of "cognitive reappraisal" of places over time that demonstrates the importance of considering how personal stressor appraisal and coping habits change across the life course and in response to changing contexts.

A place-based notion of stress also suggests that access to resourceful attributes in the environment that may support coping must not be assumed by the mere co-location of an individual and a resource. On this note, Bernard et al. (2007) recently proposed a concept of how agency and local opportunity structures mediate access to resources in the neighbourhood (i.e., local) environment. For example, Schieman (2005) recently described complex heterogeneity in access to social support for elderly populations living in disadvantaged neighbourhoods in the District of Columbia and in Maryland. Black women were more likely to be supported than residents of other racial/ethnic backgrounds, though only in areas with high residential stability (i.e., low turnover). On the other hand, White men and women were less likely to receive support, specifically in areas with low stability. Given growing interest in reducing *social* disparities in CD, the accessibility of resources by individuals should be conceptualized not only in terms of availability and proximity, but also their affordability (see Chap. 7).

For example, Kwan (2008) recently applied a notion of "time geography" (see Hägerstrand 1970) to understand how "emotional geographies" reflect the fears of anti-Muslim hate violence of an American Muslim woman as she moves through Columbus, Ohio before and shortly after the September 11th attacks in 2001. This includes an analysis of places that were perceived to be dangerous and, therefore, inaccessible by this woman, including her mosque – a regular place of worship (i.e., a resource) for the woman – and many public spaces, and associated changes in routine behaviours. Work describing poorer birth outcomes among Arabic named women in California before and after the September 11th attacks supports the notion that such perceived discrimination may have resulted in stress-related population health impacts (Lauderdale 2006).

As described above, the implications of a place-based notion of stress are complex. However, they can facilitate a more realistic account for the heterogeneity of the stress experience across the different types of individuals that utilize specific places. Since a given setting may include individuals carrying out activities related to work, study, play and domesticity (especially places with very mixed land use, like the urban core of a major city), there may be multiple perceptions of the stressful attributes of this place across activity mode groups. Further, each activity group can be comprised of individuals with different sociodemographic characteristics that may also affect such perception (e.g., employees filling a range of job types in a typical workplace). An analogous lesson could be developed around the expectation of differential access to resources in the local environment, in spite of availability and proximity.

In this way, and with respect to the stress process, the responses to a stressor (or group of stressors) may differ between individuals of different activity mode and/or social position because of both unique perceptions of the same stressor and differential access to (healthy and unhealthy) resources for coping. Since people's time activity tends to follow a daily or semi-regular routine, responses to the same stressors over time in the course of domesticity, work, school and recreation may result in behavioural repetition (e.g., type and intensity) that could become habit over time (e.g., Folkman et al. 1986). This is supported by a large body mental health research suggesting that chronic stress is related to the development of addictions to alcohol, tobacco and other drugs (e.g., Lloyd and Turner 2008; Turner and Lloyd 2003, 2004) as a coping mechanism. On a related note, our understanding of how coping works also suggests that the healthfulness of coping habits will be shaped, in part, by the healthfulness (or lack thereof) of resources perceived to be accessible in the local environments of individuals. This may help explain why healthier coping responses appear to be more prevalent in individuals with higher socioeconomic position (Billings and Moos 1981). However, drawing on the notion of cognitive reappraisal, it's worth noting that places – but also people's concept of a place – can change over time, with implications for the appraisal of stressors and coping resources by individuals.

6.5   Environmental Stressors and Resources

Our understanding of the place-based stress experience facilitates the identification of environmental attributes that stress and support populations experiencing or at risk for CD epidemics, particularly to the extent that specific subpopulations share in their *perception* of environmental stressors and perceived *accessibility* of environmental resources. For example, a place-based notion of stress may help explain why a neighbourhood disorder index was recently shown to be predictive of altered stress hormone levels among African American children, but not European American children, in Alabama (Dulin-Keita et al. 2010). In turn, preventive efforts to ameliorate persistent disparities in chronic disease among African Americans in this region (e.g., Howard et al. 2011) may focus on understanding how and why the lives of African American children, in particular, are stressful. This may include the assessment of specific environmental stressors that ought to be addressed, as well as environmental resources that are culturally appropriate and accessible.

A broad approach to identifying environmental stressors and resources can be informed by the growing discourse on how environments can "get under the skin" and affect CD pathology (Taylor et al. 1997). For example, in reflecting on their examination of health promoting and damaging features in the west of Scotland, Macintyre et al. (2002) suggested five features of local areas that could influence health of different people in different ways: (1) the physical environment; (2) built environments; (3) the provision of services; (4) sociocultural features; and (5) the reputation of an area. As described above, similar groups of people who utilize or experience these features in similar ways may be susceptible to related stressors and access related resources in similar ways, while there may be differences in how these features represent stressors and resources between population groups of more disparate socioeconomic position.

In general, environmental *stressors* directly present demands to be appraised and coped with and they can also contextualize the perception of other environmental and personal stressors. For example, in simple terms (i.e., ignoring the process of cognitive reappraisal mentioned above), an individual who has previously been exposed to violence (i.e., an individual-level stressor) may find living in a high crime neighbourhood more stressful than someone who has never been personally affected by violence as a result of their perception of danger in the local environment, as conveyed by the local media and word of mouth. It is also worth noting that individuals may find environmental stressors more difficult to control than personal stressors since they are often determined by structural forces, such as urban planning processes in government.

Environmental *resources* can buffer the negative effects of stress by offering appropriate, accessible services to cope with stress in the short and long-term, including networks for social support and care provision (e.g., a support group or free clinic for first time, single mothers); by facilitating healthy or unhealthy coping behaviours that may translate into habits over time (e.g., physical activity or smoking); by presenting preferable and restorative environments (Ulrich 1984); and in relation to other social and cultural resources (Cohen and McKay 1984; Matheson et al. 2006). Similarly, the absence of resources may also contribute to chronic stress by reducing the effectiveness of coping. Note that this definition allows that the presence of environmental resources that facilitate unhealthy coping behaviours (e.g., convenient access to cheap tobacco products) may help buffer the emotional and physiological impact of stress, but could still contribute to chronic disease.

A multidisciplinary discourse has examined characteristics of the natural, built and social environment that may represent environmental stressors and resources that influence coping (e.g., Aneshensel and Sucoff 1996; Elliott 2000; Kessler 1979; O'Campo et al. 2009; Seeman and McEwen 1996; Stockdale et al. 2007). The natural environment includes living and non-living things that occur naturally, including chiefly soil ("green space"), water ("blue space") and air. For example, the perception of a polluted environment has been described as a stressor (Cutchin 2007; Luginaah et al. 2002), while green spaces are often discussed in terms of their restorative effect on the mind (e.g., Mitchell and Popham 2008; Ulrich 1984).

The built environment relates to constructions and services for human activity, for example, buildings, roads and water management systems. Evans et al. (2001) demonstrated associations between residential crowding and airplane noise with socioemotional distress and elevated psychophysiological stress among children. On the other hand, accessible, affordable child care services in a neighbourhood may act as a resource for families coping with a stressful job or financial limitations, while areas with better walkability and availability of healthy foods may also help buffer stress (Mujahid et al. 2008).

The social environment has been defined differently by various institutions. The National Library of Medicine (2010) in the United States uses the broad definition of "the aggregate of social and cultural institutions, forms, patterns, and processes that influence the life of an individual or community." Yen and Syme (1999) specify that the social environment includes "groups to which we belong, the neighbourhoods in which we live, the organization of our workplaces, and the policies we create to order our lives." Macintyre et al. (2002) have also written about the "collective dimension" of place effects on health, which appears to be synonymous with an effect of the social environment on health. Kessler (1979) implied that a stressful or less stressful social environment can affect the perception of personal or other environmental stressors. For example, stressful social environments may embody social disorder (Dulin-Keita et al. 2010) including crime (Wright 2006) or political violence (Giacaman et al. 2007). On the other hand, social environments may provide resources that support healthy or unhealthy coping behaviours (e.g., by embodying social norms). A high prevalence of trust or social cohesion may be resourceful in different ways for individuals coping with stress (Mujahid et al. 2008), while "smoke-free building" laws may support healthy coping behaviours among those who normally smoke cigarettes. In immigrant communities that are segregated from the rest of society, chronic stress may be higher in children as they struggle through the process of acculturation (e.g., learning a second language while trying to maintain academic achievement) (Thomas 1995). At the same time, evidence suggests that Hispanic immigrants who reside in neighbourhoods with a high density of fellow immigrants may actually have lower risk for asthma than non-immigrants in these neighbourhoods and compared to Hispanics immigrants in neighbourhoods with low density of immigrants (Cagney et al. 2007). It is suggested that this protective effect may occur due to increased social capital formed among Hispanic immigrants, which may explain the so-called "Latino Paradox."

While places are described above in terms of built, natural and social characteristics, this is merely for purposes of demonstration. In conceptualizing analyses and interpreting results, social epidemiologists should recognize that there is often broad overlap when placing actual perceived stressors and resources into such categories. For example, some environmental features may be both man-made and natural, such as parks, noise and air pollution. In another example, a range of services were established for expectant mothers by the Homerton University Hospital in the Hackney area of London that reduced ethnic disparities in infant mortality (Cox 2010). In particular, a helpline staffed by trained midwives improved accessibility to expert care, while another program connected expectant mothers to local mothers trained to provide "peer education support." Anecdotal evidence suggests that the provision of social support was a key benefit to users of both services. In this example, these local services could be viewed as resourceful attributes of both the built and social environment.

A given setting may also be comprised of multiple stressors (Evans and English 2002) and/or resources of interest. For example, high density transportation corridors (think of a major intersection in an urban area) can not only determine the walkability and safety for pedestrians, but can feature high traffic-related pollution that may be perceived as harmful, and noise that may act as an irritant. Further, multiple attributes of a place may need to be accounted for in order to understand the perception of that place by individuals; for example, a *safe* park could be restorative, while an *unsafe* park could be a source of stress. Finally, it should also be noted that individuals may perceive a given environmental characteristic as both stressful and resourceful. Yen et al. (2007) conducted focus groups with women about the resources and hazards in their neighbourhood and found, for example, that fast food restaurants were seen as both a hazard due to their poor nutritional content, but also as an affordable and convenient way to feed their family. The authors described such attributes under the theme of "resource-hazard conflicts."

6.6   A Systems View

A systems view of how environmental attributes that characterize a place help shape chronic stress (a physiological-behavioural-emotional process) and CD can help integrate knowledge on this topic from a variety of disciplines (Diez-Roux 2007). Whereas more mechanistic interpretations of reality often utilize approaches characterized by *reductionism, linearity* and *hierarchy* to clarify broadly generalizable relationships that are ostensibly not endogenous, this chapter has described the experience of stress and chronic disease pathology as being in a type of *complex adaptive system* with environmental attributes, where population health outcomes are an emergent property of specific places (or rather, the sum of places that an individual may routinely encounter) (Jayasinghe 2011). Curtis (2004) suggests that frameworks describing complex systems can help focus attention on the "connections between the different parts of the system as well as on individual component parts," and that such models bring a clearer understanding of how factors that "have not always conventionally been considered as part of the 'health system'" can contribute to problems of health inequality.

The conceptual framework presented in Fig. 6.1 describes two key pathways linking environmental determinants of stress to CD, along with the potential for other pathways of endogeneity, confounding and effect modification that should particularly concern social epidemiologists. As mentioned earlier, places and environmental attributes of relevance are not limited to residential neighbourhoods and

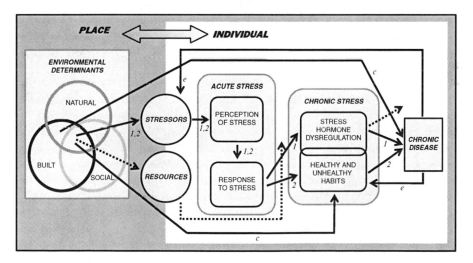

Fig. 6.1 Place-based stress and chronic disease: a systems view of environmental determinants. *Solid arrows* indicate the pathways that relate environmental determinants of stress to chronic diseases via primarily physiologic changes in response to stress hormone dysregulation (*1*) and in relation to healthy and unhealthy habits related to coping (*2*), pathways of endogeneity (*e*), and pathways of confounding (*c*), while *dashed arrows* that cross *solid arrows* indicate effect modification

can include contexts related to other types of activity (e.g., work, study and play). It is also worth noting that while the pathways presented in Fig. 6.1 may be key mechanisms of social disparities in CD, the system presented is neutral with respect to individual- and area-level social status. For example, the socioeconomic position of individuals and the socioeconomic status of places are not made explicit in the framework; rather, the framework makes explicit some key factors in the system that social statuses may be associated with. By describing this system, the framework can be used to study place-based stress in specific settings or with specific populations, while also facilitate the examination of broader questions such as, why are some populations more susceptible to stress-related disparities and in what settings?

The first broad pathway described in Fig. 6.1 is one often cited as a plausible mechanism for why chronic diseases may be elevated in areas of low socioeconomic status (Evans and English 2002; McEwen and Gianaros 2010; Taylor et al. 1997). It describes the accumulation of stress in response to environmental and personal stressors leading to allostatic overload and the dysregulation of key mechanisms for chronic disease psychopathology such as the sympathetic-adrenal-medullary and hypothalamic-pituitary-adrenocortical systems. Further, to the extent that stressful environmental characteristics may coexist with environmental hazards directly related to CD (e.g., areas of high traffic density could indicate the perception of a stressor like noise and exposure to toxins in traffic-related pollution), a growing body of environmental epidemiology implies the importance of accounting for these potentially strong relationships with CD as potential confounders of stress-related effects (Shankardass et al. 2010). Furthermore, in addition to direct effects of environmental hazards on CD pathology, growing evidence suggests that chronic stress may increase susceptibility for CD in relation to certain hazards. For example, recent studies suggest that chronic stress related to exposure to violence or crime increase susceptibility to air pollution in the onset of childhood asthma (e.g., Clougherty et al. 2007; Shankardass et al. 2009, 2010).

The second pathway described in Fig. 6.1 differs from the first in the manifestation of chronic stress that can lead to CD pathology; namely, the transactional model and the relational notion of place-based stress suggest that coping behaviours (influenced by personal coping types) in response to repeated activity in the same (or similar) stressful places may lead to habitual healthy and unhealthy behaviours, which can also directly affect risk for CD over time. There is also growing evidence of some relationship between emotional and physiological consequences of hormone dysregulation related to chronic stress and the uptake of certain health behaviours. For example, McEwen (2008) describes implications of chronic stress for sleep disturbance and hunger, which may negatively impact physical activity and diet, while macronutrient selection (in particular, consumption of high fat diets) has been described in terms of both emotionally and physiologically ameliorative effects in response to chronic stress (Yin et al. 2005; Fachin et al. 2008; Teegarden and Bale 2008; Dallman et al. 2003; Nguyen-Rodriguez et al. 2008). Again, chronic stress may also increase susceptibility for CD to some types of health behaviours, such as smoking (e.g., Shankardass et al. 2009).[5] It is also worth noting that having a chronic disease can lead to changes in health behaviours (e.g., the uptake of healthier diet or smoking reduction following a heart attack) as well as represent a personal source of stress for individuals (e.g., Ruo et al. 2003). Therefore, pathways of endogeneity ought to be considered when examining relationships between stress and chronic disease, particularly in terms of behavioural pathways and the psychological burden of illness.

The framework also highlights the role of resources, both environmental and personal, as potential modifiers of the translation from acute to chronic stress since evidence suggests that chronic stress is less likely to develop over time if resources are available in order to effectively cope with stressful events (McEwen and Gianaros 2010). While the role of environmental resources in coping with perceived stress and buffering negative physiological impacts is well described, the potential for specific types of resources to shape healthy and unhealthy coping behaviours is less often articulated (e.g., Weaver et al. 2008).

Finally, a bi-directional relationship between *individuals* embedded within *places* is emphasized in the framework since the experience of stress is impacted by an individual's environment, and individuals also play a role in conceiving and per-ceiving their places. Furthermore, places may change over time and individuals may also reappraise the meaning they ascribe to places, including how certain attributes represent stressors and resources. Additionally, to represent the contribution of stressors and resources at both the personal and environmental levels,[6] these factors are depicted as crossing the boundary of place and individual.

6.7 Implications for Social Epidemiology

This chapter uses a narrative review and proposes a conceptual framework to describe a place-based experience of stress in order to account for a complex relationship with the onset of multiple CD. In doing so, two key pathways for understanding the role of stress in sociospatial disparities in CD are highlighted that integrate ecosocial, psychosocial and materialist explanations: (1) physiological dysfunction related to allostatic *overload*, and (2) healthy and unhealthy habits that are the outcome of a largely emotional-behavioural process of coping with perceived stressors. Several specific pathways of potential confounding, endogeneity and effect modification are also identified by the framework. In these ways, the framework helps to clarify

---

[5] Incidentally, while the relevance of environmental confounders for both of these pathways depends on the co-incidence of stressful and hazardous or otherwise unhealthy environments, the literature on environmental justice highlights many examples where this confluence does exist in areas of low socioeconomic status (e.g., Morello-Frosch and Lopez 2006).

[6] Interestingly, Pearlin (1999) describes primary and secondary stressors to distinguish how an environmental stressor experienced at a specific place and time can contribute to personal stress at a later point in time. On the other hand, it is less clear to what extent environmental resources from one context are relevant to secondary appraisal of stressors in other settings.

potential mechanisms by which social inequities may be embodied as inequalities in disparities in CD (Aneshensel 2005; Kaufman and Cooper 1999; Krieger 2001). Further work is required to confirm, clarify and correct the system described in Fig. 6.1 in order to validate the above-described pathways.

By guiding social epidemiologists toward an understanding of environmental attributes as harmful and/or supportive to specific populations of interest, the framework can facilitate the control of sociospatial disparities in CD using interventions that target *populations* at high lifetime risk for multiple CD or *places* where there is a high prevalence of multiple CD or where stressful conditions such as poverty persist (Thoits 2010). In this way, just as clinical epidemiologists have informed evidence-based approaches to care-giving protocols that minimize what are essentially individual differences in the treatment of CD, social epidemiologists have an important role to play by informing urban or community development approaches that double as population health interventions (and vice versa) (see Chap. 15). For example, public health and urban planning actors can work together on a local scale to identify and minimize stressors and ensure that appropriate resources are accessible by at-risk populations.[7] Communities under stress, or experiencing a high burden of CD, may need to be engaged under such approaches to identify potentially important environmental modifications both to ameliorate stressors and to provide resources to specific populations. In turn, further work would be required to evaluate the effectiveness of such local approaches to prevent CD outcomes and disparities in comparison to other disease-specific approaches to prevention.

Further work is required to integrate a place-based conceptualization of stress-related mediation of CD disparities with a life course perspective (Thoits 2010). In their synthesis of the stress process and the life course perspective, Pearlin and Skaff (1996) commented on how studies of stress are "essentially studies of changing lives: changing conditions having the potential to affect people adversely, changing responses to these conditions, and changing consequences for well-being." Pearlin (1999) further argues that the sources, mediators and manifestations that comprise the stress process – and determine the experience of stress – "entail the many factors that over time can connect the inner lives of individuals to the larger social systems of which they are a part." Interestingly, Wheaton and Clarke (2003) noted that the early childhood environment was a better predictor of adult mental health status than current neighbourhood for individuals with relatively low parental education, which highlights the relevance of considering broader patterns of mobility across the life course to identify environmental determinants of chronic stress specific to certain critical periods. A body of evidence also suggests that stress *mediators* – both biological and behavioural (Karoly 1993; Riggs et al. 2007; Farah et al. 2006; Dunn 2010; McEwen and Seeman 1999; McEwen and Stellar 1993; Maccari et al. 2003; Weinstock 2001; Wright 2011) – may be partly determined by characteristics *in utero* and of the early life environment that may be stressors

---

[7] At the same time, studies examining environmental determinants of stress and CD of specific places and smaller populations can lead to broadly generalizable theory about these relationships to facilitate an increasingly detailed understanding of these relationships.

themselves (Evans and English 2002). In particular, there is a growing understanding of how early life environments may shape stress appraisal "phenotypes" (Dunn 2010; McEwen 2006) and behavioural coping habits (Umberson et al. 2008).

On a related note, in assessing how environmental attributes may represent *sources* of chronic stress, it will be important to account for differences in both the perception of and response to stressors (including differential access to resources for coping) as well as exposure to stressors and access to resources across the multiple places that account for people's daily activities (Pearlin et al. 2005; Wheaton and Clarke 2003). Further, since people routinely spend significant amounts of time outside of the home – in places of work, study and recreation – key stressors experienced outside of the home may drive sociospatial disparities in CD between non-residential environments in some cases (e.g., Shankardass et al. 2010).

Unfortunately, there is currently very little evidence that validates environmental stressors and resources, especially with the type of population specificity implied by a place-based notion of stress or specificity with respect to critical periods and cumulative exposure to these determinants implied by a life course perspective. Given the fundamentally subjective nature of environmental stressors and resources described in this chapter, social epidemiologists can aim to understand how the attributes of *specific* settings (e.g., a persistently low-income neighbourhood with low residential stability and a high proportion of recent immigrants in Toronto, Ontario) rather than attributes associated with vague neighbourhood types (e.g. low-income neighbourhoods), help shape the experience of stress and CD outcomes of the different types and ages of individuals that utilize these spaces (e.g., workers and residents of high and low socioeconomic status).

Conventional approaches to characterize places that use convenient administrative data, such as the use of census data to construct poverty indices or mapping the locations of health clinics to calculate proximity to such resources across study populations, may not provide enough detail about meaningful idiosyncrasies to adequately account for variation in the perception and accessibility of environmental stressors and resources. Indeed, such objective features of places have to be understood as imprecise measures when applied to a diverse population group. For example, this may help account for observed differences in stress hormone responses across children of different racial/ethnic backgrounds living in "low socioeconomic" neighbourhoods (Dulin-Keita et al. 2010). Rather, social epidemiologists may utilize methods capable of accounting for locally-informed perspectives of stressors and resources in the environment. For example, concept mapping has recently been used to identify how environmental attributes specific to Toronto neighbourhoods contribute to good and poor mental well-being (O'Campo et al. 2009). Here, a process of "structured conceptualization" was used by Toronto residents of high and low socioeconomic status to identify, group and rate neighbourhood attributes; diagrams were developed to demonstrate inter-relationships between specific attributes and broader domains with good and poor mental well-being (O'Campo et al. 2009).

Social epidemiologists should also consider the implications of a place-based, life course approach to this topic for how the *manifestations* of acute and chronic stress are measured. Figure 6.1 emphasizes the importance of assessing both physiological and behavioural manifestations over time. Further, as stress becomes experienced chronically, it may be relevant to identify precisely when physiological dysfunction – what has been termed "allostatic overload" (McEwen 2008) – occurs, and what (if any) the associated implications for behavioural coping habits are. In terms of measurement, then, we may be interested in tracking the cumulative "wear and tear" of perceiving and responding to stressors as they occur in units that we can compare and contrast across individuals. This suggests the value of efforts to examine cumulative allostatic load using an index of biomarkers as well as work on conceptualizing and validating telomere length as a marker for the biological "weathering" individuals experience as a result of cumulative hardship over the life course. Further, we might expect time to be a modifier of how allostasis is associated with physiological and behavioural actions at some point in the long-term.

Finally, and perhaps most fundamentally, in facilitating the types of research outlined above, social epidemiologists will need to adopt an analytical perspective that assumes that there may be multiple "social consequences" (Aneshensel 2005) of places for multiple chronic stress pathways, including mediation of CD outcomes by both physiological and behavioural-emotional processes. Due to the likelihood of complex inter-relationships between these pathways, empirical evidence may need to be derived using mixed methods approaches that integrate quantitative and qualitative approaches to foster more intensive analysis. For example, Kwan's (2008) aforementioned approach of using geographic information systems (GIS) and in-depth interviews to construct and interpret "emotional geographies" can lead to a clearer understanding of how specific types of individuals may be at risk for various chronic stress sequelae across a changing landscape, including how one's perception of places changes over time and the emotional and behavioural implications of such changes. Elsewhere in this volume, Rhodes et al. present a series of case studies that describe complex relationships between macro-level physical, social, policy and economic influences as well as HIV risk at the individual level (see Chap. 10). This includes the use of "complementary" approaches to reconcile divergent qualitative and quantitative evidence (Slonim-Nevo and Nevo 2009) that intensively reveal (for example) policing practices experienced by sex workers in Serbia and injection drug users in Russia as stressors contributing to unhealthy behaviours that increase risk for HIV.

Acknowledgements The author thanks Patricia O'Campo and James Dunn for their thoughtful and constructive advice.

References

Adam TC, Hasson RE, Ventura EE et al (2010) Cortisol is negatively associated with insulin sensitivity in overweight Latino youth. J Clin Endocrinol Metab 95:4729–4735

Adler NE, Stewart J (2010) Health disparities across the lifespan: meaning, methods, and mechanisms. Ann N Y Acad Sci 1186:5–23

Almeida DM, Neupert SD, Banks SR (2005) Do daily stress processes account for socioeconomic health disparities? J Gerontol B Psychol Sci Soc Sci 60(Spec 2):34–39

Aneshensel CS (2005) Research in mental health: social etiology versus social consequences. J Health Soc Behav 46:221–228

Aneshensel C (2010) Neighbourhood as a social context of the stress process. In: Avison W, Aneshensel C, Schieman S, Wheaton B (eds) Advances in the conceptualization of the stress process: essays in honor of Leonard I. Pearlin. Springer, New York

Aneshensel CS, Sucoff CA (1996) The neighborhood context of adolescent mental health. J Health Soc Behav 37:293–310

Auchincloss AH, Diez-Roux AV (2008) A new tool for epidemiology: the usefulness of dynamic-agent models in understanding place effects on health. Am J Epidemiol 168:1–8

Avison W, Aneshensel C, Schieman S et al (eds) (2010) Advances in the conceptualization of the stress process: essays in honor of Leonard I. Pearlin. Springer, New York

Baum A, Garofalo JP, Yali AM (1999) Socioeconomic status and chronic stress. Does stress account for SES effects on health? Ann N Y Acad Sci 896:131–144

Bernard P, Charafeddine R, Frohlich K et al (2007) Health inequalities and place: a theoretical conception of neighbourhood. Soc Sci Med 65:1839–1852

Billings AG, Moos RH (1981) The role of coping responses and social resources in attenuating the stress of life events. J Behav Med 4:139–157

Bruce MA, Beech BM, Sims M et al (2009) Social environmental stressors, psychological factors, and kidney disease. J Invest Med 57:583–589

Buzzelli M, Jerrett M (2007) Geographies of susceptibility and exposure in the city: environmental inequity of traffic-related air pollution in Toronto. Can J Regional Sci 30:195–210

Cagney KA, Browning CR, Wallace DM (2007) The Latino paradox in neighborhood context: the case of asthma and other respiratory conditions. Am J Public Health 97:919–925

Cannon W (1915) Bodily changes in pain, hunger, fear and rage: an account of recent researches into the function of emotional excitement. Appleton, New York

Carlson ED, Chamberlain RM (2005) Allostatic load and health disparities: a theoretical orientation. Res Nurs Health 28:306–315

Chandola T, Britton A, Brunner E et al (2008) Work stress and coronary heart disease: what are the mechanisms? Eur Heart J 29:640–648

Chen E, Hanson MD, Paterson LQ et al (2006) Socioeconomic status and inflammatory processes in childhood asthma: the role of psychological stress. J Allergy Clin Immunol 117:1014–1020

Chrousos GP, Gold PW (1992) The concepts of stress and stress system disorders. Overview of physical and behavioral homeostasis. JAMA 267:1244–1252

Clougherty JE, Kubzansky LD (2009) A framework for examining social stress and susceptibility to air pollution in respiratory health. Environ Health Perspect 117:1351–1358

Clougherty JE, Levy JI, Kubzansky LD et al (2007) Synergistic effects of traffic-related air pollution and exposure to violence on urban asthma etiology. Environ Health Perspect 115:1140–1146

Cohen S, McKay G (1984) Social support, stress and the buffering hypothesis: a theoretical analysis. In: Baum A, Taylor S, Singer J (eds) Handbook of psychology and health, vol 4. Lawrence Erlbaum, Hillsdale

Cohen S, Kessler RC, Gordon LU (1995) Strategies for measuring stress in studies of psychiatric and physical disorders. In: Cohen S, Kessler RC, Gordon LU (eds) Measuring stress: a guide for health and social scientists. Oxford University Press, New York

Cohen L, Davis R, Cantor J et al (2007) Reducing health care costs through prevention. Prevention Institute and The California Endowment, Oakland

Cox P (2010) Reducing infant mortality due to health inequalities. Paper presented at the 18th international conference on health promoting hospitals and health services. 14–16 Apr 2010, Manchester

Creatore MI, Gozdyra P, Booth GL (2007) Socioeconomic status and diabetes. In: Neighbourhood environments and resources for healthy living – a focus on diabetes in Toronto. ICES Atlas. Institute for Clinical Evaluative Sciences, Toronto

Cummins S, Curtis S, Diez-Roux AV et al (2007) Understanding and representing 'place' in health research: a relational approach. Soc Sci Med 65:1825–1838

Curtis S (2004) Health and inequality: geographical perspectives. Sage, London

Cutchin MP (2007) The need for the "new health geography" in epidemiologic studies of environment and health. Health Place 13:725–742

Daar AS, Singer PA, Persad DL et al (2007) Grand challenges in chronic non-communicable diseases. Nature 450:494–496

Dallman MF, Pecoraro N, Akana SF et al (2003) Chronic stress and obesity: a new view of "comfort food". Proc Natl Acad Sci U S A 100:11696–11701

Dankwa-Mullan I, Rhee KB, Stoff DM (2010) Moving toward paradigm-shifting research in health disparities through translational, transformational, and transdisciplinary approaches. Am J Public Health 100:S19–S24

Dave ND, Xiang L, Rehm KE et al (2011) Stress and allergic disease. Immunol Allergy Clin N Am 31:55–68

de Vriendt T, Moreno LA, De Henauw S (2009) Chronic stress and obesity in adolescents: scientific evidence and methodological issues for epidemiological research. Nutr Metab Cardiovasc Dis 19:511–519

Diez-Roux AV (2007) Integrating social and biologic factors in health research: a systems view. Ann Epidemiol 17:569–574

Diez-Roux AV, Mair C (2010) Neighborhoods and health. Ann N Y Acad Sci 1186:125–145

Diez-Roux AV, Nieto FJ, Muntaner C et al (1997) Neighborhood environments and coronary heart disease: a multilevel analysis. Am J Epidemiol 146:48–63

Dulin-Keita A, Casazza K, Fernandez JR et al (2010) Do neighbourhoods matter? Neighbourhood disorder and long-term trends in serum cortisol levels. J Epidemiol Community Health 24 Aug 2010 [Epub ahead of print]

Dunn JR (2010) Health behavior vs the stress of low socioeconomic status and health outcomes. JAMA 303:1199–1200

Elliott M (2000) The stress process in neighborhood context. Health Place 6:287–299

Epel E, Lapidus R, McEwen B et al (2001) Stress may add bite to appetite in women: a laboratory study of stress-induced cortisol and eating behavior. Psychoneuroendocrinology 26:37–49

Evans GW, English K (2002) The environment of poverty: multiple stressor exposure, psychophysiological stress, and socioemotional adjustment. Child Dev 73:1238–1248

Evans GW, Lercher P, Meis M et al (2001) Community noise exposure and stress in children. J Acoust Soc Am 109:1023–1027

Fachin A, Silva RK, Noschang CG et al (2008) Stress effects on rats chronically receiving a highly palatable diet are sex-specific. Appetite 51:592–598

Farah MJ, Shera DM, Savage JH et al (2006) Childhood poverty: specific associations with neurocognitive development. Brain Res 1110:166–174

Folkman S, Lazarus RS, Gruen RJ et al (1986) Appraisal, coping, health status, and psychological symptoms. J Pers Soc Psychol 50:571–579

Gee GC, Payne-Sturges DC (2004) Environmental health disparities: a framework integrating psychosocial and environmental concepts. Environ Health Perspect 112:1645–1653

Giacaman R, Shannon HS, Saab H et al (2007) Individual and collective exposure to political violence: Palestinian adolescents coping with conflict. Eur J Public Health 17:361–368

Hägerstrand T (1970) What about people in regional science? Pap Reg Sci Association 24:7–21

Hayward K, Colman R (2003) The tides of change: addressing inequity and chronic disease in Atlantic Canada: a discussion paper. Public Health Agency of Canada, Halifax

Hertzman C, Wiens M (1996) Child development and long-term outcomes: a population health perspective and summary of successful interventions. Soc Sci Med 43:1083–1095

Hill TD, Ross CE, Angel RJ (2005) Neighborhood disorder, psychophysiological distress, and health. J Health Soc Behav 46:170–186

Holmes ME, Ekkekakis P, Eisenmann JC (2009) The physical activity, stress and metabolic syndrome triangle: a guide to unfamiliar territory for the obesity researcher. Obes Rev 11:492–507

House JS, Landis KR, Umberson D (1988) Social relationships and health. Science 241:540–545

Howard VJ, Kleindorfer DO, Judd SE et al (2011) Disparities in stroke incidence contributing to disparities in stroke mortality. Ann Neurol 69:619–627

Hughes CC, Sherman SN, Whitaker RC (2010) How low-income mothers with overweight pre-school children make sense of obesity. Qual Health Res 20:465–478

Iqbal Kring SI, Barefoot J, Brummett BH et al (2011) Associations between APOE variants and metabolic traits and the impact of psychological stress. PLoS One 6:e15745

Jayasinghe S (2011) Conceptualising population health: from mechanistic thinking to complexity science. Emerg Themes Epidemiol 8:2

Jerrett M, Finkelstein M (2005) Geographies of risk in studies linking chronic air pollution exposure to health outcomes. J Toxicol Environ Health A 68:1207–1242

Juster RP, McEwen BS, Lupien SJ (2009) Allostatic load biomarkers of chronic stress and impact on health and cognition. Neurosci Biobehav Rev 35:2–16

Karoly P (1993) Mechanisms of self-regulation: a systems view. Annu Rev Psychol 44:23–52

Kaufman JS, Cooper RS (1999) Seeking causal explanations in social epidemiology. Am J Epidemiol 150:113–120

Kawachi I, Kennedy BP, Glass R (1999) Social capital and self-rated health: a contextual analysis. Am J Public Health 89:1187–1193

Kessler RC (1979) Stress, social status, and psychological distress. J Health Soc Behav 20:259–272

Kivimaki M, Head J, Ferrie JE et al (2006) Work stress, weight gain and weight loss: evidence for bidirectional effects of job strain on body mass index in the Whitehall II study. Int J Obes (Lond) 30:982–987

Korte SM, Koolhaas JM, Wingfield JC et al (2005) The Darwinian concept of stress: benefits of allostasis and costs of allostatic load and the trade-offs in health and disease. Neurosci Biobehav Rev 29:3–38

Krieger N (2001) Theories for social epidemiology in the 21st century: an ecosocial perspective. Int J Epidemiol 30:668–677

Krieger N, Alegria M, Almeida-Filho N et al (2010) Who, and what, causes health inequities? Reflections on emerging debates from an exploratory Latin American/North American workshop. J Epidemiol Community Health 64:747–749

Kwan M (2008) From oral histories to visual narratives: re-presenting the post-September 11 experiences of the Muslim women in the United States. Soc Cult Geo 9:653–669

Larrat EP, Zierler S (1993) Entangled epidemics: cocaine use and HIV disease. J Psychoact Drugs 25:207–221

Lauderdale DS (2006) Birth outcomes for Arabic-named women in California before and after September 11. Demography 43:185–201

Laugero KD, Falcon LM, Tucker KL (2011) Relationship between perceived stress and dietary and activity patterns in older adults participating in the Boston Puerto Rican Health Study. Appetite 56:194–204

Lazarus RS, Folkman S (1984) Stress, appraisal, and coping. Springer Publishing, New York

Lloyd DA, Turner RJ (2008) Cumulative lifetime adversities and alcohol dependence in adolescence and young adulthood. Drug Alcohol Depend 93:217–226

Luginaah IN, Taylor SM, Elliott SJ et al (2002) Community reappraisal of the perceived health effects of a petroleum refinery. Soc Sci Med 55:47–61

Lynch JW, Kaplan GA, Salonen JT (1997) Why do poor people behave poorly? Variation in adult health behaviours and psychosocial characteristics by stages of the socioeconomic lifecourse. Soc Sci Med 44:809–819

Maccari S, Darnaudéry M, Morley-Fletcher S et al (2003) Prenatal stress and long-term consequences: implications of glucocorticoid hormones. Neurosci Biobehav Rev 27:119–127

Macintyre S, Ellaway A, Cummins S (2002) Place effects on health: how can we conceptualise, operationalise and measure them? Soc Sci Med 55:125–139

Mällo T, Matrov D, Kõiv K et al (2009) Effect of chronic stress on behavior and cerebral oxidative metabolism in rats with high or low positive affect. Neuroscience 164:963–974

Marmot M, Singh-Manoux A (2005) Role of socialization in explaining social inequalities in health. Soc Sci Med 60:2129–2133

Maschke C, Hecht K (2004) Stress hormones and sleep disturbances: electrophysiological and hormonal aspects. Noise Health 6:49–54

Matheson FI, Moineddin R, Dunn JR et al (2006) Urban neighborhoods, chronic stress, gender and depression. Soc Sci Med 63:2604–2616

Matheson FI, Moineddin R, Glazier RH (2008) The weight of place: a multilevel analysis of gender, neighborhood material deprivation, and body mass index among Canadian adults. Soc Sci Med 66:675–690

McEwen BS (1998) Protective and damaging effects of stress mediators. N Engl J Med 338:171–179

McEwen BS (2006) Protective and damaging effects of stress mediators: central role of the brain. Dialogues Clin Neurosci 8:367–381

McEwen BS (2008) Central effects of stress hormones in health and disease: understanding the protective and damaging effects of stress and stress mediators. Eur J Pharmacol 583: 174–185

McEwen BS, Gianaros PJ (2010) Central role of the brain in stress and adaptation: links to socio-economic status, health, and disease. Ann N Y Acad Sci 1186:190–222

McEwen BS, Seeman T (1999) Protective and damaging effects of mediators of stress. Elaborating and testing the concepts of allostasis and allostatic load. Ann N Y Acad Sci 896:30–47

McEwen BS, Stellar E (1993) Stress and the individual. Mechanisms leading to disease. Arch Intern Med 153:2093–2101

Mitchell R, Popham F (2008) Effect of exposure to natural environment on health inequalities: an observational population study. Lancet 372:1655–1660

Morello-Frosch R, Lopez R (2006) The riskscape and the color line: examining the role of segregation in environmental health disparities. Environ Res 102:181–196

Morello-Frosch R, Shenassa ED (2006) The environmental "riskscape" and social inequality: implications for explaining maternal and child health disparities. Environ Health Perspect 114:1150–1153

Mujahid MS, Diez-Roux AV, Shen M et al (2008) Relation between neighborhood environments and obesity in the multi-ethnic study of atherosclerosis. Am J Epidemiol 167:1349–1357

National Library of Medicine (2010) Medical subject headings. National Library of Medicine and the National Institutes of Health. http://www.ncbi.nlm.nih.gov/mesh/68012931. Accessed 10 Dec 2010

Nguyen-Rodriguez ST, Chou CP, Unger JB et al (2008) BMI as a moderator of perceived stress and emotional eating in adolescents. Eat Behav 9:238–246

O'Campo P, Salmon C, Burke J (2009) Neighbourhoods and mental well-being: what are the pathways? Health Place 15:56–68

Orpana HM, Lemyre L, Gravel R (2009) Income and psychological distress: the role of the social environment. Health Rep 20:21–28

Pearlin LI (1989) The sociological study of stress. J Health Soc Behav 30:241–256

Pearlin LI (1999) The stress process revisited: reflections on concepts and their interelationships. In: Aneshensel CS, Phelan J (eds) Handbook on the sociology of mental health. Plenum Press, New York

Pearlin LI, Skaff MM (1996) Stress and the life course: a paradigmatic alliance. Gerontologist 36:239–247

Pearlin LI, Lieberman MA, Menaghan EG et al (1981) The stress process. J Health Soc Behav 22:337–356

Pearlin LI, Schieman S, Fazio EM et al (2005) Stress, health, and the life course: some conceptual perspectives. J Health Soc Behav 46:205–219

Riggs NR, Sakuma KK, Pentz MA (2007) Preventing risk for obesity by promoting self-regulation and decision-making skills: pilot results from the PATHWAYS to health program (PATHWAYS). Eval Rev 31:287–310

Rod NH, Gronbaek M, Schnohr P et al (2009) Perceived stress as a risk factor for changes in health behaviour and cardiac risk profile: a longitudinal study. J Intern Med 266:467–475

Ruo B, Rumsfeld JS, Hlatky MA et al (2003) Depressive symptoms and health-related quality of life: the heart and soul study. JAMA 290:215–221

Sayer A (1992) Method in social science: a realist approach. Routledge, London

Schieman S (2005) Residential stability and the social impact of neighbourhood disadvantage: a study of gender and race-contingent effects. Soc Forces 83:1031–1064

Seeman TE, McEwen BS (1996) Impact of social environment characteristics on neuroendocrine regulation. Psychosom Med 58:459–471

Selye H (1936) A syndrome produced by diverse nocuous agents. Nature 138:32

Selye H (1956) The stress of life. McGraw-Hill, New York

Selye H (1975) Confusion and controversy in the stress field. J Hum Stress 1:37–44

Shankardass K, McConnell R, Jerrett M et al (2009) Parental stress increases the effect of traffic-related air pollution on childhood asthma incidence. Proc Natl Acad Sci U S A 106:12406–12411

Shankardass K, Jerrett M, Milam J et al (2010) Social environment and asthma: associations with crime and no child left behind programmes. J Epidemiol Community Health 11 Nov 2010 [Epub ahead of print]

Singh-Manoux A, Ferrie JE, Chandola T et al (2004) Socioeconomic trajectories across the life course and health outcomes in midlife: evidence for the accumulation hypothesis? Int J Epidemiol 33:1072–1079

Slonim-Nevo V, Nevo I (2009) Conflicting findings in mixed methods research: an illustration from an Israeli study on immigration. J Mix Methods Res 3:109–128

Steinberger J, Daniels SR, Eckel RH et al (2009) Progress and challenges in metabolic syndrome in children and adolescents: a scientific statement from the American Heart Association Atherosclerosis, Hypertension, and Obesity in the Young Committee of the Council on Cardiovascular Disease in the Young; Council on Cardiovascular Nursing; and Council on Nutrition, Physical Activity, and Metabolism. Circulation 119:628–647

Steptoe A (2006) Psychobiological processes linking socioeconomic position with health. In: Siegrist J, Marmot M (eds) Social inequalities in health: new evidence and policy implications. Oxford University Press, Oxford

Steptoe A, Willemsen G (2004) The influence of low job control on ambulatory blood pressure and perceived stress over the working day in men and women from the Whitehall II cohort. J Hypertens 22:915–920

Stockdale SE, Wells KB, Tang L et al (2007) The importance of social context: neighborhood stressors, stress-buffering mechanisms, and alcohol, drug, and mental health disorders. Soc Sci Med 65:1867–1881

Taylor SE, Repetti RL, Seeman T (1997) Health psychology: what is an unhealthy environment and how does it get under the skin? Annu Rev Psychol 48:411–447

Teegarden SL, Bale TL (2008) Effects of stress on dietary preference and intake are dependent on access and stress sensitivity. Physiol Behav 93:713–723

Thoits PA (2010) Stress and health: major findings and policy implications. J Health Soc Behav 51:S41–S53

Thomas T (1995) Acculturative stress in the adjustment of immigrant families. J Soc Distress and the Homeless 4:131–142

Tsatsoulis A, Fountoulakis S (2006) The protective role of exercise on stress system dysregulation and comorbidities. Ann N Y Acad Sci 1083:196–213

Tsiotra PC, Tsigos C (2006) Stress, the endoplasmic reticulum, and insulin resistance. Ann N Y Acad Sci 1083:63–76

Turner R (2010) Understanding health disparities: the promise of the stress process model. In: Avison W, Aneshensel C, Schieman S et al (eds) Advances in the conceptualization of the stress process: essays in honor of Leonard I. Pearlin. Springer, New York

Turner RJ, Lloyd DA (2003) Cumulative adversity and drug dependence in young adults: racial/ethnic contrasts. Addiction 98:305–315

Turner RJ, Lloyd DA (2004) Stress burden and the lifetime incidence of psychiatric disorder in young adults: racial and ethnic contrasts. Arch Gen Psychiatry 61:481–488

Ulrich RS (1984) View through a window may influence recovery from surgery. Science 224:420–421

Umberson D, Liu H, Reczek C (2008) Stress and health behaviour over the life course. Adv Life Course Res 13:19–44

Weaver K, Campbell R, Mermelstein R et al (2008) Pregnancy smoking in context: the influence of multiple levels of stress. Nicotine Tob Res 10:1065–1073

Weinstock M (2001) Alterations induced by gestational stress in brain morphology and behaviour of the offspring. Prog Neurobiol 65:427–451

Wheaton B (1994) Sampling the stress universe. In: Avison W, Gotlib I (eds) Stress and mental health: contemporary issues and prospects for the future. Plenum Press, New York

Wheaton B, Clarke P (2003) Space meets time: integrating temporal and contextual influences on mental health in early adulthood. Am Sociol Rev 68:680–706

Wright RJ (2006) Health effects of socially toxic neighborhoods: the violence and urban asthma paradigm. Clin Chest Med 27:413–421

Wright RJ (2011) Epidemiology of stress and asthma: from constricting communities and fragile families to epigenetics. Immunol Allergy Clin North Am 31:19–39

Wright RJ, Cohen RT, Cohen S (2005) The impact of stress on the development and expression of atopy. Curr Opin Allergy Clin Immunol 5:23–29

Yen IH, Syme SL (1999) The social environment and health: a discussion of the epidemiologic literature. Annu Rev Public Health 20:287–308

Yen IH, Scherzer T, Cubbin C et al (2007) Women's perceptions of neighborhood resources and hazards related to diet, physical activity, and smoking: focus group results from economically distinct neighborhoods in a mid-sized U.S. city. Am J Health Promot 22:98–106

Yin Z, Davis CL, Moore JB et al (2005) Physical activity buffers the effects of chronic stress on adiposity in youth. Ann Behav Med 29:29–36

Chapter 7
How Goes the Neighbourhood? Rethinking Neighbourhoods and Health Research in Social Epidemiology

Ketan Shankardass and James R. Dunn

Contents

7.1 Introduction 138
7.2 From Risk Factors to Mechanisms 140
7.3 Fundamental Causes and Social Mechanisms of Causation 143
7.4 Beyond Multilevel Modelling 146
7.5 Complex Understandings of Place and Health Are Inhibited
     by Crude Approaches to Space 147
7.6 Explaining Neighbourhood Effects in Social Epidemiology 150
References 152

Abstract In this chapter, we describe how social epidemiology has been proficient at describing patterns in neighbourhood health inequalities and even in modelling them in a sophisticated fashion, but has been less capable at fostering an understanding of how these effects relate to the social mechanisms of causation that underlie such inequalities at multiple levels – including with respect to neighbourhoods and more macrosocial contexts. We argue that this paradigm has to be shifted to improve the translation of research about neighbourhoods and health into effective health equity interventions, and we outline some specific ways for social epidemiologists to supplement their approach to research. We thereby problematize the social epidemiologic treatment of neighbourhoods as simple containers as a way of clarifying

K. Shankardass (✉)
Department of Psychology, Wilfrid Laurier University,
75 University Avenue West, N2L 3C5, Waterloo, ON, Canada
e-mail: KShankardass@wlu.ca

J.R. Dunn
Department of Health, Aging and Society, McMaster University,
Kenneth Taylor Hall 226, 1280 Main Street West, Hamilton, ON L8S 4L8, Canada
e-mail: jim.dunn@mcmaster.ca

P. O'Campo and J.R. Dunn (eds.), *Rethinking Social Epidemiology:*
Towards a Science of Change, DOI 10.1007/978-94-007-2138-8_7,
© Springer Science+Business Media B.V. 2012

how neighbourhood effects may reflect complex fundamental and proximate causes of health disparities. We also describe four assumptions of commonly used, multilevel models that ought to be closely considered when using this approach to study social mechanisms of causation. Finally, we argue that more diverse use of theory in the study of neighbourhood effects can help social epidemiologists embrace complexity in their research, and we review key recent (and not so recent) geographic perspectives on neighbourhoods and health that can be utilized to put "space in its place" and to better understand why some neighbourhoods are less healthy than others.

Abbreviations

GIS   Geographic information systems

7.1   Introduction

Social epidemiologists have been active contributors to the large and growing literature on the effect that attributes of local residential environments, or neighbourhoods, have on a variety of health (e.g., health, health behaviours and healthy child development) and social outcomes (e.g., youth delinquency, crime and deviance, political behaviour, employment outcomes and incomes) (see O'Campo 2003; Kawachi and Berkman 2003; Diez-Roux 2007; Diez-Roux and Mair 2010). A unifying feature of this kind of research is that it seeks to understand how, why and to what extent features of the neighbourhood shape individual outcomes over and above the effect of other individual-level factors. This research has been made possible by a variety of developments in the past 15–20 years, including advances in hierarchical modelling techniques, availability of related software, sophistication and power of desktop computing capacity, widespread availability of geo-coded databases that allow nesting of individual subjects in their area of residence, and characterization of that neighbourhood context with routinely collected and other data.

In this chapter, we describe how social epidemiology has been proficient at describing patterns in neighbourhood health inequalities and even in modelling them in a sophisticated fashion, but has been less capable at fostering an understanding of how these effects relate to the social mechanisms of causation that underlie such inequalities at multiple levels – including with respect to neighbourhoods and more macrosocial contexts. We argue that this paradigm has to be shifted to improve the translation of research about neighbourhoods and health into effective health equity interventions, and we outline some specific ways for social epidemiologists to supplement their approach to research. We thereby problematize the social epidemiologic treatment of neighbourhoods as simple containers as a way of clarifying how neighbourhood effects may reflect complex fundamental and proximate causes of health disparities. We also describe four assumptions of commonly used, multilevel models that ought to be closely considered when using this approach to study social mechanisms of causation. Finally, we argue that more diverse use of theory in the study of neighbourhood effects can help social epidemiologists embrace complexity in their research, and we review key recent (and not so recent) geographic perspectives on neighbourhoods and health that can be utilized to put "space in its place" (Badcock 1984) and to better understand why some neighbourhoods are less healthy than others.

Since long before the recent wave of interest in neighbourhoods and health research began in the late 1990s, social epidemiologists, health geographers and others have documented area variations in health status, largely using ecological study designs (Department of Health and Social Security 1980; Kitagawa and Hauser 1973; Phillimore et al. 1994). Of course a common (and valid) criticism of such analyses is that they really reflect the characteristics of individuals in the population in those areas in aggregate – the *composition* of the area – rather than anything about the particular place and time of the study (i.e., the *context*). But with the advent of new databases and statistical techniques, it has been possible to distinguish purely *compositional* effects at the neighbourhood level from cases where *contextual* effects appear to be relevant (see Macintyre et al. 1993, 2002; Cummins et al. 2007). This has led to a proliferation of research examining a variety of different neighbourhood characteristics and their relationship, controlling for individual factors, to a variety of different health outcomes, including general health status, mental health, chronic disease risk factors and outcomes, and mortality (Diez-Roux and Mair 2010; Kim 2008; Mair et al. 2008; Pickett and Pearl 2001; Rajaratnam et al. 2006; Riva et al. 2007). In terms of the attributes of neighbourhoods that have been considered, studies have largely focused on the role of absolute and relative deprivation, segregation, social capital and income inequality. Because of data constraints, these attributes are usually constructed based on the aggregation of compositional data (e.g., social capital as a neighbourhood average of an individual-level rating of trust in neighbours) (Hamano et al. 2010), often based on census data. However, there has also been some examination of more "irreducible" measures, including experimentation with the use of systematic social observation to directly measure attributes of neighbourhoods, like social and physical disorder (Parsons et al. 2010; Schaefer-McDaniel et al. 2010; Rajaratnam et al. 2006; O'Campo and Caughy 2006).

In response to growing concern for the negative societal impact and injustice of social and health inequity (Commission on Social Determinants of Health 2008; Marmot 2010), there is greater interest in approaches to planning and interventions that ameliorate differences in health between and within neighbourhoods by addressing the social determinants of health. For example, the Healthy Bodegas Initiative of New York City involves multiple programs aiming to address the problem of inner city food deserts, including by encouraging the availability of healthy and affordable food choices in local corner stores (Department of Health and Mental Hygiene 2010). This initiative suits growing acknowledgement that health status is not simply determined by individual factors (Evans 2004; Macintyre et al. 2002), such as behaviour or socioeconomic status. There is evidence suggesting that behaviours are significantly conditioned by environmental factors, such as the availability of convenience foods (Alter and Eny 2005; Glazier and Booth 2007) and environmental stressors (Duncan et al. 1999; Weaver et al. 2008).[1] There are also highly relevant related findings about more upstream determinants of health, including that being poor in a concentrated poverty neighbourhood is worse for health than being poor in more mixed neighbourhoods (Diez-Roux 2001; Brooks-Gunn et al. 1993), a phenomenon called "deprivation amplification" (Macintyre et al. 2002). The findings of research on neighbourhoods and health, in short, suggest an opportunity for intervention at the supra-individual level, which is highly promising for the magnitude of its potential public health impact (see Rose's (1985) "radical" approaches to population health). Despite this potential, there are still a number of challenges for social epidemiologic neighbourhoods and health research that seeks to have an impact on health and well-being.

7.2   From Risk Factors to Mechanisms

Social epidemiologists have long been interested not only in describing health inequities, but also in understanding how and why they occur (see Graham et al. 1963). While social epidemiology has excelled at identifying the characteristics of unhealthy neighbourhoods and the magnitude of neighbourhood health disparities (i.e., *where* is intervention required?), less attention has been paid to a theoretical explanation of the social mechanisms of causation, including *why* some neighbourhoods are unhealthy and *how* (and *which*) interventions can improve health (and for *whom*).

As sophisticated empirical analyses of neighbourhood differences in health have become easier (e.g., due to developments in geographic information systems (GIS) and multilevel modelling), neighbourhood-level inequalities have been identified for a range of health outcomes and in many different settings (Diez-Roux and Mair 2010; Kim 2008; Mair et al. 2008; Pickett and Pearl 2001; Rajaratnam et al. 2006; Riva et al. 2007). To be clear, social epidemiology has made valued contributions to the identification of attributes that characterize unhealthy places, including socio-economic (e.g., history of deprivation or segregation), social (e.g., low collective efficacy, crime) and physical aspects (e.g., high traffic density). By identifying specific health disparities, this type of *extensive* research can be useful for resource allocation (e.g., where should governments be focusing efforts at ameliorating

---

[1] As a result of the potential relationship between contextual and compositional factors, it is worth noting that the magnitude of neighbourhood inequality in health has likely been underestimated, given the common practice of reporting contextual effects that have been controlled for individual level compositional factors, such as behavioural (e.g., smoking) and environmental (e.g. air pollution) risk factors that may be on the pathway of social mechanisms of causation (read: social determinants) (Diez-Roux and Mair 2010; Dunn 2010; Macintyre et al. 2002).

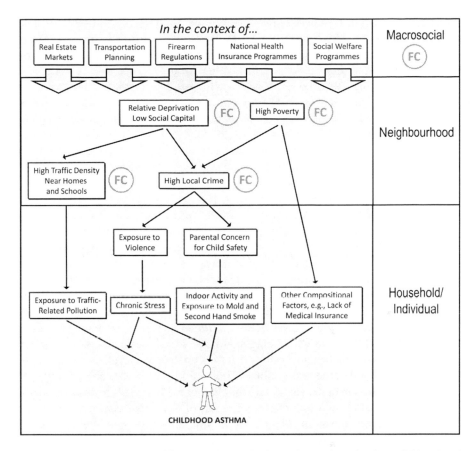

Fig. 7.1 Fundamental causes (FC) and social mechanisms of causation related to neighbourhood disparities in childhood asthma

population health disparities), as well as for generating hypotheses to better understand disparities. Yet, such studies often leave us with a largely superficial understanding of hazard, since the empirical evidence supporting a neighbourhood "risk factor" can often plausibly reflect a range of etiologic hypotheses that involve multiple social mechanisms of causation (see example in Fig. 7.1). Thus, the hazards associated with neighbourhood effects in specific places are often not broadly generalizable to neighbourhoods in other settings.

There has been a less critical, less *intensive* examination of specific mechanisms by which these neighbourhood risk factors "get under the skin" (e.g., O'Campo et al. 2009). By failing to provide a compelling explanation of how neighbourhood effects work, the ability to transform research into actionable information to support interventions to reduce health disparities across neighbourhoods is hindered. The limitation of a superficial understanding of the relationship between neighbourhoods and health can be further illustrated by considering the extent to which randomized neighbourhood interventions may *not* be ideal for generating evidence about causal relationships between neighbourhood risk factors and health, in spite of their apparent benefits (see Oakes 2004). By design, such experimental studies aim to ignore the differences in the context of neighbourhoods being examined by randomly allocating interventions and adjusting for differences between intervention and control neighbourhoods to account for residual confounding; therefore, these types of studies emphasize the importance of causal mechanisms unrelated to such idiosyncracies. Yet, in order to translate successful neighbourhood interventions to other settings, it is increasingly acknowledged that the phenomena of interest (i.e., how and why the intervention was successful) need to be understood in terms of a specific context, including the population, place and time (see Yin 1999). For example, McLaren et al. (2006) compare numerous attempts to translate the success of community-based efforts in North Karelia, Finland in the early 1970s to reduce chronic heart disease in other parts of the world. They contrast the extent to which subsequent interventions have and have not recognized the unique context of the original intervention in adapting the design, while discussing implications for the appropriateness and success of such transplanted interventions. A concrete understanding that embraces, rather than ignores, the idiosyncrasies of context can help social epidemiologists better understand the reasons why specific interventions and natural experiments work or don't work, and why specific associations between neighbourhood and individual level factors are found. In turn, the meaning of neighborhood effects in terms of within-neighbourhood social mechanisms of causation and their relation to fundamental causes that may operate at a level above the neighbourhood (discussed in the next section) (Link and Phelan 1995) can be clarified.

As a demonstration of the value and limitation of evidence that focuses on neighbourhood risk factors, consider the recent report of a positive association between local crime rates and the onset of childhood asthma across communities in Southern California (Shankardass et al. 2010). Analysis suggests that part of this relationship could be explained by the presence of higher levels of traffic-related air pollution around the homes of children living in higher crime communities. Such air pollution is believed to contribute to the formation of asthma in children (Jerrett et al. 2008; McConnell et al. 2010; Gauderman et al. 2005; Sarnat and Holguin 2007). But a large majority of the association related to the crime rate remained unexplained after controlling for the effect of air pollution, indicating that there may be other reasons why there is a higher risk for asthma onset in areas with high crime. *Exposure to violence* in the local environment has often been identified as a determinant of childhood asthma onset and morbidity in other American settings (Gupta et al. 2010; Sternthal et al. 2010; Subramanian and Kennedy 2009). Such extensive work is accompanied by a body of more intensive research, including, importantly, conceptual work that validates neighbourhood crime as an environmental stressor leading to multiple physiological and behavioural responses in children and adults that can contribute to the development of childhood asthma (Clougherty and Kubzansky 2009; Morello-Frosch and Shenassa 2006; Cohen et al. 2008; Stafford et al. 2007; Suglia et al. 2008, 2010; Wright 2006; Wright et al. 2004). Further, some evidence indicates that chronic stress may increase susceptibility to certain environmental pollutants (e.g., traffic-related pollution and second-hand smoke) (Shankardass et al. 2009; Clougherty et al. 2007). Thus, a plausible explanation for why crime in Southern California communities may increase risk for childhood asthma has been articulated, though it rests on a narrative review of evidence from a range of studies and settings.

At the same time, important details about why local crime rates are associated with asthma in some settings remain unclear, which therefore limits the design of interventions. For instance, can we assume that crime is a stressor for children living in settings other than those that have been studied, where the nature of criminal activities or factors related to social or personal resilience toward exposure to violence (i.e., that may buffer chronic stress) may be different (Pearlman 2009)? Or might crime rates be a proxy for some other, possibly more broadly generalizable mechanism related to low social capital and high relative deprivation (Darrow 2009; Kawachi et al. 1999; Kennedy et al. 1998; Hsieh and Pugh 1993), which may be a salient component of social mechanisms of causation that produce stressful neighbourhood environments for children? Is there enough evidence in order to make the case that the reduction of crime rates in Southern California or elsewhere would be an efficient, possibly cost-effective way to address the dual burden of and inequities in childhood asthma *and* violent crime, or could a combination of clinical interventions and harsher sentencing for criminals (for example) accomplish the same goals – a particularly relevant question in terms of the political will to address these issues?

7.3   Fundamental Causes and Social Mechanisms of Causation

Evidence of social disparities in health implies that there may be some fundamental causes of health inequalities – as Marmot and Singh-Manoux (2005) put it, the "causes of the causes" – that cannot be addressed *solely* by intervening on individual-level risk factors (House et al. 1990, 1994; Link and Phelan 1995).[2] By focusing on developing a clearer understanding of the processes and pathways that link risk factors at the individual level to pathology (if usually from an mainly biological perspective), a key product of clinical epidemiology has been a more comprehensive understanding of how pharmaceutical and other interventions can improve the human system with efficacy and efficiency. In a similar way, if social epidemiology is to contribute to the design and re-design of healthy neighbourhoods, more clarity is needed on the precise mechanisms that link fundamental causes to

---

[2] We do not mean to imply that neighbourhood health disparities can be completely explained by fundamental causes. The agency of individuals should always be considered in trying to understand the extent to which specific social mechanisms of causation are relevant to these disparities. The frameworks of Bernard et al. (2007), discussed in this chapter, and of Shankardass, discussed in Chap. 6, are examples of how we can conceive of the synergy between agency and fundamental causes.

social determinants of health and health disparities, and on how neighbourhood contexts may be integral to social mechanisms of causation that include fundamental causes at and above the neighbourhood level (as in Fig. 7.1).

Sir Bradford Hill (1965) suggested that the key, underlying question about causality is whether "the frequency of the undesirable event B will be influenced by a change in the environmental feature A." He also implied that, in some circumstances, the question of how such an influence occurs will need to be understood in great detail ("*How* such a change exerts that influence may call for a great deal of research") (Hill 1965). Research about neighbourhoods and health, especially that concerned with how to intervene on the impact of fundamental causes with an understanding of the relevant social mechanisms that may determine success or failure, certainly applies to Hill's latter point, in part because of the unique contexts that neighbourhoods encompass and are embedded within. Neighbourhoods can be defined in terms of a great number of *built*, *natural* and *social* environmental attributes,[3] and these attributes are often complex and dynamic. Further, many different types of people – of varying social class but also undertaking different types of activity – utilize neighbourhood spaces, which highlights the question of who specifically experiences the deleterious effects of neighbourhoods when a disparity is described.

At the same time, neighbourhood spaces are part and parcel of broader places, such as cities, countries and the rest of the world, all with their own social, political, economic and environmental attributes. Put another way, in light of our interest in developing solutions to problems of health equity, neighbourhoods have to, at least in some respects, be viewed as functional units of society at large. For example, neighbourhoods are often explicitly designated as planning units within cities (e.g., *Major* and *Minor Health Planning Areas* in the City of Toronto). In turn, the processes by which neighbourhoods are thought to influence disease, injury and wellness may be "structured" by factors outside of the neighbourhood (e.g., by municipal or provincial strategies and/or funding for affordable housing, by unregulated pollution emissions that drift into a neighbourhood from other areas) (see Kjellstrom and Mercado 2008; Macintyre et al. 2002; Morello-Frosch and Lopez 2006; see also Chap. 9). That forces at higher levels of analysis than the neighbourhood level help define neighbourhood properties is consistent with the description by Chicago School sociologists of neighbourhood effects on health that persist over time in spite of local residential turnover (Park et al. 1925; Sampson 2003). For example, although our focus in this chapter is on residential neighbourhoods, it is clear that individuals may routinely move through multiple neighbourhoods of various types related to activities of work, study, play and domesticity. To the extent

---

[3] The natural environment includes living and non-living things that occur naturally, including, chiefly, soil ("green space"), water ("blue space") and air. The built environment relates to constructions and services for human activity; for example, buildings, roads and water management systems. The social environment has been defined by Yen and Syme (1999) as including "groups to which we belong, the neighborhoods in which we live, the organization of our workplaces, and the policies we create to order our lives."

that there may be similarities in such time-activity patterns reproduced by residents of a particular neighbourhood (e.g., in so-called "bedroom communities" where many residents commute to jobs outside of the neighbourhood) (Kwan 2009), there is a suggestion that extra-neighbourhood factors can be expected to determine differences in health across neighbourhoods.

As a result of the multiple levels of context that may be relevant to social mechanisms of causation within neighbourhoods, as well as the stratified populations that may occupy these spaces, neighbourhood health disparities are potentially related to multiple, overlapping and bi-directional mechanisms that link people to their neighbourhoods, which are in turn embedded within larger social, political and economic structures (as in Fig. 7.1). Due to the complexity of these mechanisms, social epidemiologists should expect that there might be multiple fundamental causes (of both the necessary and sufficient type) that contribute to specific neighbourhood health disparities.

Referring back to the example of social disparities in childhood asthma in Southern California, we can consider how the specific effect of local crime on asthma onset might be explained by a complex set of specific mechanisms related to fundamental causes (Fig. 7.1). Growing evidence suggests that neighbourhood violence represents a psychological stressor for children, while recent evidence suggests that chronic stress and exposure to environmental toxins may act synergistically in causing childhood asthma (Clougherty et al. 2007; Shankardass et al. 2009). Incidentally, this may be expected to result in within-neighbourhood heterogeneity in the impact of air pollution on asthma (Jerrett and Finkelstein 2005). At the same time, parents in areas of high crime could also be more likely to keep their children indoors out of concern for their safety, thus increasing exposure to indoor environmental toxins that may cause asthma (Rosenfeld et al. 2010). Both of these mechanisms – exposure to violence leading to chronic stress and parental concern for child safety increasing exposure to household hazards – may be driven by some more fundamental cause or causes of crime at the community level related to relative deprivation, low social capital and the availability of firearms (Darrow 2009; Kawachi et al. 1999; Kennedy et al. 1998; Hsieh and Pugh 1993). The environmental justice literature (Morello-Frosch and Shenassa 2006) also demonstrates how low social capital or high deprivation areas may feature a higher level of traffic-related pollution, another important contributor to the formation of childhood asthma. Of course, even with this level of understanding of potentially important causes and mechanisms related to effects of crime on childhood asthma, a clearer understanding of these relationships would be required in order to identify effective and efficient interventions.

In short, while it is straightforward to conceive of neighbourhoods as simple containers of social, economic and physical phenomena that may affect health, what is required to move this area of inquiry to a next stage of development is greater attention to the neighbourhood and the phenomena that constitute it, as well as extra-neighbourhood factors, as actively structuring peoples' health opportunities (Macintyre et al. 2002) in a dynamic interplay with the human agency of the neighbourhood's residents and visitors or users (Bernard et al. 2007).

7.4   Beyond Multilevel Modelling

As social epidemiologists shift attention to social mechanisms of causation, we can identify some specific areas requiring focus by considering the limitations of the multilevel modelling approach that is often used to study neighbourhoods and health. Although these models represent a significant advancement in our ability to examine so-called "neighbourhood effects," its exclusive use, or even its primacy in the inferences we draw about links between neighbourhoods and health, significantly constrains the explanations that are possible for a number of reasons. Like most models, the ones produced by this technique embody a number of assumptions about the nature of the phenomenon that simplify it significantly.

First, multilevel modelling of neighbourhoods and health assumes the universal primacy of residential location as the salient level for exposure to health risks and access to health resources for all individuals in such studies. Yet, many individuals lead very mobile lives and in many cases leave their residential neighbourhoods in diurnal patterns of movement related to activities of work, study, play and domesticity. Given the unique balance and type of such activities for different types of individuals, places of residence may be a more or less important context for health.

Second, multilevel modelling, when it parcels overall individual variance into variance that can be explained at the individual level and variance that can be explained at the contextual level, treats the former as primordial and the latter, quite literally, as residual. Conceptually, it is possible to sustain an argument that the neighbourhood factors should be the primordial part of the modelling and the individual the residual. The notion of fundamental causes involving structural and intermediate determinants of health (Whitehead and Dahlgren 2006) implies that individuals are shaped by their contexts, and the tendency to describe geographic or group-level differences in health in terms of individual attributes has been critiqued as the "atomistic fallacy" (Diez-Roux 1998; Schwartz 1994; Subramanian et al. 2009).

Third, multilevel models are often used with the assumption that they will contribute to an explanation for neighbourhood effects. Given that the explanations of interest to social epidemiologists are complex, it should be recognized that these models generally facilitate a narrow view – explanation of individual variance by discrete neighbourhood constructs – and then only meaningfully so in the context of a rigorous theoretical framework and sophisticated measures that accurately capture the salient dynamics of interest. Earlier work with multilevel models has often been geared towards the simpler task of identifying the relevance of *non-compositional* explanations for neighbourhood disparities in health (e.g., "Are neighbourhoods important for this outcome?"). As a result, neighbourhood socioeconomic characteristics based on convenient census data (e.g., median household income) are often utilized accompanied by *ad hoc*, data-driven theorizing where there are multiple possible explanations of interest (e.g., Oliver et al. 2007). Often this amounts to no more than speculation about all the possible meanings that a particular census measure may have for the phenomenon of study. In realist terminology, this is called "naïve empiricism" (Sayer 1992). The problem with it is not so much where the analysis begins – many great scientific insights have been developed through exploratory analysis – but it's where the analysis stops, with much of the explanation left (again) to speculation about what the finding may mean followed by a recommendation of further research. In other words, there is little capacity to probe the relevance of precise social mechanisms of causation.

A fourth issue for explanation in epidemiologic neighbourhood effects studies is what Oakes (2006) calls "structural confounding," the chief component of which is, essentially, the absence of a complete array of *counterfactuals* available in reality, making the interpretation of multilevel models challenging. In other words, it means that when doing multilevel neighbourhood studies, there are too few low-income people living in high-income neighbourhoods and too few high-income people living in low-income neighbourhoods (each of these is a counterfactual) to make reliable statements about causation. This absence of counterfactuals, of course, is not evidence that phenomena like deprivation amplification do not exist, only that the tool social epidemiology has available and has made the implicit gold standard for causal inference is unable to reliably detect such causal relationships. This limitation implies that greater pluralism of methods and a different notion of explanation are needed in social epidemiology (as argued in Chap. 2).

7.5   Complex Understandings of Place and Health Are Inhibited by Crude Approaches to Space

Cutchin (2007) notes that while social epidemiology has recently begun to explore a wide range of what we are referring to as social mechanisms of causation (e.g., involving socioeconomic stratification, social capital, social networks, discrimination and segregation), "the conceptual and methodological approaches remain those of (traditional) epidemiology." Given the complex mechanisms by which neighbourhood contexts can drive inequalities in health (see Link and Phelan 1995; Macintyre et al. 2002; Materia and Baglio 2005; Bernard et al. 2007; Cummins et al. 2007; Kjellstrom and Mercado 2008; Putnam and Galea 2008), social epidemiologists may benefit by conceptualizing their work in terms of a more detailed theoretical understanding of the neighbourhood processes that comprise specific places, as well as other mechanisms pertaining to macrosocial determinants of neighbourhood spaces.

For example, the urban theorists Logan and Molotch (2007) have described "durable differences among places" driven by market forces in concert with "conflicting interests, contested plans and policy choices" concomitant with growth. Such differences (or "stratification") determine health opportunity and risk for residents by affecting the ability to "participate in the surrounding systems of power and privilege" and "hold back the deleterious impacts of development" (Logan and Molotch 2007). In reference to the earlier example of childhood asthma disparities in Southern California, this mechanism may help to explain why minority and high poverty neighbourhoods in this region bear over twice the traffic density compared with other neighbourhoods in the region and a disproportionate level of stationary sources of air pollution (Houston et al. 2004; Morello-Frosch et al. 2002). It may also explain why schools with less local air pollution are attended by a dispropro-tionately more White student body, whereas the most polluted school environments contained 92% minority students (Pastor et al. 2002). To be sure, a growing chorus suggests that social epidemiology ought to shake hands with political economy more often (Macintyre et al. 2002; Materia and Baglio 2005; Putnam and Galea 2008; Kjellstrom and Mercado 2008; Szreter and Woolcock 2004).

In order to further demonstrate how social epidemiology can use theory to problematize current practice and arrive at more concrete understandings of why neighbourhood health inequalities occur, we present a critical analysis of key assump-tions about space and health that have often been made by social epidemiologists.

Cummins et al. (2007) recently proposed a "relational" approach to understand-ing place in health research that challenges us to account for not only the "processes and interactions occurring between people and places and over time," but also for the "dynamic and changing characteristics of places and the place-to-place mobility of populations on a daily basis, and over the life-course." In contrast to the complex relationship between space and health that is implied, we can look back and describe two key assumptions that much previous descriptive work on neighbourhoods and health has made that imply a simpler relationship. For example, a common use of multilevel models and GIS has been to nest individuals within static residential environments and to assign specific neighbourhood characteristics, such as high deprivation, low social capital or distance to a hazard or resource. Here, anyone who resides within a geographic neighbourhood boundary, or at a specific distance to a neighbourhood hazard or resource, is broadly assumed to bear equal risk for the health outcome of interest, and these neighbourhood exposures are assumed to be primarily important. Health geographers have long offered theories that would problematize this assumption, especially for the purpose of understanding who within a neighbourhood is more likely to be exposed to hazards, who may benefit from local resources and whether some may be at risk or have access to resources outside of the neighbourhood (Gesler 1992; Wolch and Dear 1987).

The first specific assumption is that proximity to a hazardous exposure or resource, as defined by neighbourhood of residence and/or Euclidian distance, translates to equal exposure to that hazard or access to that resource. For example, although there is some evidence from ecological studies showing that populations living proximate to concentrations of fast food restaurants have poorer health (Alter and Eny 2005), fast food consumption habits are complex (Yen et al. 2007). There is no evidence that proximity *necessarily* means these populations are large con-sumers of fast food, or that people who do not live proximate to fast food cannot be large consumers of it. Indeed, it is possible that it is fast food restaurants' location relative to people's frequently travelled routes, as opposed to their residential location, that is the greater determinant of their fast food consumption. Similarly, proximity to a recreation centre does not necessarily mean that someone has access to it; the hours of operation, the price or other personal constraints (like child care) may prohibit them from using the facility for physical activity (Bernard et al. 2007). Proximity, in other words, which is relied upon heavily in existing studies of neighbourhood effects, does not *necessarily* imply exposure to a health risk or access to a health resource. To make this assumption is akin to the ecological fallacy problem that is a fundamental concern of epidemiology.

In reference to the use of GIS for social science research, Anselin (2000) suggests a need to "go beyond dealing with Euclidean space and physical geographical locations to include location in "'social' and 'perceptual' space (social distance, economic distance)." Bernard et al. (2007) suggest that the opportunity structures facing individuals within neighbourhoods are complicated by processes that determine the distribution of key resources. These processes, they argue, are governed by more than just proximity, including by price, rights and informed reciprocity. The resources (authoritative and allocative) are related to five domains (economic, institutional, physical, community organisations and local sociability) and the individuals in question are active agents in acquiring resources (Bernard et al. 2007). A similar framework could be developed to demonstrate how exposure to hazards within a neighbourhood may be complex. For example, in Chap. 6, a framework is proposed to imply that social disparities in chronic disease are partly mediated as a result of how environmental stressors, which can be reflected in the built, natural and social attributes of neighbourhoods are differentially perceived and coped with by various population groups. In this way, theory can offer a more complex understanding of the forces that shape neighbourhood social dynamics.

By implying that different social communities can have very different relationships with the risks and resources within a neighbourhood, the theoretical framework of Bernard et al. (2007) facilitates a more mechanistic understanding of grand theories of fundamental cause, such as social capital, in terms of "spatial externalities" (e.g., economic policies made at the city or province level) and non-geographic communities (e.g., religious institutions), that comprise supportive social and physical environments for health and health equity (Sampson 2003). In turn, this can help us design studies to test hypotheses about why certain people within certain neighbourhoods are at risk for poor health, and how interventions can be designed and evaluated in a way to promote effectiveness. For example, research has suggested that individuals living in disadvantaged neighbourhoods may end up with particularly high rates of obesity as a result of unhealthy diet, and dietary habits are thought to be partly determined by the quality of the local food environment (Davis and Carpenter 2009).

Yet, the framework put forward by Bernard et al. (2007) predicts that interventions to improve access to healthy, affordable foods will require a broader understanding of how policies, economies, programmatic interventions and grassroots action intersect in specific neighbourhoods. For example, the purpose of the Healthy Bodegas Initiative, implemented by the Department of Health and Mental Hygiene in New York City, has been to combat obesity by increasing access to healthy foods in inner-city neighbourhoods dominated by bodegas (read: corner stores) that offer easy access to predominantly unhealthy foods (Department of Health and Mental

Hygiene 2010). Yet, this program was explicitly designed to account for the market forces that bodega owners operate within by way of a key objective being to work with community organizations and residents to increase demand for these foods. Perhaps because of this practical and complex approach to the intervention, the intervention has resulted in both an increase in the uptake of healthy foods by community residents and also the continued availability of these foods at bodegas (Emerson 2009; The Community Development Project of the Urban Justice Center 2009).

The second assumption that traditional risk factor-based research into neighbourhoods and health has often made is that we can understand a person's risk or access by considering the characteristics of their residential neighbourhood alone. Specifically, there has not been much attention paid to the movement of individuals, both within and outside of their residential neighbourhoods (including for work, school, errands, etc.) (see Sampson et al.'s (2002) call to account for the role of "routine activities"). Such time activity has implications for personal experience and, ultimately, access and exposure (Kwan 2009; Hägerstrand 1970), and may be determined structurally within society. Thus above-mentioned evidence that traffic-related pollution plays a role in the development of childhood asthma (Jerrett et al. 2008; Gauderman et al. 2005; Sarnat and Holguin 2007) includes evidence demonstrating independent contributions of exposure at the residential and school location to overall risk for incidence (McConnell et al. 2010).

Kwan (2008) recently applied a similar notion of "time geography" (see Hägerstrand 1970) to understand how "emotional geographies" describe an American Muslim woman's affective response as she moves through Columbus, Ohio (United States) in the context of growing anti-Muslim hate violence in the period following the September 11th attacks. Given the recent evidence mentioned earlier that suggests a synergistic relationship between chronic stress and traffic-related pollution on the development of childhood asthma, an understanding of emotional geographies may be important for developing interventions for susceptible population groups.

7.6 Explaining Neighbourhood Effects in Social Epidemiology

What we are suggesting in the foregoing demands a different notion of what constitutes "explanation" in social epidemiology, as described in Chap. 2. A key goal for social epidemiologists should be to participate more fully in unravelling the pathways by which neighbourhood environments affect health – to reveal key processes and pathways that drive complex inequalities and to contribute to initiatives to remedy those inequalities. A related question is, when we observe an association between a neighbourhood-level variable and an individual-level outcome, what does it mean? In this chapter we have argued that the use of theories capable of conceptualizing neighbourhoods in terms of its local residents and wider societal structures can be of great use to researchers interested in exploring the social mechanisms of causation that operate through these environments. In turn, while neighbourhoods have traditionally been treated as a unit of analysis by social epidemiology, we argue that they ought to also be intensively studied in their own right.

Such intensive research can help us move from the description of inequalities occurring in neighbourhood "containers," within which residents have varying levels of risk for illness or disease, to an appreciation of the ways in which society at large and neighbourhood users jointly determine population health and well-being.

Two examples illustrate this potential nicely. First, Klinenberg (2003) examines the social dynamics of two socioeconomically similar neighbourhoods with divergent mortality patterns attributable to the 1996 Chicago heat wave (as described in Chap. 8). Similarities asides, he finds that the neighbourhood with the greater number of deaths was one characterized by high levels of crime, social isolation, poor social capital and a lack of community gathering spaces (retail streetscapes, churches, etc.), while the neighbourhood with the better outcomes fared more favourably on these dynamics. The outcome, therefore, was that vulnerable people, especially seniors living alone, were too afraid to leave their apartments and were not connected into a social network that had people checking on them, so they stayed in their apartments, without air conditioning, and died as a result. Second, Hunter (2007, 2010) seeks to explain patterns of HIV infection in KwaZulu-Natal province of South Africa (as described in Chap. 2). In so doing, he goes well beyond simple *post hoc* conjectures about the possible mechanisms for patterns of HIV infection and tries to understand the embodiment of inequality in emotions and everyday practices, including love, economic insecurity and employment, and in patterns of regional migration.

While the development of theories and concepts about neighbourhoods and health will often come from within the health research field, it should be noted that researchers from other disciplines (including sociology, geography, economics and anthropology) have already attempted to describe the complex dynamics of neighbourhoods, and that these perspectives may be very useful to epidemiology (as demonstrated in the multidisciplinary narrative review presented in Chap. 6 and in the application of diverse theory to explain health inequalities in Chaps. 8 and 10). Although challenging, the rise in popularity of place-based policy making suggests that this is a relevant endeavour for modern social epidemiology.

Moving toward the study of broader social mechanisms of causation has implications for the professional practice of epidemiology. For example, the nature of medical publishing encourages very short articles with a heavy emphasis on the statistical analysis, study limitations and remaining uncertainty, while the way in which health researchers are rewarded in their career progress (e.g., priority placed on quantity of publications with impact factor as dominant measure of quality) encourages a focus on studies that aim to test specific pathways rather than more complex and potentially broader mechanisms (as discussed in Chap. 2). Over time, research has therefore focused on replicating discrete and de-contextualized neighbourhood pathways, but seldom is attention paid in the published literature to a richer explanation of the mechanisms at work in the relationship between neighbourhoods and health (unless it comes from an allied discipline like medical sociology), in part because there is no reward system for it. This represents a significant constraint on the practical impact and relevance of social epidemiology to making a difference.

In summary, the process and pathways by which neighbourhoods can determine health inequalities are numerous and non-linear, and there are limitations to the level of understanding about fundamental causes that can be gleaned without some measure of intensive research. Where social disparities in health are demonstrated (empirically or otherwise) or where planning of healthy neighbourhoods is the goal, concrete research into complex mechanisms of causation are valuable for the development of effective interventions.

References

Alter DA, Eny K (2005) The relationship between the supply of fast-food chains and cardio-vascular outcomes. Can J Public Health 96:173–177

Anselin L (2000) The link between GIS and spatial analysis: GIS, spatial econometrics and social science research. J Geograph Syst 2:11–15

Badcock B (1984) Unfairly structured cities. Blackwell, Oxford

Bernard P, Charafeddine R, Frohlich KL et al (2007) Health inequalities and place: a theoretical conception of neighbourhood. Soc Sci Med 65:1839–1852

Brooks-Gunn J, Duncan G, Klebanov P et al (1993) Do neighbourhoods influence child and adolescent development? Am J Sociol 99:353–395

Clougherty JE, Kubzansky LD (2009) A framework for examining social stress and susceptibility to air pollution in respiratory health. Environ Health Perspect 117:1351–1358

Clougherty JE, Levy JI, Kubzansky LD et al (2007) Synergistic effects of traffic-related air pollution and exposure to violence on urban asthma etiology. Environ Health Perspect 115:1140–1146

Cohen RT, Canino GJ, Bird HR et al (2008) Violence, abuse, and asthma in Puerto Rican children. Am J Respir Crit Care Med 178:453–459

Commission on Social Determinants of Health (2008) Closing the gap in a generation: health equity through action on the social determinants of health. Final report of the Commission on Social Determinants of Health, World Health Organization, Geneva

Cummins S, Curtis S, Diez-Roux AV et al (2007) Understanding and representing "place" in health research: a relational approach. Soc Sci Med 65:1825–1838

Cutchin MP (2007) The need for the "new health geography" in epidemiologic studies of environment and health. Health Place 13:725–742

Darrow C (2009) Crime: its cause and treatment. Kaplan Publishing, New York

Davis B, Carpenter C (2009) Proximity of fast-food restaurants to schools and adolescent obesity. Am J Public Health 99:505–510

Department of Health and Mental Hygiene (2010) New York city healthy bodegas initiative 2010 report, Department of Health and Mental Hygiene, New York

Department of Health and Social Security (1980) Inequalities in health: report of a research working group, Department of Health and Social Security, London (Black report)

Diez-Roux AV (1998) Bringing context back into epidemiology: variables and fallacies in multi-level analysis. Am J Public Health 88:216–222

Diez-Roux AV (2001) Investigating neighbourhood and area effects on health. Am J Public Health 91:1783–1789

Diez-Roux AV (2007) Neighborhoods and health: where are we and were do we go from here? Rev Epidemiol Sante Publique 55:13–21

Diez-Roux AV, Mair C (2010) Neighborhoods and health. Ann N Y Acad Sci 1186:125–145

Duncan C, Jones K, Moon G (1999) Smoking and deprivation: are there neighbourhood effects? Soc Sci Med 48:497–505

Dunn JR (2010) Health behavior vs the stress of low socioeconomic status and health outcomes. JAMA 303:1199–1200

Emerson C (2009) A food policy for New York. Gotham Gazette, Citizens Union Foundation, New York

Evans GW (2004) The environment of childhood poverty. Am Psychol 59:77–92

Gauderman WJ, Avol E, Lurmann F et al (2005) Childhood asthma and exposure to traffic and nitrogen dioxide. Epidemiology 16:737–743

Gesler W (1992) Therapeutic Landscapes: medical issues in light of the new cultural geography. Soc Sci Med 34:735–746

Glazier RH, Booth GL (2007) Neighbourhood environments and resources for healthy living – a focus on diabetes in Toronto: ICES Atlas. Institute for Clinical Evaluative Sciences, Toronto

Graham S, Levin ML, Lilienfeld AM et al (1963) Ethnic derivation as related to cancer at various sites. Cancer 16:13–27

Gupta RS, Zhang X, Springston EE et al (2010) The association between community crime and childhood asthma prevalence in Chicago. Ann Allergy Asthma Immunol 104:299–306

Hamano T, Fujisawa Y, Ishida Y, et al (2010) Social capital and mental health in Japan: a multilevel analysis. PLoS One 5:e13214

Hägerstrand T (1970) What about people in regional science? Pap Reg Sci 24:7–21

Hill AB (1965) The environment and disease: association or causation? Proc R Soc Med 58:295–300

House JS, Kessler RC, Herzog AR et al (1990) Age, socioeconomic status, and health. Milbank Q 68:383–411

House JS, Lepkowski JM, Kinney AM et al (1994) The social stratification of aging and health. J Health Soc Behav 35:213–234

Houston D, Wu J, Ong P et al (2004) Structural disparities of urban traffic in Southern California: implications for vehicle-related air pollution exposure in minority and high-poverty neighborhoods. J Urban Affairs 26:565–592

Hsieh CC, Pugh MD (1993) Poverty, income inequality, and violent crime: a meta-analysis of recent aggregate data studies. Crim Just Rev 18:182–202

Hunter M (2007) The changing political economy of sex in South Africa: the significance of unemployment and inequalities to the scale of the AIDS pandemic. Soc Sci Med 64:689–700

Hunter M (2010) Love in the time of AIDS: inequality, gender, and rights in South Africa. Indiana University Press, Bloomington

Jerrett M, Finkelstein M (2005) Geographies of risk in studies linking chronic air pollution exposure to health outcomes. J Toxicol Environ Health Part A 68:1207–1242

Jerrett M, Shankardass K, Berhane K et al (2008) Traffic-related air pollution and asthma onset in children: a prospective cohort study with individual exposure measurement. Environ Health Perspect 116:1433–1438

Kawachi I, Berkman L (eds) (2003) Neighborhoods and health. Oxford University Press, New York

Kawachi I, Kennedy BP, Wilkinson RG (1999) Crime: social disorganization and relative deprivation. Soc Sci Med 48:719–731

Kennedy BP, Kawachi I, Prothrow-Stitha D et al (1998) Social capital, income inequality, and firearm violent crime. Soc Sci Med 47:7–17

Kim D (2008) Blues from the neighborhood? Neighborhood characteristics and depression. Epidemiol Rev 30:101–117

Kitagawa E, Hauser P (1973) Differential mortality in the United States: a study in socioeconomic epidemiology. Harvard University Press, Cambridge

Kjellstrom T, Mercado S (2008) Towards action on social determinants for health equity in urban settings. Environ Urban 20:551–574

Klinenberg E (2003) Heat wave: a social autopsy of disaster in Chicago. University of Chicago Press, Chicago

Kwan MP (2008) From oral histories to visual narratives: re-presenting the post-September 11 experiences of the Muslim women in the United States. Soc Cult Geo 9:653–669

Kwan MP (2009) From place-based to people-based exposure measures. Soc Sci Med 69:1311–1313

Link BJ, Phelan J (1995) Social conditions as fundamental causes of disease. J Health Soc Behav 35(extra issue):80–94

Logan JR, Molotch HL (2007) Urban fortunes: the political economy of place, 20th anniversary edition. University of California Press, Berkeley

Macintyre S, Maciver S, Sooman A (1993) Area, class and health: should we be focusing on places or people? J Soc Policy 22:213–234

Macintyre S, Ellaway A, Cummins S (2002) Place effects on health: how can we conceptualise, operationalise and measure them? Soc Sci Med 55:125–139

Mair C, Diez-Roux AV, Galea S (2008) Are neighbourhood characteristics associated with depressive symptoms? A review of evidence. J Epidemiol Community Health 62:940–946, 948 p following 946

Marmot M (2010) Fair society, healthy lives: a strategic review of health inequalities in England post-2010. The Marmot Review, London

Marmot M, Singh-Manoux A (2005) Role of socialization in explaining social inequalities in health. Soc Sci Med 60:2129–2133

Materia E, Baglio G (2005) Health, science, and complexity. J Epidemiol Community Health 59:534–535

McConnell R, Islam T, Shankardass K et al (2010) Childhood incident asthma and traffic-related air pollution at home and school. Environ Health Perspect 118:1021–1026

McLaren L, Ghali L, Lorenzetti D et al (2006) Out of context? Translating evidence from the North Karelia project over place and time. Health Educ Res 22:414–424

Morello-Frosch R, Lopez R (2006) The riskscape and the color line: examining the role of segregation in environmental health disparities. Environ Res 102:181–196

Morello-Frosch R, Pastor Jr. M, Porras C et al (2002) Environmental justice and regional inequality in southern California: implications for future research. Environ Health Perspect 110:149–154

Morello-Frosch R, Shenassa ED (2006) The environmental "riskscape" and social inequality: implications for explaining maternal and child health disparities. Environ Health Perspect 114:1150–1153

O'Campo P (2003) Invited commentary: advancing theory and methods for multilevel models of residential neighborhoods and health. Am J Epidemiol 157:9–13

O'Campo P, Caughy M (2006) Measures of residential community contexts. In: Oakes M, Kaufman J (eds) Methods in social epidemiology. Jossey-Bass, San Francisco

O'Campo P, Salmon C, Burke J (2009) Neighbourhoods and mental well-being: what are the pathways? Health Place 15:56–68

Oakes JM (2004) Causal inference and the relevance of social epidemiology. Soc Sci Med 58:1969–1971

Oakes JM (2006) Commentary: advancing neighbourhood-effects research – selection, inferential support and structural confounding. Int J Epidemiol 35:643–647

Oliver L, Dunn JR, Kohen D et al (2007) Do neighbourhoods influence the readiness to learn of kindergarten children in Vancouver? A multilevel analysis of neighbourhood effects. Environ Plan A 39:848–868

Park RE, Burgess EW, McKenzie RD (1925) The city. University of Chicago Press, Chicago

Parsons JA, Singh G, Scott AN et al (2010) Standardized observation of neighbourhood disorder: Does it work in Canada? Int J Health Geogr 9:6

Pastor M, Sadd JL, Morello-Frosch R (2002) Who's minding the kids? Pollution, public schools, and environmental justice in Los Angeles. Soc Sci Quart 83:263–280

Pearlman DN (2009) Neighborhood-level risk and resilience factors: an emerging issue in childhood asthma epidemiology. Expert Rev Clin Immunol 5:633–637

Phillimore P, Beattie A, Townsend P (1994) Widening inequality of health in northern England, 1981–91. BMJ 308:1125–1128

Pickett KE, Pearl M (2001) Multilevel analyses of neighbourhood socioeconomic context and health outcomes: a critical review. J Epidemiol Community Health 55:111–122

Putnam S, Galea S (2008) Epidemiology and the macrosocial determinants of health. J Public Health Policy 29:275–289

Rajaratnam JK, Burke JG, O'Campo P (2006) Maternal and child health and neighborhood context: the selection and construction of area-level variables. Health Place 12:547–556

Riva M, Gauvin L, Barnett TA (2007) Toward the next generation of research into small area effects on health: a synthesis of multilevel investigations published since July 1998. J Epidemiol Community Health 61:853–861

Rose G (1985) Sick individuals and sick populations. Int J Epidemiol 14:32–38

Rosenfeld L, Rudd R, Chew GL et al (2010) Are neighborhood-level characteristics associated with indoor allergens in the household? J Asthma 47:66–75

Sampson RJ (2003) Neighborhood-level context and health: lessons from sociology. In: Kawachi I, Berkman L (eds) Neighborhoods and health. Oxford University Press, New York

Sampson RJ, Morenoff JD, Gannon-Rowley T (2002) Assessing "neighborhood effects" social processes and new directions in research. Annu Rev Sociol 28:443–478

Sarnat JA, Holguin F (2007) Asthma and air quality. Curr Opin Pulm Med 13:63–66

Sayer A (1992) Method in social science: a Realist approach, 2nd edn. Routledge, London

Schaefer-McDaniel N, Caughy MO, O'Campo P et al (2010) Examining methodological details of neighbourhood observations and the relationship to health: a literature review. Soc Sci Med 70:277–292

Schwartz S (1994) The fallacy of the ecological fallacy: the potential misuse of a concept and the consequences. Am J Public Health 84:819–824

Shankardass K, McConnell R, Jerrett M et al (2009) Parental stress increases the effect of traffic-related air pollution on childhood asthma incidence. Proc Natl Acad Sci USA 106:12406–12411

Shankardass K, Jerrett M, Milam J et al (2010) Social environment and asthma: associations with crime and No Child Left Behind programmes. J Epidemiol Community Health 11 Nov 2010 [Epub ahead of print]

Stafford M, Chandola T, Marmot M (2007) Association between fear of crime and mental health and physical functioning. Am J Public Health 97:2076–2081

Sternthal MJ, Jun HJ, Earls F et al (2010) Community violence and urban childhood asthma: a multilevel analysis. Eur Respir J 36:1400–1409

Subramanian SV, Kennedy MH (2009) Perception of neighborhood safety and reported childhood lifetime asthma in the United States (U.S.): a study based on a national survey. PLoS One 4:e6091

Subramanian SV, Jones K, Kaddour A et al (2009) Revisiting Robinson: the perils of individualistic and ecologic fallacy. Int J Epidemiol 38:342–360

Suglia SF, Ryan L, Laden F et al (2008) Violence exposure, a chronic psychosocial stressor, and childhood lung function. Psychosom Med 70:160–169

Suglia SF, Staudenmayer J, Cohen S et al (2010) Posttraumatic stress symptoms related to community violence and children's diurnal cortisol response in an urban community-dwelling sample. Int J Behav Med 17:43–50

Szreter S, Woolcock M (2004) Health by association? Social capital, social theory, and the political economy of public health. Int J Epidemiol 33:650–667

The Community Development Project of the Urban Justice Center (2009) Food fight: expanding access to affordable and healthy food in downtown Brooklyn. Families United for Racial and Economic Equality, New York

Weaver K, Campbell R, Mermelstein R et al (2008) Pregnancy smoking in context: the influence of multiple levels of stress. Nicotine Tob Res 10:1065–1073

Whitehead M, Dahlgren G (2006) Levelling up (part 1): a discussion paper on concept and principles for tackling social inequities in health. Studies on social and economic determinants of population health, No. 2. WHO Regional Office for Europe, Copenhagen

Wolch JR, Dear MJ (1987) Landscapes of despair: from deinstitutionalization to homelessness. Princeton University Press, Princeton

Wright RJ (2006) Health effects of socially toxic neighborhoods: the violence and urban asthma paradigm. Clin Chest Med 27:413–421

Wright RJ, Mitchell H, Visness CM et al (2004) Community violence and asthma morbidity: the inner-city asthma study. Am J Public Health 94:625–632

Yen IH, Syme SL (1999) The social environment and health: a discussion of the epidemiologic literature. Annu Rev Public Health 20:287–308

Yen IH, Scherzer T, Cubbin C et al (2007) Women's perceptions of neighborhood resources and hazards related to diet, physical activity, and smoking: focus group results from economically distinct neighborhoods in a mid-sized U.S. city. Am J Health Promot 22:98–106

Yin RK (1999) Enhancing the quality of case studies in health services research. Health Serv Res 34:1209–1224

Chapter 8
Application of Two Schools of Social Theory to Neighbourhood, Place and Health Research

Irene H. Yen, Janet K. Shim, and Airín D. Martínez

Contents

8.1	Introduction	158
8.2	Conflict Theory	162
8.3	Interactionist Theory	166
8.4	Neighbourhood-Health Mechanisms – Social Capital and Physical Disorder	168
8.5	Future Research Directions for Neighbourhood-Health Research	170
8.6	Conclusions	171
	References	172

Abstract There is an increasing interest in neighbourhoods in the public health and epidemiology literature. Conventional epidemiologic investigations of neighbourhood health associations have primarily used census and administrative data to describe neighbourhoods. These studies report that people who live in neighbourhoods with higher proportions of people with low incomes or who are unemployed are in poorer health than people who live in neighbourhoods with lower proportions of people with low incomes. It is difficult to translate these sorts of findings into policy or practice. These limitations motivate us to ask how different questions

I.H. Yen (✉)
Department of Medicine, University of California, San Francisco, 3333 California Street, Suite 335, Box 0856, San Francisco, CA 94143-0856, USA
e-mail: irene.yen@ucsf.edu

J.K. Shim
Department of Social and Behavioral Sciences,University of California, San Francisco, 3333 California Street, Suite 455, San Francisco, CA 94118, USA
e-mail: janet.shim@ucsf.edu

A.D. Martínez
W. K. Kellogg Postdoctoral Fellow, Community Track Program Johns Hopkins Bloomberg School of Public Health, 624 N. Broadway, HH 753 Baltimore, MD 21205
e-mail: amartine@jhsph.edu

P. O'Campo and J.R. Dunn (eds.), *Rethinking Social Epidemiology: Towards a Science of Change*, DOI 10.1007/978-94-007-2138-8_8,
© Springer Science+Business Media B.V. 2012

might be formulated to understand neighbourhood-health connections in such a way as to move into solution-focused research. In this chapter, we suggest that understanding and applying social theory to neighbourhood-health research questions provokes us to ask different sorts of questions than have been posed by most epidemiologists thus far. We provide some examples of how two sociological paradigms, conflict and interactionist theories, suggest different questions, which then warrant different methods of investigation. To the extent that epidemiology has uncovered mechanisms that connect neighbourhoods to people's health, the most investigated mechanisms are social capital and physical disorder. We take up the specific research in this area with the lens of sociological paradigms.

Abbreviations

CDC   Centers for Disease Control and Prevention

8.1   Introduction

Sociologists and geographers have long identified the importance of place, both literal and symbolic, in influencing people's lives (Siegrist 2000). Similar to the term "community," "place" can be defined by webs of relationships and shared identities, though no community or place is homogeneous (Etzioni 1997; Minkler 2004). Recent work by social epidemiologists, however, has explored the important contextual role of geographic area in determining disease outcomes (Yen and Syme 1999; Diez-Roux 2001) and identifying resources such as services, businesses and recreation or hazards such as crime, graffiti, traffic and environmental toxins. One of the first epidemiologic studies of the effects of place showed that people living in a federally designated poverty area within Alameda County, California experienced an age-sex all-cause mortality rate 47% higher than people in a non-poverty area, even after adjusting for multiple confounders (Haan et al. 1987). Subsequent epidemiologic analyses have documented area effects on a wide variety of health-related variables such as physical activity, depression, hypertension, tuberculosis, atherosclerosis and kidney disease (Yen and Kaplan 1998, 1999b; Acevedo-Garcia 2001; Diez-Roux 2001; Diez-Roux et al. 2003; Cubbin and Winkleby 2005; Merkin et al. 2007).

Policymakers and foundations are looking to neighbourhoods as one of the key social determinants of health, which could be an important intervention point to address health disparities, a current priority in the United States. For example, the largest health foundation in California, The California Endowment, has a program area in disparities and within that area a focus on diabetes and obesity. One report that emerged from this focus area is on engaging communities to change nutrition and physical activity environments. PolicyLink, an American national policy advocacy organization, recently created the Center for Health and Place and in 2007 released a report entitled *Why Place Matters: Building the Movement for Healthy Communities* (Bell and Rubin 2007). An American public television documentary series called *Unnatural Causes*, another example, which aired in the spring of 2008, focused on health disparities and featured a segment on place and health connections.

Neighbourhood and place research in epidemiology is growing rapidly with the availability of geospatial data and accompanying quantitative methods (e.g., multilevel modeling that takes into consideration spatial autocorrelation). In spite of this rapid growth, if we look at the current body of literature with an eye toward taking the sum total of the findings and making policy or designing programs, it would be difficult to do so. The key limitations are the study designs (predominantly cross-sectional), the reliance on census or administrative data and the often limited scope of the questions such research addresses, all of which constrains the ability to translate findings into policy or program content. The majority of published studies rely on cross-sectional data. Epidemiologists and social scientists are troubled by cross-sectional studies because of the limitation of assigning cause and effect. A study reports that people who live in a poor neighbourhood (i.e., a neighbourhood with a high proportion of poor people) were more likely to have heart disease than people who lived in a non-poor neighbourhood. To an epidemiologist, the simple association of these two characteristics does not provide the information to understand how the poor neighbourhood would cause heart disease in the resident. Epidemiologists could speculate that a poor neighbourhood is less safe, so a person who lives there is not as comfortable walking in the neighbourhood and gets less exercise. Also, epidemiologists might hypothesize that a poor neighbourhood causes stress for its residents, which can lead to increased vulnerability to chronic diseases. Social scientists are particularly troubled by the issue of selection. They might argue that with only cross-sectional data, it is not possible to determine that the neighbourhood environment causes poor health. People with certain characteristics might sort themselves into neighbourhoods and the factors that influence the sorting may cause health problems.

Another issue with the current body of neighbourhood-health research is the reliance on administrative definitions of neighbourhood (e.g., census tracts or dissemination areas). Administrative definitions are problematic because rarely do these correspond with historically recognized neighbourhoods and neighbourhoods as residents actually conceive of and move through them (Coulton et al. 2001; Yen et al. 2007; Smith et al. 2010). Using administrative boundaries to define neighbourhoods makes administrative data the obvious way to characterize the economic circumstances of the residents (e.g., percentage of people with incomes below the poverty level, percentage of female-headed households with children under age 18, percentage of adults who are unemployed). Knowing that living where a high proportion of people have poverty-level incomes might be associated with poorer health is difficult to translate into a policy.

Should the policy be to disperse people with lower incomes or increase the incomes of the people who have low incomes? Indeed, the former has been tried in the United States in the well-documented HOPE IV program and evaluation that provided vouchers to people who were eligible to live in public or subsidized housing (Greenbaum 2002; Clampet-Lundquist 2004; Popkin et al. 2004; Kleit 2005).

A panel study of nearly 900 HOPE IV program participants surveyed their health in 2001, 2003 and 2005. At baseline, panel study respondents were in far worse health than other low-income households, reporting high rates of poor perceived health, asthma and depression (Popkin et al. 2002). Respondents who had moved to private market housing with vouchers were living in better housing in neighbourhoods that were safer. In contrast, those who remained in their original units or had moved to another traditional public housing development did not experience these improvements in their circumstances (Buron et al. 2007; Comey 2007; Popkin and Cove 2007). Regardless of the new living circumstances, HOPE VI participants did not report improvements in their health in 2005 (Manjarrez et al. 2007). We are not aware of another intervention of this sort and maintain that, in general, using policy to direct where people live such that people with low incomes are dispersed among people with higher incomes is not a policy that most governments would entertain.

While there have been impressive contributions in the neighbourhood-health research literature, there remains several conceptual and methodological challenges that could benefit from the contribution of other sociological theory and concepts (Macintyre et al. 2002; O'Campo 2003; Bernard et al. 2007). Consider, for example, the question of causal direction: Do multiple liquor outlets increase the likelihood of violent crime or do people with violent inclinations tend to move to areas with liquor outlets? Or do both violent crime and liquor outlets depend on a third factor, a factor that may differ by local community resources versus demands, which may call for distinctly different intervention strategies? Sociological theories regarding the effects of local and cultural context on behaviours, risks and social environment can help guide the choice of sophisticated social epidemiologic models (Kaplan and Lynch 1999; Marmot 1999; Kaplan 2004). Such coupling of theories with methods could provide crucial information about neighbourhood issues to advance scholarship with regard to directionality, for example, and move into solution-focused research.

In this chapter we explore how two sociological paradigms can help direct research on neighbourhoods or place and health, with particular attention to how they can help uncover mechanisms that are amenable to policy actions or strategies for addressing health disparities. By way of illustration, we root our exploration in an extended consideration of two adjacent neighbourhoods featured in Eric Klinenberg's (2003) *Heat Wave: A Social Autopsy of Disaster in Chicago*. We chose this example because the book explicitly aims to show how "natural" disasters are far more social and, therefore, preventable than is often presumed and because the work has figured prominently in public debates about the health consequences of social isolation. There is other examples we could have selected. After we illustrate key concepts from the two sociological paradigms with Klinenberg's work, we examine social capital as a potential mechanism that links neighbourhoods to health. In particular, sociological concepts are used to extend the notion of social capital beyond how it has been conventionally used and understood in epidemiologic research. We argue that the consideration of the highlighted sociological theories and others can lead to a better understanding of the social processes that underlie the significance of neighbourhoods to health and that such understandings in turn may provide clearer directions for thinking about ways to promote health through neighbourhood-based interventions.

Other than the identification of the composition of an area as a risk factor for poor health, another factor that has been identified as an important neighbourhood characteristic is social capital. Neighbourhood social capital manifests, in part, as the relationships one forms in one's neighbourhood whether with other residents or with service providers. There are several definitions of social capital, each emphasizing different qualities (Lochner et al. 1999). The sociologist Pierre Bourdieu (1983, 1986) introduced the concept of social capital as the actual and potential resources that one has access to by virtue of belonging to a group; thus, social capital resides in the connections and relationships one has with others. The political scientist Robert Putnam (1993) subsequently argued that "social capital is a feature of social organizations such as networks, norms and trust that facilitates coordination and cooperation for mutual benefit." Expanding on Putnam's work, Sampson et al. (1997) argue that a key function of social capital is "collective efficacy," comprised of two related concepts: "social cohesion," defined as norms of trust, and "informal social control" defined as the willingness to intervene to stop negative neighbourhood activity. To develop the findings on neighbourhood social capital into policy or practice, it has to be understood how social capital is created and maintained. Later in the chapter, we will provide an example of research into social capital informed by theoretical frameworks.

During the historic 1995 heat wave that hit much of the Midwestern United States, North Lawndale and Little Village, two adjacent neighbourhoods in Chicago, had very different mortality rates: North Lawndale's was unusually high, while Little Village's was unusually low. Why? Conventional epidemiologic approaches would likely look at the demographics of the people who had died. Men have higher mortality rates than women so perhaps North Lawndale had many more old people than Little Village or had older men. In fact, neither was the case. Poor people have higher mortality rates than non-poor; perhaps North Lawndale had more poor people than Little Village. This hypothesis was indeed found to be true; in 1990, median family income was $14,000 and 44% of the residents lived under the poverty line in North Lawndale. The corresponding figures for Little Village were $23,000 and 22%, respectively. Were there racial and/or ethnic differences in the two neighbourhoods? African Americans have higher mortality rates than Whites for heart diseases, stroke, cancer, asthma, influenza and pneumonia, diabetes and homicide (Office of Minority Health 2009). In fact, North Lawndale had a majority African Americans living in the neighbourhood, while Little Village had a majority of Latinos living in the neighbourhood. This might be the end of the conventional epidemiologic investigation with the conclusion that the higher mortality in the wake of the heat wave in North Lawndale was due to the higher proportion of poor people and African American residents.

Yet with this conclusion, what sort of strategies can we develop within solution-focused options to prevent a similar outcome in the future? Dispersing the impoverished and African American populations is clearly neither feasible nor desirable, and it sidesteps a host of important etiologic questions about the connections between place, race and health. Multiple additional questions could be articulated and investigational strategies pursued based on the information of the different socioeconomic and racial and/or ethnic compositions of the two neighbourhoods. For example, why did the African Americans in North Lawndale die at higher rates than the Latinos in Little Village? What is it about living in a neighbourhood with a high proportion of poor people and African American residents that puts an individual at higher risk of mortality when a natural disaster occurs? Or was there something about the physical environment or available resources in the North Lawndale neighbourhood? What resources did residents living in Little Village have that helped them to survive? Or are there causes that could be found in the histories of the two neighbourhoods that could explain both their differing socio-economic and racial compositions as well as their disparate mortality rates? Pursuing these questions can provide evidence to guide the design of meaningful programs or interventions.

Klinenberg applied a number of concepts informed by larger social theory paradigms to determine a research program to answer the questions posed above. These concepts draw from both conflict theory and interactionist theory, two major sociological theoretical paradigms that are not mutually exclusive. Below we provide a brief overview of key concepts within these paradigms with a focus on those paradigms that would be relevant for investigations of neighbourhood, place and health relations.

8.2   Conflict Theory

The *conflict paradigm* in sociology contends that the organization of society can be understood and analyzed as the outcome of power struggles for material and ideological resources. Material resources are the physical things that people need to survive (e.g., shelter, food) or those that they wish to possess (e.g., leather jacket, air conditioning). Ideological resources are ideas, beliefs and practices that help people acquire increased access to material things and/or to power and prestige. This paradigm asserts that conflict is inherent in any society because society is always stratified into status groups that have differential access to resources, including those that promote well-being and higher status. Traditionally, this paradigm asserts that People with the most resources are those who control production, specifically the "means of production" or the non-human inputs that produce wealth (e.g., factories, technology and tools). Karl Marx (1978), one of the early conflict theorists, highlighted the unequal distribution of the means of production – for instance, between the factory owner and the worker – as the fundamental tension in capitalist societies. Contemporary conflict theorists emphasize that society is stratified along more complex conceptions of class (Olin Wright 1996) as well as other dimensions including political affiliation (Weber 1956), race and ethnicity (Blauner 1972) and gender (Hartmann 1976).

The interplay between *structure* and *agency* is a key empirical question from the perspective of conflict theory. Agency is associated with individuals' ability to create ideas and intervene (to variable degrees) in the social circumstances in which they live. However, people's freedom and creativity to produce new ideas, objects and actions are conditioned by their particular historical moment, their structural positions and their differential access to resources (Marx 1978). This circumstance is the influence and effects of structure. Although a neighbourhood might be poor, what are the opportunities and obstacles encountered by an individual who would like to organize a community group that might then promote social capital and create a basis for neighbourhood-level changes? A good example comes from the work of Yonas and colleagues (2007) in Baltimore. They interviewed "prominent neighbourhood individuals" in neighbourhoods that were at low and high risk for youth violence. A group of mothers in a high-risk area organized themselves and their neighbours to speak out against and fight the violence. Residents perceived these efforts to be somewhat effective in reducing violence. Moreover, the events aimed at reducing youth violence gave neighbours a chance to meet and support each other.

Interdependent processes such as *political economy, ideology* and *hegemony* influence the interplay of structure and agency. These three processes maintain the stratification of society and the unequal distribution of material and ideological resources (Scott 1996). *Political economy* refers to the interdependent relationships linking economic to political systems, in which legislative, regulatory and political institutions and processes determine how production is organized and what is distributed and how. Simultaneously, economic power and privilege shape decision making on policies, programs and other institutional actions. For example, the concept of political economy can be used to uncover the political and economic forces that create specific employment opportunities (e.g., location of a stadium for professional sports events or attracting a corporation to locate its headquarters), educational opportunities (e.g., philanthropic dollars from executives who support charter school expansion) and environmental harms (e.g., sites of hazardous waste facilities and spatial concentrations of liquor and fast food outlets) in a neighbourhood with downstream consequences for community resources and health.

The conflict paradigm also contends that social stratification in resources, power and status is maintained not through sheer force alone but also through ideological processes. Within this paradigm, *ideology* refers to the prevailing political and cultural ideas of the society. The dominant ideologies of a time and place are not neutral ideas as they help to legitimate the prevailing social order and hierarchy as natural, proper, taken-for-granted and difficult to change. Moreover, an analysis of ideological processes is important because it pays attention to how certain ideas, concepts, understandings of a situation and discourses are mobilized in the struggle for resources and power. Weber (1958) defined *power* as "the ability to impose one's will on another, even when the other objects." In this view, power is always a social relationship rather than an intrinsic characteristic of a group, and the distribution of power, in turn, determines the shape and degree of stratification, inequality and the distribution of life chances. Moreover, power relations can also be thought of as embedded within institutional arrangements of a society and not only in the overt or intentional actions of one group against another.

Finally, closely related to the notion of ideology is the concept of *hegemony*, which refers to the representation of the interests of the ruling class as universal interests (Gramsci 1929). For example, democracy and equality are held up as ideals of all citizens yet can be interpreted and practiced in ways that largely serve the ruling class. Hegemonic domination depends upon the capacity to elicit and manufacture consent among the masses through control of social and cultural ideas as well as institutions. That is, it requires the production and maintenance of ways of thinking and understanding the world that legitimate the prevailing, unequal social order. In general, ideologies and hegemony benefit the ruling class by shaping people's understanding of the world they live in as a natural way of life.

To demonstrate the potential empirical applicability of concepts discussed in this section, let us return to the Chicago heat wave example. In July 1995, temperatures soared, and 739 more Chicago residents died between July 14 and July 20 than in a typical week for that month. The United States' Centers for Disease Control and Prevention (CDC) conducted an intensive matched pair study of decedents and paired cases to controls selected within walking distances from the decedent's residence. The reported results observe that the more vulnerable residents were those who did not leave home daily, had a medical problem, were confined to bed, lived alone or who lacked air conditioning, access to transportation and nearby social contacts (Semenza et al. 1996). However, as Klinenberg argued, the CDC's study design precluded the ability to identify neighbourhood or regional differences in heat wave mortality: "The CDC study directs the attention of public health agencies to the particular set of individuals who are most vulnerable to heat-related problems, but not to the places where such problems are likely to be concentrated."

In contrast, Klinenberg used social ecology, what he calls a "political economy of vulnerability" and the notion of "symbolic violence" as an analytic lens that enabled him to take account of neighbourhood-level determinants and effects that he believed led to geographic concentrations of mortality during the heat wave. His analysis served to illustrate the roles that political economy, ideology and hegemony played in producing the disparate mortality between North Lawndale and Little Village. He identified these two neighbourhoods intentionally, seeking out two places with similar demographic features but with divergent consequences from the heat wave. The similarities include similar microclimates, same number of seniors, same proportion of seniors living alone and same proportion of seniors living in poverty. North Lawndale experienced a mortality rate of 40 per 100,000 residents; whereas, Little Village experienced a rate of 4 per 100,000. Historically and visually, the two communities are "worlds apart." North Lawndale had been a neighbourhood that had attracted immigrants who worked in nearby manufacturing plants. When those plants closed, the economic foundation of the neighbourhood was severely compromised. As workers relocated, the population base to support local retail and services eroded. The area had lost 60% of its residents between 1960 and 1990, and those who had moved away were less able to support their elderly family members who remained. By 1995, the year of the heat wave, North Lawndale was characterized by abandoned buildings, commercial depletion, violent crime, degraded infrastructure and family dispersion. In addition to these characteristics, there had been a disintegration of the safety net of social services and programs that could have mitigated excess mortality.

On the other hand, Little Village had busy streets, lively commercial activity and a low crime rate. The activity in the streets drew people out, including seniors, promoting social interactions with neighbours, shop keepers and community service providers. Unlike the population decline of North Lawndale, Little Village grew by 30% between 1970 and 1990. In 1996, people described Little Village to Klinenberg as "booming." There were people in the streets from the morning until 9:30 p.m. in the evening on most days. During the heat wave, older people sought refuge in the air-conditioned stores in the main commercial center, something they often did on ordinary summer days. Some residents described the neighbourhood as too crowded, but a positive side effect of this density was that people were rarely alone. Also, the majority Latino residents often relied on the proximity of the older generation, usually grandmothers, to provide affordable child care. The ongoing connections within generations meant that seniors were not isolated in Little Village.

Klinenberg's investigation into the histories of these two neighbourhoods shows his application of the concepts of political economy and ideology within the conflict theory paradigm. Examples of the political economic factors include investment of private resources (e.g., the sites of manufacturing facilities), accompanying economic opportunities (e.g., a base for small businesses near residential areas where workers settle) the subsequent decline when manufacturing facilities close, and the distribution of social services and programs. Locating a factory is a decision with inherent tensions. More than one location would be considered and when a decision is made, the locations that were not chosen lost the opportunities associated with having a factory in their midst (and would also "lose" the exposure to any pollutants that the factory will produce or other negative effects). Factory owners might consider whether there is nearby housing for workers or if transportation between nearby housing and the factory is suitable. Once a factory is built and operational it will serve to promote other business opportunities, such as lunch vendors for the workers. Broader economic circumstances may lead to factory closures, such as competition from overseas labour. These decisions are rarely informed by economic factors alone; rather, they are shaped by politicized ideologies about what kinds of neighbourhoods have a better economic climate, labour market and client customer base. Thus economic decisions and political processes operate together to produce markedly different kinds of neighbourhoods that, in turn, influence the actions and behaviours of their residents in different ways.

Moreover, supporting and sustaining the stratified political economy within North Lawndale and the contrasting history of Little Village were rhetorical responses to the heat wave that exemplify the significance of ideology and hegemony. Klinenberg chronicled how Chicago's political leaders repeatedly emphasized that "government alone cannot do it all." This message was intended to help justify government cutbacks in social services and investments in poor communities and implied that not only did communities need to step up but also that individuals needed to take better heed of expert advice to protect themselves against the effects of the heat wave. This line of discourse helped to construct a particular ideological understanding of the nature of "the problem" – the failure of communities and individuals to help themselves. To the extent that those in political power convinced the public that failures on the part of neighbourhoods and individuals were indeed the cause of excess mortality from the heat wave, this logic sustained the prevailing unequal social order, contributed to hegemonic domination and ultimately helped to *socially* produce racially disproportionate deaths from "natural" disasters like the 1995 heat wave.

Klinenberg's application of theory and subsequent analysis showed how a catastrophic event revealed underlying fissures, such as gaps in services and social pathology, which caused disproportionate mortality. Rather than individual-level characteristics of age, sex or race and/or ethnicity, his analysis exposed institutional and social mechanisms to be responsible for the geographic concentrations of excess deaths and, in so doing, highlighted the connections between neighbourhood and health, all made visible through attending to theoretical concepts associated with the conflict perspective.

8.3   Interactionist Theory

In this section, we describe concepts within the interactionist paradigm. By using the term *interactionist* we refer to scholarship in the tradition of symbolic interactionism as well as other frameworks and perspectives that emphasize interpretations and meanings of social actions and interactions. The interactionist paradigm is most focused on meaning-making and interactions among human beings. Within this broad paradigm (which is not mutually exclusive of the conflict paradigm), the social world is seen as consisting of fluid, contingent meanings created by people, which need to be understood within their own material and imagined contexts. Imagined contexts are the collective memories and actions that people share about a particular place or experience (Anderson 1991). The primary goal of the interactionist paradigm is to understand the social world and its collectivities (i.e., representations of multiple groups) by examining how people construct and act in their social worlds. While there are multiple varieties of interpretive approaches, they share the perspective that the social world is produced and reproduced through constant engagement with others and oneself, made possible through language and shared understandings and interpretations. Interactionist theorists do not assume that the meanings of things are inherent or intrinsic to those things, but rather they are mutually and collectively constructed and defined and can be redefined as humans interact with one another (Blumer 1969; Strauss 1993).

Interactionist theorists analyze and examine how history and power shape identities, how people ascribe meanings to and interpret their physical and social environments and the situations that face them, how those meanings and interpretations then shape people's actions toward each other and their environments and how cultural, economic, and political practices arise and are maintained within society. Researchers working within the interactionist paradigm have historically been primarily concerned with the micro and meso level of human activity and the constant social interactions that create, "build up" and sustain organizations, institutions, social worlds and ideologies or discourses (i.e., ways of representing). More recently, however, scholars have used the kinds of questions that animate the interactionist paradigm to trace the relationships between the micro, meso and macro levels of social action. These kinds of research aim to illuminate how personal and social identities, meanings and arenas of human interaction and practice both shape, and are shaped, by social structures and institutions at the macro level.

Application of the interactionist paradigm leads to a somewhat different set of questions than have been asked so far: What meanings do we ascribe to things, people, groups, acts and events? Where do these meanings come from, and how do we continually shape and reinterpret them? How do we then take those meanings and use them as the basis for how we act toward things? How does human action contribute to the production and reproduction of what we see and experience as "society"? What are the relationships of human actions to social structures and institutions?

The potential applications of these questions to exploring neighbourhood-health relations are numerous, as Klinenberg's case study of North Lawndale and Little Village helps to demonstrate. North Lawndale residents commonly described the area as "bombed out," while, in contrast, Little Village residents characterized their neighbourhood as "booming." In Little Village, seniors, as everyone else, would often be in the streets or on hot summer days in stores or senior centers with air conditioning. The fear of crime and the desolation of abandoned buildings kept the seniors of North Lawndale in their homes isolated from each other and other North Lawndale residents. As Klinenberg chronicles, political and economic disinvestment in North Lawndale was motivated in part by the elites' constructions of the "inner city" and "black neighbourhoods" as bad places to do business and as populated by undeserving residents. Residents, in turn, thought North Lawndale was not the kind of place to raise kids and so younger adults who could leave moved away, leaving the elderly and poor residents behind. These discourses about this particular neighbourhood – and the material consequences they had on economic and political decisions about locating businesses and services and on families' choices – show how meanings attributed to North Lawndale were jointly shaped alongside actions at the structural all the way down to the individual level.

Sampson and Raudenbush (2004) described complex findings with regard to perceptions and direct observations of disorder in Chicago neighbourhoods, which corroborates the interrelationship between the material circumstances of neighbourhoods and the ways in which they are perceived. Social structure was a more powerful predictor of perceived disorder than observed disorder. They suggested that "residents supplement their knowledge with prior beliefs informed by racial stigmatization."

Without asking and understanding residents' answers to the questions of the perceptions, interpretations and meanings that motivate their own actions, programs intended to improve neighbourhoods and enhance their health-promoting characteristics or designed to bring communities together for the same purpose may be irrelevant, ineffective or even counterproductive. In fact, as we turn to the specific example of social capital below, we see how one study revealed how difficult it was for people to have social capital in an impoverished area because of fear, distrust and the physical design of housing.

8.4   Neighbourhood-Health Mechanisms – Social Capital and Physical Disorder

The quantitative literature for neighbourhood-health associations points most commonly and consistently to social capital, civic engagement and physical disorder as plausible mechanisms for how a neighbourhood is associated with health (Cattell 2001; Ross and Mirowsky 2001; Lochner et al. 2003; Sampson 2009). Leyden (2003) reported that people living in more walkable neighbourhoods (i.e., proximity to services) were more likely to know their neighbours, participate politically, have greater trust and faith in people and be more socially engaged. Studies have shown that greater levels of social capital are related to increased physical activity (Greiner et al. 2004; Kim et al. 2006). In quantitative literature, social capital is measured with survey questions about social networks, number of friends, membership in organizations and the like. Initially epidemiologists, among other researchers interested in social capital, investigated simple associations that suggested that having more friends, being a member of more organizations and other measures of social capital were related to better health. Later social scientists pointed out that having fewer, rather than greater, contacts in certain settings could be better for health, drawing conclusions in part from William Julius Wilson's (1990) descriptions of impoverished areas of Chicago. O'Brien and colleagues (2003) also found this to be the dynamic for African American children, ages 3 and 4 years old. That is, children in poor neighbourhoods had fewer behavioural problems if their parents did not know many neighbours compared to children in the same poor neighbourhoods whose parents knew more neighbours. In non-poor neighbourhoods, the association was the opposite; children whose parents did not know neighbours had more behavioural problems than the children of parents who knew many neighbours did.

Moreover, with access to geospatial data, studies can now characterize neighbourhoods in greater detail, offering findings that can contribute to better articulating the relationships between social capital, physical disorder and health. A recent quantitative study tested the hypotheses that parks would facilitate social interactions and cooperation, alcohol outlets would interfere with the development of trust and operation and fast food outlets would negatively affect collective efficacy and interpersonal interactions (Cohen et al. 2008). The authors specifically used collective efficacy as their measure of social capital. Collective efficacy, measured with a validated survey tool, is an aggregate measure of individual perceptions of "social cohesion among neighbours combined with the willingness to intervene on behalf of the common good" (Sampson et al. 1997). The authors verified their hypotheses that parks would facilitate social interactions and cooperation and that alcohol outlets would interfere with the development of trust. However, fast food outlets and collective efficacy were not linearly associated. The authors speculated that fast food outlets might very well serve both local residents and commuters such that the effects of local people congregating could be offset by the presence of outsiders. In conclusion, the authors suggest that urban design, operating through social cohesion mechanisms, does have implications for health.

However, it is not always clear how current knowledge about these mechanisms can translate into strategies for solutions, as it is often the case that more fundamental social processes and histories operate to produce neighbourhoods with low levels of social capital and high levels of social disorder. Moreover, while social capital and social networks had been identified with positive health, it is not clear what sort of networks (e.g., strong or weak, homogeneous or heterogeneous) were most effective for creating social capital with positive effects for health. Cattell (2001) conducted qualitative research in two housing projects in East London to examine poverty, neighbourhood and health and well-being and to consider the role of social networks and social capital. She selected two areas that were economically deprived with dissimilar opportunities for participation. She interviewed 35–37 residents from each area and approximately 15 non-residents who worked in the two areas. Her research questions included: (1) What is the mediating role of social networks in the relationship between poverty and health and place and health? (2) Does the local neighbourhood context affect network formation and the genesis of social capital? (3) Is participation a major source of social capital? and (4) What are the processes by which health can benefit from involvement? Cattell described how the social interactions and residents' perceptions were affected by the physical geography (e.g., location of major roads, railways and docks), housing design and the social and economic structure in the neighbourhoods. The housing design directly affected social networks and social capital in that it could support or hinder neighbour interactions and "helping each other out" with regard to child watching.

Cattell also found that the majority of people in both areas who did not join activities and organizations were constrained by poverty, feelings of defeatism and the neighbourhood's reputation. Suspicion negatively affected social capital: "Lack of neighbourhood trust can add to a mother's financial problems and have implications for health. As a resident explained: 'It's difficult to manage, but if your child doesn't look smart someone might call the social services in and say the child is being neglected. So if you buy winter shoes for the child, you may have to go without food.'" She concluded that "the predominant expectation of 'you look after your own'...is both evidence of social capital – of the 'thick trust' kind – and a block to wider social trust."

Thus, Cattell's study shows that social capital, networks and trust may be operating in far more complicated relationships than conventionally thought and that these factors could not be investigated using conventional statistical analysis. They do not seem to express varying aspects of a more or less singular phenomenon, at least in this case, and there are sometimes unintended consequences to the kinds of ties that are widely seen as being beneficial. Moreover, it was clear that the availability of opportunities for interaction and participation was simply not enough. The two neighbourhoods had dissimilar opportunities for residents to make connections with one another, but the levels of participation were similarly low.

We would argue here that using the two theoretical paradigms described above could expand the questions social epidemiologists might ask of Cattell's findings and have the potential to improve upon and make more nuanced sense of some of these findings. Other questions researchers might pursue could include asking residents: What do you see as social capital or physical disorder? (This question is suggested as a way to find out the meaning of social capital or physical disorder to people in addition to the identification of specific sources of it and should be written using phrases that are more meaningful to the study subjects.) More specific questions to delve into the ways residents generate social capital or the level of social capital in an area could include: Who do you go to for help when you are sick? The application of the concept of political economy would further provoke questions of other actors who influence how the resources are distributed among and within neighbourhoods such that the role and perspective of political leaders, civic leaders and business people would become part of an investigation into the way social capital or physical disorder is generated, maintained and distributed. Examples of resources include grocery stores (i.e., where they are located), work opportunities and schools. Examples of disorder include economic or ethnic segregation, redlining or government disinvestment. If we learn the decision makers' shared and competing ideologies regarding resource distribution and health held by these leaders and residents, this knowledge can be used to create communication campaigns and interventions (e.g., promote locating a grocery store where one is needed). By taking an interactionist approach, it can be understood how people take care of themselves in and through their own neighbourhood or, in other neighbourhoods, by examining their actions. We have used this approach in a qualitative study of older adults, asking them where they go for their usual activities and what being healthy means to them. This study highlighted how much time older adults spend outside their neighbourhoods in other "activity spaces," a concept previously identified by sociologists and geographers (Matthews 2008).

8.5   Future Research Directions for Neighbourhood-Health Research

One of the authors, Irene Yen, is an epidemiologist who has conducted conventional epidemiologic research into the association between and influence of neighbourhood environments on health (Yen and Kaplan 1998, 1999a; Yen et al. 2006, 2008). As she has become familiar with social theory, this has changed her thinking and approach to the research. Rather than rely on survey tools, she has developed skills in qualitative research methodologies (Yen et al. 2007).

For a project on the influence of neighbourhood environment on the health of older adults, she began with intensive interviews. These interviews were guided, in part, by a concept about connectedness to neighbourhood developed by geographer Graham Rowles. Rowles' (1983) term for this connectedness is "placement attachment." Place attachment emerges from peoples' sense of a places' social and physical "insidedness." Social insidedness comes from everyday social exchanges over long periods of time resulting in integration into the social fabric and an over-arching identification with a locale that is largely unconscious. Physical insidedness comes from familiarity and routine behaviours within specific settings. Place attach-ment is a concept consistent with the interactionist paradigm, featuring interrela-tionships of people and meaning-making. Some of the questions asked included: What do you do in your neighbourhood? Where do you spend time? Do you like your neighbours? Why or why not? In addition to learning about the potential importance of other locations for the well-being of older adults, as mentioned above, the study highlighted how a neighbourhood changing over time affects these older adults. Many people stay in one place or "age in place," while similarly-aged neigh-bours move away, and younger people move into the area. The older adults feel a social distance and unfamiliarity with these people, even though they may have lived in the neighbourhood for decades.

Other future work that Irene Yen is currently exploring is moving into the policy arena. There is a policy called "Complete Streets" being promoted in the United States by a coalition of urban planners, public health experts, transportation plan-ners and the American Association of Retired Persons (a national, senior advocacy organization). Complete Streets policies are road design guidelines that make roads accessible for people of all ages. They are location specific and highlight the need for sidewalks for walking, bike lanes for cyclists, transit stops for people without cars and the like.

8.6   Conclusions

We hope that the examples provided above demonstrate how the application of sociological paradigms leads to asking different questions in order to move neigh-bourhood-health research into solution-focused research. These paradigms help us analyze the fundamental processes that shape neighbourhoods and their residents and, thereby, understand the *conditions* under which particular solutions and/or interventions do or do not make sense.

In addition to highlighting how the application of social theory could change the direction of research on neighbourhoods and places and how they affect health, the examples we present suggest the value of natural experiments, or investigating phenomena as they occur, as in the case of the terrible 1995 heat wave in Chicago. Other examples that are pertinent at time of this writing include the effect of the mortgage foreclosure crisis in the United States, including neighbourhood trans-formation as people moved in during "The Housing Bubble" and then moved out when they could not keep their homes, as well as the rebuilding of New Orleans after hurricane Katrina. These examples also highlight the importance of place-specific investigations and the contribution of understanding the historical processes over time.

Application of social theory also highlights different methods than traditional epidemiologic survey and statistical approaches. Klinenberg used direct observation (walking in the different neighbourhoods), interview (talking with residents and business owners), content analysis (reading newspaper articles) and historical records to investigate the differences between the two Chicago neighbourhoods. Cattell, similarly, used a variety of ethnographic and qualitative methods in her study.

References

Acevedo-Garcia D (2001) Zip code-level risk factors for tuberculosis: neighborhood environment and residential segregation in New Jersey, 1985–1992. Am J Public Health 91:734–741

Anderson B (1991) Imagined communities: reflections on the origin and spread of nationalism. Verso, New York

Bell J, Rubin V (2007) Why place matters: building the movement for healthy communities. PolicyLink, Oakland

Bernard P, Charafeddine R, Frohlich KL et al (2007) Health inequalities and place: a theoretical conception of neighborhood. Soc Sci Med 65:1839–1852

Blauner R (1972) Racial oppression in America. Harper and Row, New York

Blumer H (1969) Symbolic interactionism: perspective and method. University of California Press, Berkeley

Bourdieu P (1983) Ökonomisches Kapital, kulturelles Kapital, soziales Kapital. In: Krechel R (ed) Soziale Ungleichheiten (Soziale Welt), Sonderheft 2 [German]. Otto Schartz & Co, Goettingen

Bourdieu P (1986) The forms of capital. In: Richardson JG (ed) Handbook of theory and research for the sociology of education. Greenwood, New York

Buron L, Levy D, Gallagher M et al (2007) Housing choice vouchers: how HOPE VI families fared in the private market. HOPE VI: where do we go from here? The Urban Institute, Washington, DC

Cattell V (2001) Poor people, poor places, and poor health: the mediating role of social networks and social capital. Soc Sci Med 52:1501–1516

Clampet-Lundquist S (2004) HOPE VI relocation: moving to new neighborhoods and building new ties. Hous Policy Debate 15:415–447

Cohen DA, Inagami S et al (2008) The built environment and collective efficacy. Health Place 14:198–208

Comey J (2007) HOPE VI'd and on the move HOPE VI: where do we go from here? The Urban Institute, Washington, DC

Coulton CJ, Korbin J, Chan T et al (2001) Mapping residents' perceptions of neighborhood boundaries: a methodological note. Am J Community Psychol 29:371–383

Cubbin C, Winkleby MA (2005) Protective and harmful effects of neighborhood-level deprivation on individual-level health knowledge, behavior changes, and risk of coronary heart disease. Am J Epidemiol 162:559–568

Diez-Roux AV (2001) Investigating neighborhood and area effects on health. Am J Public Health 91:1783–1789

Diez-Roux AV, Merkin SS et al (2003) Area characteristics, individual-level socioeconomic indicators, and smoking in young adults: the coronary artery disease risk development in young adults study. Am J Epidemiol 157:315–326

Etzioni A (1997) The new golden rule: community and morality in a Democratic society. Profile, London

Gramsci A (1929) Selections for the prison notebooks. International Publishers, New York

Greenbaum S (2002) Report from the field: social capital and deconcentration: theoretical and policy paradoxes of the HOPE VI Program. N Am Dialogue 5:9–13

Greiner KA, Li C, Kawachi I et al (2004) The relationships of social participation and community ratings to health and health behaviors in areas with high and low population density. Soc Sci Med 59:2303–2312

Haan M, Kaplan GA, Camacho T (1987) Poverty and health. Prospective evidence from the Alameda County study. Am J Epidemiol 125:989–998

Hartmann H (1976) Capitalism, patriarchy, and job segregation by sex. Signs 1:137–168

Kaplan GA (2004) What's wrong with social epidemiology, and how can we make it better? Epidemiol Rev 26:124–135

Kaplan GA, Lynch JW (1999) Socioeconomic considerations in the primordial prevention of cardiovascular disease. Prev Med 29:S30–S35

Kim D, Subramanian SV, Gortmaker SL et al (2006) US state- and county-level social capital in relation to obesity and physical inactivity: a multilevel, multivariable analysis. Soc Sci Med 63:1045–1059

Kleit RG (2005) HOPE VI new communities: neighborhood relationships in mixed-income housing. Environ Plann A 37:1413–1441

Klinenberg E (2003) Heat wave: a social autopsy of disaster in Chicago. University of Chicago Press, Chicago

Leyden KM (2003) Social capital and the built environment: the importance of walkable neighborhoods. Am J Public Health 93:1546–1551

Lochner K, Kawachi I et al (1999) Social capital: a guide to its measurement. Health Place 5:259–270

Lochner KA, Kawachi I et al (2003) Social capital and neighborhood mortality rates in Chicago. Soc Sci Med 56:1797–1805

Macintyre S, Ellaway A, Cummins S (2002) Place effects on health: how can we conceptualise, operationalise and measure them? Soc Sci Med 55:125–139

Manjarrez CA, Popkin SJ, Guernsey El (2007) Poor health: adding insult to injury for HOPE VI families. HOPE VI: where do we go from here? The Urban Institute, Washington, DC

Marmot M (1999) Epidemiology of socioeconomic status and health: are determinants within countries the same as between countries? Ann N Y Acad Sci 896:16–29

Marx K (1978) The German Ideology. In: Tucker RC (ed) The Marx-Engels reader, 2nd edn. The Norton Press, New York

Matthews SA (2008) The salience of neighborhood: some lessons from sociology. Am J Prev Med 34:257–259

Merkin SS, Roux AV, Coresh J et al (2007) Individual and neighborhood socioeconomic status and progressive chronic kidney disease in an elderly population: the cardiovascular health study. Soc Sci Med 65:809–821

Minkler M (2004) Community organizing and community building for health. Rutgers University Press, New Brunswick

O'Brien CM, O'Campo PJ, Muntaner C (2003) When being alone might be better: neighborhood poverty, social capital, and child mental health. Soc Sci Med 57:227–237

O'Campo P (2003) Invited commentary: advancing theory and methods for multilevel models of residential neighborhoods and health. Am J Epidemiol 157:9–13

Office of Minority Health (2009) African American Profile. U.S. Department of Health and Human Services. http://minorityhealth.hhs.gov/templates/browse.aspx?lvl=2&lvlID=51. Accessed 8 Sept 2010

Popkin SJ, Cove E (2007) Safety is the most important thing: how HOPE VI helped families. HOPE VI: where do we go from here? The Urban Institute, Washington, DC

Popkin SJ, Levy DK, Harris LE (2002) HOPE VI panel study: baseline report. The Urban Institute, Washnington, DC

Popkin SJ, Katz B, Cunningham M et al (2004) A decade of HOPE VI: research findings and policy challenges. Urban Institute and Brookings Institution, Washington, DC

Putnam RT (1993) Making Democracy work: civic traditions in modern Italy. Princeton University Press, Princeton

Ross CE, Mirowsky J (2001) Neighborhood disadvantage, disorder, and health. J Health Soc Behav 42:258–276

Rowles GD (1983) Geographical dimensions of social support in rural Appalachia. In: Rowles GD, Ohta RJ (eds) Aging and milieu: environmental perspectives on growing old. Academic, New York

Sampson RJ (2009) Disparity and diversity in the contemporary city: social (dis)order revisited. Br J Sociol 60:1–31; discussion 33–38

Sampson RJ, Raudenbush SW (2004) Seeing disorder: neighborhood stigma and the social construction of "broken windows". Soc Psychol Q 67:319–342

Sampson RJ, Raudenbush SW, Earls F (1997) Neighborhoods and violent crime: a multilevel study of collective efficacy. Science 277:918–924

Scott J (1996) Stratification and power: structures of class, status and command. Polity Press, London

Semenza JC, Rubin CH, Falter KH et al (1996) Heat-related deaths during the July 1995 heat wave in Chicago. N Engl J Med 335:84–90

Siegrist J (2000) Place, social exchange and health: proposed sociological framework. Soc Sci Med 51:1283–1293

Smith G, Gidlow C et al (2010) What is my walking neighborhood? A pilot study of English adults' definitions of their local walking neighborhoods. Int J Behav Nutr Phys Act 7:34

Strauss A (1993) Continual permutations of action. Aldine de Gruyter, New York

Weber M (1956) Social Action. In: Roth G, Wittich C (eds) Economy and society: an outline of interpretive sociology. University of California Press, Berkeley

Weber M (1958) From Max Weber: essays in sociology. Oxford University Press, Oxford

Wilson WJ (1990) The truly disadvantaged: the inner city, the underclass, and public policy. University of Chicago Press, Chicago

Wright O (1996) Class counts: comparative studies in class analysis. Cambridge University Press, Cambridge

Yen IH, Kaplan GA (1998) Poverty area residence and prospective change in physical activity level: evidence from the Alameda County study. Am J Public Health 88:1709–1712

Yen IH, Kaplan GA (1999a) Neighborhood social environment and risk of death: multilevel evidence from the Alameda County study. Am J of Epidemiol 149:898–907

Yen IH, Kaplan GA (1999b) Poverty area residence and change in depression and perceived health status. Int J of Epidemiol 28:90–94

Yen IH, Syme SL (1999) The social environment and health: a discussion of the epidemiologic literature. Annu Rev Public Health 20:287–308

Yen IH, Yelin EH, Katz P et al (2006) Perceived neighborhood problems and quality of life, physical functioning, and depressive symptoms among adults with asthma. Am J Public Health 96:873–879

Yen IH, Scherzer T, Cubbin C et al (2007) Women's perceptions of neighborhood resources and hazards related to chronic disease risk factors: focus group results from economically diverse neighborhoods in a mid-sized US city. Am J Health Promot 22:98–106

Yen IH, Yelin E, Katz P et al (2008) Impact of perceived neighborhood problems on change in asthma-related health outcomes between baseline and follow-up. Health Place 14:468–477

Yonas MA, O'Campo P, Burke JG et al (2007) Neighborhood-level factors and youth violence: giving voice to the perceptions of prominent neighborhood individuals. Health Educ Behav 34:669–685

Chapter 9
Locating Politics in Social Epidemiology

Carles Muntaner, Carme Borrell, Edwin Ng, Haejoo Chung, Albert Espelt,
Maica Rodriguez-Sanz, Joan Benach, and Patricia O'Campo

Contents

9.1   Introduction 176
9.2   Why Politics Matters to Social Epidemiology 177
9.3   Politics in Social Epidemiology: Ubiquitous Yet Overlooked 179
9.4   Politics as a Social Determinant of Health: Epidemiologic Evidence 182
9.5   Considerations Regarding Comparative Political Studies
       in Social Epidemiology 191
       9.5.1   The Problem of A-Historicism in Time-Series Analyses
            of Historical Processes 191
       9.5.2   The "Small N" Problem, Statistical Power, Omitted Variables
            and Sensitivity Analyses 193
9.6   The Missing Link in Political Epidemiology: Social Class 194
9.7   Bringing Politics Back into Epidemiology 195
9.8   Conclusions 195
References 197

C. Muntaner (✉)
Bloomberg Faculty of Nursing and Dalla Lana School of Public Health, University of Toronto,
155 College Street, 6th floor, ON M5T 3M7, Toronto, Canada
e-mail: carles.muntaner@utoronto.ca

C. Borrell
Agència de Salut Pública de Barcelona, Plaça Lesseps 1, 08023 Barcelona, Spain
e-mail: cborrell@aspb.cat

E. Ng
Dalla Lana School of Public Health, University of Toronto, 155 College Street,
6th floor, ON M5T 3M7, Toronto, Canada
e-mail: edwin.ng@utoronto.ca

H. Chung
College of Health Sciences, Korea University, 704 Justice Building, Jeongneung 3-dong,
Seongbuk-gu, Seoul 136-703, Republic of Korea
e-mail: hpolicy@korea.ac.kr

P. O'Campo and J.R. Dunn (eds.), *Rethinking Social Epidemiology:*
Towards a Science of Change, DOI 10.1007/978-94-007-2138-8_9,
© Springer Science+Business Media B.V. 2012

Abstract Recent social epidemiologic research has focused on the impact of politics, expressed as political traditions or parties and welfare state characteristics, on population health. Guided by a political economy of health and welfare regimes framework, this chapter synthesizes this growing body of evidence and locates 73 empirical and comparative studies on politics and health meeting our inclusion criteria. Two major research programs – welfare regimes and democracy – and two emerging programs – political tradition and globalization – are identified. Primary findings include: (1) left and egalitarian political traditions on population health are the most salutary, consistent and substantial; (2) the health impacts of advanced and liberal democracies are also positive and large; (3) welfare regime studies, primarily conducted amongst wealthy countries, find that Social Democratic regimes tend to fare best with absolute health outcomes yet inconsistently in terms of relative health inequalities; and (4) globalization defined as dependency indicators such as trade, foreign investment and national debt is negatively associated with population health.

Abbreviations

OECD Organization for Economic Cooperation and Development

9.1 Introduction

This chapter analyzes the emerging area of politically-oriented, empirical studies in the population health literature (Bambra et al. 2005; Beckfield and Krieger 2009; Navarro and Shi 2001). In doing so, we explore the intersection between political science, sociology and social epidemiology and we present a review on how politics

A. Espelt
Agència de Salut Pública de Barcelona, Plaça Lesseps 1, 08023 Barcelona, Spain
e-mail: aespelt@aspb.cat

M. Rodriguez-Sanz
Servei de Sistemes d'Informació Sanitària, Agència de Salut Pública de Barcelona,
Plaça Lesseps 1, 08023 Barcelona, Spain
e-mail: mrodri@aspb.cat

J. Benach
GREDS/EMCONET, Universitat Pompeu Fabra, Passeig Circumval lació 8,
08003 Barcelona, Spain
e-mail: joan.benach@upf.edu

P. O'Campo
Centre for Research on Inner City Health www.crich.ca and Dalla Lana School of Public Health,
Saint Michael's Hospital and University of Toronto, 209 Victoria, 3rd floor, Toronto,
Ontario M5B 1C6, Canada
e-mail: O'CampoP@smh.ca

shapes population health in a global context. This book chapter is adapted from a paper published in *Sociology of Health and Illness* (2011, 33(6):946–964. License Number: 2746021315671, John Wiley and Sons).

The status of epidemiology as a socio-natural science is still debated (Krieger 2001). Yet epidemiology is social by definition. The death of an organism is a biological fact, but dying from drinking contaminated water or from a gunshot wound are social facts as well, making the study of population health a biosocial (or socio-natural) science. The problem does not reside, then, in the adequacy of social (economic, cultural and *political*) explanations in epidemiology. Rather, it is the systematic shunning of politics (and economics and culture) that is surprising.

During the twentieth century, Milton Terris, an eminent epidemiologist, always considered epidemiology "social" and thus found the term "social epidemiology" redundant (M. Terris, personal communication 2000). However, growth in the substantive knowledge, including new methods, models and problems and the number of scholars devoted to the study of social determinants of health justifies today's separate term "social epidemiology" (Berkman and Kawachi 2000) and "political epidemiology" as one of its constituent areas of study.

9.2 Why Politics Matters to Social Epidemiology

The role of politics and policies in applied social epidemiology (i.e., a branch of public health) is hard to ignore. It is indeed central to implement and evaluate policies aimed at reducing health inequalities. In fact, the discipline of social epidemiology, by being overly descriptive and focused on methods, becomes almost irrelevant to policy efforts to reduce social inequalities in health (see Chap. 13). Its focus is mainly the description of inequalities and rarely (if ever) the study of the policies or programs that might reduce them. It has become a comfortable "apolitical" field of study (e.g., poor neighbourhoods are associated with poor diet or bad "health behaviours," "social capital" is associated with worse self-rated health, lack of autonomy at work and job insecurity leading to poor mental health and so on) (Muntaner et al. 1999, 2002, Muntaner 2004; Navarro et al. 2003). Its outlook is that of a basic science, although epidemiology is, by definition, an applied science driven by the fact that disease is harmful to populations.

Yet, even when our aim is just explanation, the role of politics in shaping population health cannot be ignored either. There is no *a priori* reason why the effects of politics on health should be confined to policies. Politics can affect population health via other social processes such as, for example, grassroots organizing, social movements, wars, riots, non-government organizations, unions, strikes and protests. Moreover, policies are not randomly distributed in societies; they follow political patterns. In that sense, the causes (i.e., political and economic arrangements) of the causes (i.e., single policies) are a necessary part of a deeper explanation of social epidemiology, such as when income inequality and poverty (or indicators of economic structure) might determine proximal social determinants, such as crime rates, lack of social networks, lack of exercise facilities, lack of healthy food stores, alcohol stores, open illicit drug markets, lack of public transportation or lack of access to health care. From an empiricist perspective, the fact remains that the associations between political variables (e.g., number of "left wing" cabinet members or type of political party in government) exist even after models are adjusted for health and social policies (Chung and Muntaner 2006; Espelt et al. 2008). Even if we accept that policies are the only means by which politics have an effect, one should be interested in why certain egalitarian policies cluster together in certain societies and not in others. There are other benefits to studying comparative politics as opposed to policies alone. When we compare groups of countries based on their political traditions, welfare state types or political economy, we may understand why some countries are better overall than others in reducing inequities. The study of specific national policies does not reveal these patterns. For example, the focus on national health policies that defines most American health services research leads to a narrow set of policy alternatives and to "a lack of understanding of their political origin" (Navarro 1989). A policy approach misses why the American government still ignores "single payer" options, ignorance that likely results from the liberal political trajectory and deep class divisions of the United States, which do not lead to egalitarian universal policies (Esping-Andersen 1990).

Another benefit of considering political issues, in addition to policy concerns, in social epidemiology is that it implicates the need for intersectoral action to reduce health inequalities. It is likely that egalitarian policies involve the "synergic" effect of egalitarian policies from different sectors (e.g., health, labour market, social services). Such intersectoral effects are more likely to arise in certain political traditions than others due to political-policy coherence. In addition, the evaluation of the effect of any single policies in such context might be inadequate (i.e., cannot deal with their interaction) or very difficult to conduct due to their complexity. With regard to the effect of social democracies on class inequalities in health, the evidence is mixed (Muntaner et al. 2006; Tapia Granados 2010), although health inequalities *per se* can be a policy effect of interest as they are inequitable.

The underlying discussion about "political epidemiology" is one of technocracy versus social justice, an issue that pits supposedly value-free public health policies against policies rooted in a set of political views (e.g., egalitarianism) (Gil-González et al. 2009). Public health approaches adopting technological orientations tend to focus on the potential of policy interventions alone to improve population health. These policy decisions are guided by established bodies of knowledge in addition to credentialed expertise and skills. These decisions are made by highly knowledgeable individuals and not by individuals possessing political power. However, applying technocratic methods to social epidemiology and health policy is limited on two fronts. First, remaining value free when conducting health research is inadequate because public health scientists are explicitly committed to improving population health and reducing health inequalities. Second, myopically focusing on health policy effectiveness ignores how politics is a major social institution by which most societies distribute power and organize decision making. To advance and move beyond "just policy" approaches, it is crucial to explicitly study politics as a "fundamental" determinant and to not treat it as an afterthought.

9.3   Politics in Social Epidemiology: Ubiquitous Yet Overlooked

The roots of such contemporary scholarship can be traced back to the mid-nineteenth century with Friedrich Engels' (1958) classic treatise *The Condition of the Working Class in England*. In that work Engels developed the notion of the social production of disease and demonstrated that the politics of industrial capitalism resulted in premature mortality and unnecessary morbidity amongst the working class. Echoing this idea, Rudolph Virchow's (1985) investigation of a typhus outbreak in Upper Silesia in 1848 led him to famously conclude "disease is not something personal and special, but only a manifestation of life under (pathological) conditions…Medicine is a social science and politics is nothing else but medicine on a large scale." Contemporary empirical research looks quite different methodologically. Researchers in this area are sharply divided along two theoretical streams, which find their roots in the work of classical sociologists and which influence how politics is defined and what hypotheses are tested in population health studies.

Research guided by political economy of health and welfare regime theories has gained momentum in the extant literature. Though their role and impact has been questioned in medical sociology (Cockerham 2001), researchers working within these conflict-based perspectives emphasize the political factors beyond the immediate control of individuals that adversely affect their health. These approaches have been instrumental in highlighting the political context of health inequalities (Navarro and Shi 2001; Navarro et al. 2003), re-engaging with neo-Marxist models of class division (Coburn 2000, 2004) and testing the health effects of working-class power (Muntaner and Lynch 1999). Rather than income inequality being the fundamental determinant of health inequalities (Wilkinson and Pickett 2010), these frameworks are broader, more contextualized and sensitive to historical changes and are more sociologically relevant through their explicit focus on inequality-generating mechanisms such as social class relations (i.e., relative power between capital and labour), neo-liberal ideology (i.e., private profits versus public goods) and varieties of welfare regimes (i.e., social democratic versus liberal versus conservative). Unlike "neo-Durkheimian" approaches, the political economy of health and welfare regime frameworks, which begin their analysis with politics and endogenous consequences such as income inequality, are treated as fully implicated in society rather than as a sub-system that can be understood in isolation. For instance, Navarro et al.'s (2006) political economy of health framework illustrates how politics (expressed in terms of voting behaviour and trade union characteristics) is related to the expansion of the welfare regimes and labour market policies, which in turn affect income inequalities and population health. Regarding welfare state regimes, Eikemo et al. (2008a) confirmed the importance of politics with their finding that welfare state characteristics explain approximately half of the national-level variation of health inequalities between Scandinavian (Denmark, Finland, Norway, Sweden) and Anglo-Saxon (United Kingdom, Ireland) regimes, which report better health in comparison to Bismarckian (Austria, Belgium, France,

Germany, Luxembourg, Netherlands, Switzerland), Eastern European (Czech Republic, Hungary, Poland, Slovenia) and Southern European (Greece Italy, Portugal, Spain) countries.

This leads to the question of how researchers should approach and conceptualize politics in population health research: from a cohesion/Durkheimian perspective or from a conflict/political economy/welfare regimes perspective? Thus, sociological theory plays the crucial role in helping us determine the theoretical location and empirical focus of this chapter. We adopt a political economy of health and welfare regimes approach and contend that contemporary scholarship needs more theoretically informed research and conflict-based perspectives that examine not only the health effects of social cohesion and income inequality but the political causes of these factors as well.

To advance our understanding of the political determinants of population health, we review the extant literature devoted to identifying the political origins of population health and health inequalities amongst nations and explicitly focus on issues relevant to the sociology of health and illness: politics, welfare regimes and democracy. Before reviewing the literature, we first conceptualize politics as a key substantive theme and second make a case for comparative designs as the preferred analytical method for understanding cross-national health differences.

We understand politics at a national level as the "practice of the art or science of directing and administrating states" (McLean and McMillan 2003). Politics has been variously defined as concerned with: (1) civil government, the state and public affairs; (2) human conflict and its resolution; or (3) the sources and exercise of power. Thus, political economy of health and welfare regime approaches attempt to uncover the political forces that shape the development of welfare states and the implementation of social and health policies that, in turn, lead to social and health inequalities within and between nations. An important impetus for this research stream has been the justification for studying politics in addition to policies, which are the province of health policy (Espelt et al. 2008; 2010 Lundberg et al. 2008; Lundberg 2009; Muntaner et al. 2009). The basic argument is that there is no *a priori* reason why the effects of politics on health should be confined to policies that are, themselves, exogenous to politics (Navarro 1993). Politics may have an impact on population health by means of social movements, grassroots organizing and non-government organizations, such as not-for-profits, unions, professional and business associations (Aronson et al. 2004), blockades, embargoes, occupations and wars (Burnham et al. 2006), strikes, protests, coups or revolutions (Muntaner et al. 1999) and lobbying and may also take the form of influence peddling, insider trading, bribery and blackmail (Idrovo et al. 2010).

The link between health and political indicators such as "number of left cabinet members" or "type of political party in government" is robust adjustment for health policies, indicating that political processes other than health policies might determine population health (Chung and Muntaner 2006). Even if we accept that social and health policies are the only mediators between politics and population health, the question remains why egalitarian policies cluster together in certain societies but not in others. Policies are not conceived and implemented randomly in social systems; instead they follow predictable political patterns (Navarro and Muntaner 2004). Following the terminology of the World Health Organization's Commission on Social Determinants of Health (2008), the causes (i.e., political systems) of the causes (i.e., specific health and social policies) should be an essential part of societal mechanisms and explanations in medical sociology and social epidemiology. As determinants they should be perceived similarly to how we accept income inequality and poverty (or indicators of economic systems) as determinants of more proximal social determinants of health, such as social cohesion, green spaces, stores stacked with vegetables, functioning public transportation, good public schools or access to quality health care.

The Macro-level comparative design, which is common to political sociology, has been adopted by population health researchers as it provides an efficient way to uncover political determinants that are typically homogeneous within nations and, therefore, unassailable with national samples (Rose 2001). The strengths of the comparative method in other disciplines such as historical sociology and political sociology lend further impetus to the inclusion of politics within political economy and population health research (Esping-Andersen 1990). When we compare clusters of nations with common political backgrounds, democratic systems or welfare regimes, we gain insights into why some countries are more successful than others at improving their countries' population health or reducing health inequities (Esping-Andersen 1990; Huber and Stephens 2001).

In sum, while politics appears to be a major social determinant of population health, there have been relatively few studies in this area. For example, a recent systematic review of politics and health studies focused on four processes: (1) the transition to a capitalist economy; (2) neo-liberal restructuring; (3) development or evolution of the welfare state; and (4) political incorporation of subordinated racial/ ethnic, indigenous and gender groups (Beckfield and Krieger 2009). The authors did not examine the role of major political tradition (e.g., political ideology of party in government) in explaining cross-country levels of health nor did they probe for political tradition when examining cross-country differences in health inequalities. To address this knowledge gap, our literature review pays more attention to political traditions, including welfare regimes types and their effects on both population health and socioeconomic inequalities in health. We contend that comparing average levels of population health between countries with different political backgrounds is also of interest (Lundberg 2009) in addition to the effects of politics on socioeconomic inequalities. To this end, we synthesize the scientific evidence on the link between politics and health by means of a systematic literature review and ask three interrelated questions: (1) Does politics influence population health? (2) To what extent has empirical research been guided by political economy and welfare regimes theories? and (3) Which political-sociologic factors, processes and mechanisms are predictive of better population health outcomes? We end by discussing epistemological, theoretical and methodological issues for consideration in future studies of politics and population health.

9.4   Politics as a Social Determinant of Health: Epidemiologic Evidence

Using guidelines outlined by Pope et al. (2007), we used a two-step approach to locate articles that investigated the link between politics and population health: (1) review of electronic databases; and (2) hand search of reference lists.

First, the following three databases were searched for English language studies: *CSA Sociological Abstracts* (1953–), *PubMed* (1948–) and *ISI Web of Science* (1900–) for references until April 23, 2010. The key word search combined two groups of terms using a Boolean strategy: *democracy, welfare regime, welfare state, welfare capitalism AND health, health services, population health*. Preliminary key word searches yielded a total of 2,790 records. Two reviewers reviewed the abstracts of these records and independently identified 188 potentially relevant (not mutually exclusive) studies using our inclusion criteria: (1) presented empirical findings related with health or health services outcomes; (2) investigated cross-national political differences in health (e.g., democracy versus dictatorship, social democratic versus liberal welfare regimes); and (3) included a direct measure of one political or welfare state variable. To minimize reviewer bias, we assessed interrater reliability between the two reviewers using the Kappa coefficient. Agreement results ranged from substantial to outstanding (ISI Web of Science: $k = 0.727, p < 0.001$; Sociological Abstracts: $k = 0.839, p < 0.001$; PubMed: $k = 0.838, p < 0.001$). The full-text of these 188 studies were then reviewed by the authors and re-evaluated against our inclusion criteria to determine final eligibility. A total of 59 studies met our full inclusion criteria.

Second, the reference lists of these 59 manuscripts were hand searched for additional studies, book chapters and conference papers to capture the full range of politically-oriented, comparative health studies in the extant literature. This process identified an additional 122 potentially relevant studies in which 12 articles and two book chapters met our full inclusion criteria for a final sample of 73 core publications. Of the 310 studies retrieved for full-text review, reasons for exclusion included being non-empirical (31.0%), non-political (20.6%), non-health outcome (18.4%) and non-comparative (4.8%); other reasons included being editorials or duplicates (1.6%). Figure 9.1 presents a flow chart on our literature review selection and exclusion and inclusion process. Disagreements amongst reviewers during this process were resolved by consensus.

Each of these 73 publications was classified along one of four political themes: (1) *Democracy*, if the hypothesis tested democracy as defined and measured by the authors (see below); (2) *Globalization*, if the article examined how high-, middle- and low-income countries are integrated through global networks of trade, foreign investment and multinational corporations; (3) *Political tradition*, if the study included variables referring to the left-right political dimension (e.g., social democratic versus conservative parties in government); and (4) *Welfare state*, if the analysis included welfare state indicators (e.g., universal health coverage) but not indicators of political ideology (e.g., along the left-right dimension). These groupings were mutually exclusive. Given the emerging nature of political economy/

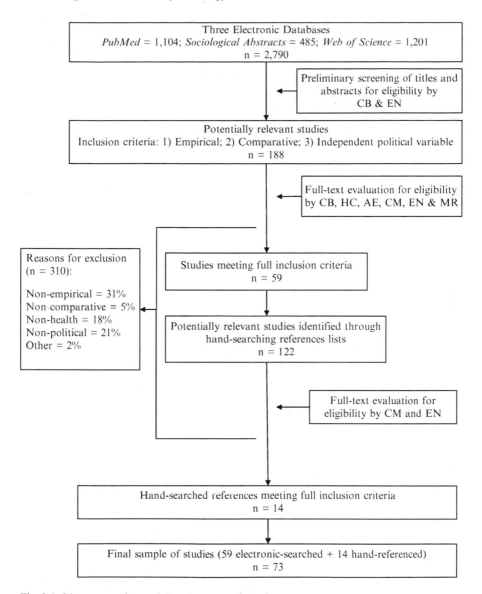

Fig. 9.1 Literature review and data abstraction flow chart

welfare regime and population health research, we provide a descriptive analysis of whether findings are supportive of political effects rather than a detailed appraisal of study quality and/or synthesis of findings across studies. A *pro forma* was developed to ensure the consistent coding and classification of the following information: year of publication (coded into 5-year intervals beginning in 1985); study objectives and hypotheses; study design (cross-sectional or longitudinal/panel/time series/ trend); unit of analysis (individual or ecological); number of countries compared (coded into 25 country increments); political variables (e.g., democracy measures, political traditions, welfare regime classifications); confounding factors; health outcomes; and main findings. To summarize the empirical findings between politics and health, studies grouped by political theme are also coded to the extent to which statistically significant associations are positive (i.e., political variable is associated with improved health) or negative (i.e., political variable is inversely associated with population health) or mixed (i.e., political variable is either unrelated or inconsistently related to health outcome).

All data was entered into SPSS version 18.0 (IBM Corporation, Somers, NY) and analyzed using basic descriptive and cross-tabulated statistics. A formal meta-analysis was not conducted owing to the heterogeneity of studies in terms of design, study populations and political and outcome measures, which limits options to aggregate findings into combined estimates.[1]

Table 9.1 presents the key characteristics of the 73 studies selected for this review. The most frequent comparative question addressed was the link between welfare states and population health or social inequalities in health (31 studies, 42.5%), followed by an interest in the beneficial health effects of democracy (26 studies, 35.6%). Less interest has been devoted to understanding how political traditions function as a determinant of population health (10 studies, 13.7%) and only six studies (8.2%) investigated the health effects of globalization.

Most reviewed studies used a cross-sectional study design (49 studies, 53.4%) with an ecological focus on countries as the unit of analysis (56 studies, 76.7%). The number of countries compared ranged from 2 to 208 with a primary focus on Organization for Economic Cooperation and Development (OECD) nations. Such a focus on wealthy countries often limited the number of countries compared to less than 24. Our review found 36 studies (49.3%) falling into this category, while 22 studies (30.1%) broadened their focus to include non-wealthy countries with country sample sizes over 100. Health outcomes tend to gravitate toward child health indicators such as infant mortality, low birth weight and under-five mortality (35 studies, 47.9%); life expectancy (24 studies, 32.9%); longstanding illness (8 studies, 11.0%); and self-perceived health (7 studies, 9.6%). The vast majority of the 73 studies were published since the turn of the century (2000–2010: 61 studies, 83.6%) with almost half of these contributions involving welfare state analyses (2000–2010: 28 studies, 45.9%), suggesting that politically oriented approaches to medical sociology and social epidemiology are heuristic research programs. Almost half (15 studies, 48.4%) of the 31 welfare state studies relied on individual-level survey data from nationally representative surveys with self-perceived health as the preferred dependent variable (25 studies, 81.0%). Conceptualizing and measuring the health effects of welfare states clustered around three dominant indicators: (1) welfare regimes (Avendano et al. 2009; Bambra et al. 2009; Bambra and Eikemo 2009; Bambra 2005, 2006; Chung and Muntaner 2007; Conley and Springer 2001; Dahl et al. 2006; Eikemo

---

[1] Summary characteristics of 73 studies on politics and health grouped by political theme are available from the authors upon request.

Table 9.1 Descriptive characteristics of 73 empirical studies on politics and health

	Number of studies	Percentage of total studies
Political themes		
Democracy	26	35.6
Globalization	6	8.2
Political tradition	10	13.7
Welfare state	31	42.5
Year of publication		
1985–1989	2	2.7
1990–1994	5	6.8
1995–1999	5	6.8
2000–2004	21	28.8
2005–2010	40	54.8
Study design		
Cross-sectional	49	53.4
Longitudinal/panel/time-series/trend	34	46.6
Unit of analysis		
Individual	17	20.0
Ecological	56	80.0
Number of countries compared		
2–24	36	49.3
25–49	6	8.2
50–74	4	5.5
75–99	5	6.8
100+	22	30.1
Health outcomes[a]		
Infant and child mortality	35	47.9
Life expectancy	24	32.9
Longstanding illness	8	11.0
Public health/health care needs/spending	4	5.5
Self-reported health	7	9.6
Other[b]	25	34.2

Notes

[a]Many articles examined multiple outcomes and, hence, the number of health outcomes (103) is greater than the number of studies. For this reason, percentages do add up to 100% and represent the proportion of health outcomes in relation to our final of 73 studies

[b]Other health outcomes included: absolute and relative health inequalities (Dahl et al. 2006; Muntaner et al. 2006); HIV/AIDS (Gizelis 2009; Menon-Johansson 2005); health care index (Bambra 2005); health conditions index (Correa and Namkoong 1992); immunization programs (Gauri and Khaleghian 2002); maternal mortality (Alvarez-Dardet and Franco-Giraldo 2006; Franco et al. 2004); mental health (Nordenmark et al. 2006; Zambon et al. 2006); mortality rate (Correa and Namkoong 1992; Lundberg et al. 2008; Safaei 2006); national health indicators (Klomp and de Haan 2008, 2009); oral health (Sanders et al. 2009); Physical Quality of Life Index (Cereseto and Waitzkin 1986; Moon and Dixon 1985); probability of dying between 15 and 65 (Adeyi et al. 1997); The Short-Form 36 (Sekine et al. 2009); women's reproductive health (Pillai and Gupta 2006; Wejnert 2008); and years of potential lost life (Elola et al. 1995)

et al. 2008a, b; Farfan-Portet et al. 2010; Grosse et al. 2010; Karim et al. 2010; Lahelma and Arber 1994; Muntaner et al. 2006; Nordenmark et al. 2006; Rostila 2007; Sanders et al. 2009; Sekine et al. 2009; Zambon et al. 2006); (2) welfare state efforts, policies and spending (Burstrom et al. 2010; Elola et al. 1995; Fayissa 2001; Lundberg et al. 2008; Ouweneel 2002; Raphael and Bryant 2004; Veenhoven and Ouweneel 1995; Veenhoven 2000; Whitehead et al. 2000); and (3) welfare governance (Klomp and de Haan 2008; Menon-Johansson 2005).

All 26 studies on democracy are ecological in focus and 16 (61.5%) are longitudinal in design. To measure the presence, depth and breadth of democracy, these studies tend to use "Polity Scores" (e.g., concomitant qualities of democratic and autocratic authorities) (Baum and Lake 2003; Besley and Kudamatsu 2006; Gauri and Khaleghian 2002; Ghobarah et al. 2004; Gizelis 2009; Houweling et al. 2005; Lake and Baum 2001; Ross 2006; Safaei 2006; Shandra et al. 2010; Tsai 2006; Wejnert 2008); "Freedom House Ratings" (e.g., degree of democracy and political freedom in nations) (Alvarez-Dardet and Franco-Giraldo 2006; Franco et al. 2004; Klomp and de Haan 2009; Pillai and Gupta 2006; Stroup 2007); democracy indexes (e.g., freedom of group opposition, political rights and legislative effectiveness) (Frey and Al-Roumi 1999; Kick et al. 1990; Lena and London 1993; London and Williams 1990; Moon and Dixon 1985); and discrete classifications (e.g., country has system in which parties lose elections) (Adeyi et al. 1997; Huber et al. 2008; Navia and Zweifel 2003; Zweifel and Navia 2000). Nevertheless, single indicators predominate and do not allow for drawing important empirical distinctions between different notions of democracy (e.g., constitutional, substantive, procedural, process-oriented).

Regarding the six studies classified under globalization, all were ecological and most investigated infant mortality (5 studies, 83.3%) over time (5 studies, 83.3%) amongst less-developed countries (5 studies, 83.3%). Though small in number, globalization studies tested for a relatively wide range of political variables: exposure and openness to international markets (Kaufman and Segura-Ubiergo 2001); capital-intensive exchange and world-system role (Moore et al. 2006); private capital flows (Rudra and Haggard 2005); commodity concentration, multinational corporate penetration and International Monetary Fund conditionality (Shandra et al. 2004); and dependency indicators such as foreign investment and debt increase (Shen and Williamson 1997, 2001). Given the small sample size it is difficult to make useful generalizations. A literature review explicitly dedicated to "globalization and health" might have retrieved a larger number of empirical studies with political variables.

The ten studies testing political tradition primarily use cross-sectional designs (8 studies, 80.0%) and used countries (8 studies, 80.0%) as units of analysis. The remaining two individual-level studies used national representative surveys (Borrell et al. 2009; Espelt et al. 2008). Ecological studies favoured child health (6 studies, 60.0%) and life expectancy (4 studies, 40.0%) as health outcomes, while the health surveys concentrated on self-perceived health and long-term illness. Political variables ranged from political-economic conditions and systems (Cereseto and Waitzkin 1986; Correa and Namkoong 1992) to left-right political dimensions (Chung and Muntaner 2006; Moene and Wallerstein 2003; Navarro et al. 2006) to

Table 9.2 Findings of 73 empirical studies on politics and health grouped by political theme

Political theme	Positive association[a] n (%)	Negative association[b] n (%)	Mixed results[c] n (%)	Total n
Democracy	21 (80.8)	3 (11.5)	2 (7.7)	26
Globalization	1 (16.7)	4 (66.7)	1 (16.7)	6
Political tradition	9 (90.0)	1 (10.0)	0	10
Welfare state	19 (61.3)	1 (3.2)	11 (35.5)	31
Total: n (%)[d]	50 (68.5)	9 (13.7)	14 (19.2)	73 (100)

Notes
[a]Political variable exerts a positive, direct or indirect effect on the population health-related outcome
[b]Political variable exerts a negative, direct or indirect effect on the population health-related outcome
[c]Political variable is either unrelated or inconsistently related to population health-related outcome
[d]Number of studies and row percentages are organized by direction of association

power resources (Muntaner et al. 2002; Navarro et al. 2003) and to political regimes and traditions (Borrell et al. 2009; Espelt et al. 2008; Navarro and Shi 2001).

Table 9.2 shows the associations found between politics and population health outcomes in the 73 studies included in this review. These outcomes, grouped by political theme, are coded along whether politics has a positive, negative or mixed association with population health and health inequalities. Overall, 68.5% of the studies reviewed were positively associated with democracy, globalization, political tradition and welfare state. Positive associations were observed most often for the effects of political tradition (9 studies, 90.0%). The strength of power resources (Navarro et al. 2003) and working class power (Muntaner et al. 2002), expressed in terms of union density, left vote and egalitarian political parties, appear to lead to strong welfare states that implement redistributive policies, reduce social inequalities and improve population health. The lone negative association involved public health expenditures being reduced by strong conservative parties in government and high levels of voter turnout (Moene and Wallerstein 2003).

Democracy was the second most consistent finding with 21 studies (80.8%) reporting a positive association, all in the expected direction (i.e., advanced levels of democracy improves population well-being), even after adjustment for national income, education and income inequality. The health effects of democracy are direct through individual income (Klomp and de Haan 2009) and the provision of basic needs (London and Williams 1990) as well as indirect through economic growth (Baum and Lake 2003) and strong political institutions (Besley and Kudamatsu 2006). Negative health outcomes were reported amongst formerly socialist countries transitioning toward democracy (Adeyi et al. 1997), middle-income countries implementing immunization programs (Gauri and Khaleghian 2002) as well as low-income groups in democratic countries with respect to infant and child mortality rates (Ross 2006). Studies reporting on the non-health effect of democracy found stronger empirical support for higher national incomes (Houweling et al. 2005) and expanding economic freedoms (Stroup 2007).

Population health differences across welfare state regimes were for the most part positive (19 studies, 61.3%) and primarily used Esping-Andersen's (1990) original country classification of Liberal/Residual, Conservative/Corporatist/ Bismarckian and Social Democratic in addition to Ferrera's (1996) addition of Southern regimes. Social Democratic regimes appear to have a salutary effect on population health and tend to narrow absolute health inequalities through the generous provision of universal welfare policies and labour market decommodification (Avendano et al. 2009; Bambra 2005, 2006; Burstrom et al. 2010; Chung and Muntaner 2007; Eikemo et al. 2008b; Lundberg et al. 2008; Nordenmark et al. 2006; Raphael and Bryant 2004; Zambon et al. 2006). However, more than any other political theme, approximately a third of welfare state studies (11 studies, 35.5%) reported inconclusive and contradictory associations regarding its effect on reducing social class inequalities in health (Dahl et al. 2006; Eikemo et al. 2008b; Muntaner et al. 2006), gender and socioeconomic differences in health (Bambra et al. 2009) and government effort and health spending (Ouweneel 2002; Veenhoven 2000; Veenhoven and Ouweneel 1995). Amongst the limited number of globalization studies, the most common finding was that international capitalism appears to be structurally detrimental to the health of less developed countries (Moore et al. 2006; Shandra et al. 2004; Shen and Williamson 1997, 2001).

According to these findings, the literature on political determinants of population health has so far been concerned with four major research problems. The first problem concerns the relation between varieties of welfare states and population health, which is earning the most attention. A standard textbook definition of welfare state is that "it involves state responsibility of securing some basic modicum of welfare for its citizens" (Esping-Andersen 1990). This idea of collective responsibility, together with social citizenship (i.e., who should be endowed of the welfare service of the government and what is the boundary) constitutes the core notion of a welfare state (Esping-Andersen 1990). These studies typically compare the population health averages or socioeconomic inequalities of countries by welfare state regime type (e.g., social democratic, liberal, conservative) (Navarro and Shi 2001). Researchers have also focused on specific components of the welfare state (e.g., social expenditures as proportion of the national budget) and examined their association with population health status across age groups and countries (e.g., Conley and Springer 2001; Lena and London 1993). Welfare state research is at the core of contemporary debates in capitalist economies on the role of the state versus the market. These sets of welfare state studies constitute a heuristic research program even if results are contradictory; redistributive welfare regimes seem to be associated with overall better average health indicators while class inequalities in health are not consistently lower in those regimes. Variability in countries (OECD, pair comparisons, middle and low income); periods (post-World War II "golden age" versus later); units of analysis (individuals versus countries); measurement of socioeconomic position (social class, education, occupation and income); and health outcomes (life expectancy, infant mortality rate and under-five mortality) might account for the lack of consistent findings. The second area of exploration is closely linked to welfare state studies but takes the model "upstream" a step further. It concerns the relation between political tradition, for example, years of government with a Labour party and population health averages or health inequalities between socioeconomic groups (e.g., Espelt et al. 2008). In fact, researchers interested in political tradition incorporate welfare regime types in their models (Chung and Muntaner 2006).

A third area of inquiry concerns the relation between democracy and population health (Franco et al. 2004). The contemporary notion of democracy is broad and encompasses the presence of democratic institutions (e.g., universal suffrage, parliament, party) that represent "good governance" (e.g., lack of corruption, civil society participation). Yet, most of these studies focus narrowly on single indicators of democracy, which were pragmatically developed by non-academic organizations. Seemingly crucial elements of liberal democracy such as the role of private campaign contributions or proportional representation are not measured or analyzed. Overall, however, we found that democratic regimes are associated with better health outcomes than non-democratic regimes, even after adjusting for national income (Franco et al. 2004).

Fourth, a few development and globalization studies have examined population health from the perspective of international politics. Although only six articles met our inclusion criteria for our review, the potential for these substantive foci is substantial (Labonte et al. 2009). The assumption that nations are politically independent units seems unrealistic, even when we limit our studies to wealthy countries (e.g., G20, NATO, World Trade Organization, World Bank, International Monetary Fund) (Muntaner and Lynch 1999). Thus, globalization studies add a layer of complexity to country comparisons as they model the political relationship between countries.

The main conclusion of our review of the epidemiologic evidence is that politics has an effect on population health with egalitarian ("left wing") political traditions producing the most affirmative results. Advanced levels of democracy are consistently related to better population health, mirroring Sen's (1999) finding that democratic governments, on average, are more accountable to their populations than non-democratic governments. Welfare regimes with long periods of Social Democratic tenure seem to have strong effects on population health and moderate effects on health inequalities. Research focused on globalization as a determinant of population health is in its infancy though some evidence suggests deleterious impacts.

For all political themes, there is a pressing need to better understand the political mechanisms of policy formation using ecologic units of analysis and longitudinal multilevel designs to strengthen evidence of policy effects at the individual level. Also, political economy of health and welfare regime frameworks would be well-served to explicitly consider the potential causal pathways linking political processes to individual health. A specific problem of this field is the relatively narrow conceptualization and measurement of "democracy." Large differences in health effects are likely to be found between: (1) the indirect representation and dual party systems that characterize liberal parliamentary democracies; and (2) the direct participatory democracy or the local participatory budgeting of, for example, the Brazilian city of Porto Alegre (Côrtes 2009). Institutional indicators such as "constitutional veto points" (e.g., the American supreme court) that make it difficult to implement major policy changes at the national level are also likely to have an influence on population health (Huber and Stephens 2001). New indicators developed by social epidemiologists reflecting different forms of democracy should be tested with respect to their relation to population health. The measurement of democracy does not correspond to *a priori* socio-epidemiologic models but rather to available indicators constructed by academics and non-government organizations with specific views of democracy (e.g., The Freedom House indicator).

Modelling political aspects of international relations remains the most under-developed set of studies perhaps because of the elaborate social modelling that these studies require. However, based on the studies published to date, three studies did test for competing macrosocial hypotheses between modernization and dependency perspectives (Shandra et al. 2004; Shen and Williamson 1997, 2001). Political science, political sociology and comparative welfare state studies commonly analyze ecologic data using time series with panel regression analysis, methods that are seldom used in political economy of health and welfare regime disciples. Nonetheless, these methods – in which a dependent variable at one time is regressed on itself at a previous time (or lagged dependent variable) and other independent variables at that same earlier point in time – should be adopted by contemporary researchers since they are the proper method for time-series data. Thus, we can estimate the effects of independent variables on change in the dependent variable between two time points making causal inferences with non-experimental data (Finkel 1995).

Welfare state research is at the core of contemporary debates in capitalist economies on the role of the state versus the market. To date, welfare state studies have demonstrated both positive and mixed health results. On one hand, Social Democratic welfare regimes committed to more egalitarian policies exhibit better population health outcomes when compared to other regime types. This finding is consistent with the well-known capacity of social democracies to reduce social inequities through the provision of universal and redistributive policies (Esping-Andersen 1990; Kenworthy 2004). On the other hand, relative health inequalities are not consistently smaller in Social Democratic countries and do not systematically differ amongst welfare regimes. Potential explanations for these mixed findings include variability of countries analyzed (exclusive focus on OECD countries); period effects (post-World War II "golden age" versus retrenchment period); units of analysis (individuals versus countries); limited measurement of socioeconomic position (education, occupation and income); and type of health outcomes examined (no disease-specific models and over-reliance on self-reported health). In addition to the narrow scope of health indicators, limited studies on period and cohort effects and studies using time series constitute other challenges of these welfare state-type studies.

The set of studies focusing on political tradition provide some evidence on the relation of political orientation to population health. Results, however, are limited to small sample sizes. Time in government and number of cabinet members from a given political orientation (Espelt et al. 2008) are promising institutional indicators of the political power associated with a given political orientation due to the objectivity of their measurement and consistency of findings in the political science literature (Huber and Stephens 2001).

9.5   Considerations Regarding Comparative Political Studies in Social Epidemiology

Based on the articles reviewed, we acknowledge that conducting macro-level, comparative quantitative studies presents some unique challenges to advancing political of economy of health approaches including a-historicism, the "small N" problem, omitted variables and missing data.

9.5.1   The Problem of A-Historicism in Time-Series Analyses of Historical Processes

Because of the specific ontological features of this field (i.e., the universe of countries contains approximately 200 units), macro-comparative political and policy analyses have always been at risk of lack of statistical power. Recently however, quality datasets of multiple time series have become available for quantitative comparative political and policy research. As a result, sample sizes can be expanded from the traditional tens of observations to hundreds. In earlier years, the field of comparative politics, in particular the comparative study of the welfare state, was approached using descriptive and prescriptive studies, while empirical social scientists regarded welfare states as a convenient source of data for testing abstract theoretical claims. Following Shalev (2007):

> Earlier works in comparative political economy tended to focus on explaining enduring cross-national differences. …The standard tools of the trade were scatter-plots, correlations and primitive cross-sectional regressions. …The turning point was a controversial cross-national regression study by Lange and Garrett (1985) . …In a final response to their critics…they suggested that the debate would only be resolved by the use of a pooled Cross-Sectional Time Series design, which in addition to furnishing a much larger number of observations would enable researchers to directly study whether the effects of changes in government composition are conditioned by national institutional contexts. …Two years later…their seminal article…turned pooled regression into the design of choice for quantitative comparative political economists.

While alternative qualitative approaches in comparative political studies such as those of Ragin (1987) had very little impact, the pooled cross-sectional approach has become the analytical method of choice in this field. Nevertheless, the mismatch between ontology and epistemology introduced by the use of the pooled cross-sectional regression method is a problem that sociology and social epidemiology cannot ignore (e.g., Hall 2002; Ragin 1987; Verba 1967). While various regression methods remain effective tools for hypothesis testing in comparative studies, they rarely provide explanations and mechanisms (Hall 2002). In Freedman's (1991) own words, "regression may provide helpful summaries of the data" but cannot "carry out much of the burden in a causal argument."

Another problem of "political studies" relates to the characteristics of social events as opposed to those, say, of experiments. Social processes occur in sequences of actions located within constraining or enabling socio-historical structures. They are often impossible to control or reproduce; it is a matter of particular social actors in particular social places and at particular social times (Abbott 1992). "It is...the portrayal of social phenomena as temporally ordered, sequential, unfolding, and open-ended 'stories' fraught with conjunctures and contingency" (Griffin 1992). The occasions we usually encounter in comparative historical analyses are where what we have are "instances" where similar processes are apparently operating but, aside from that, differ in all manner of other relevant respects – rather than "cases" – considered comparable (the same set of properties is used to describe each of the elements). As Hopkins (1982) states: "Put sharply, the cases necessary for the statistical portion of inquiry must be presumed essentially homogeneous (members of a sample of a universe); the instances necessary for the historical portion must be presumed essentially heterogeneous (members respectively of universes of one)."

For example, Social Democracies are Northern European countries and Late Democracies are Southern European countries. As a consequence of their different historical trajectory, they are characterized by different patterns of risk factors: less smoking in the South; protection via the traditional "Mediterranean diet;" and a less stressful lifestyle. In addition they have different historical trajectories in spite of their relative geographical proximity. In the post World War II period, Late Democracies suffered from non-democratic "right wing" or Fascist regimes, while Social Democracies enjoyed stable democracies. That is, countries with different political and welfare state traditions are extremely difficult to compare due to the confounding effect of cultural and economic factors or historical trajectories on population heath.

In this situation, comparing results (as in a formal statistical approach) is not sufficient. We need to explain different initial conditions and the same process in different contexts. Because of these dilemmas and the inferential limitations of quantitative analyses, the best we can hope from quantitative analyses of comparative political and policy processes is what Hempel (1965) called a "narrative sketch." Logical positivist Hempel used the terms "narrative sketch" or "explanation sketch" to convey the notion of "covering law"-type historical scientific explanation. We suggest its use in sociology and social epidemiology in a slightly looser way. While not against the concept of general law in comparative political and policy research, the quantitative analysis of pooled countries can only present a partial answer to comparative political and policy research in sociology and social epidemiology. As the "path dependence" school suggests, there is a certain amount of irreducible and unique historical path in countries, which can only be discovered and analyzed using a qualitative methods such as case studies (Huber and Stephens 2001; Shalev 2007). Therefore, while acknowledging the necessity of the empirical quantitative approach, we recommend the use of the term *narrative sketch* as an acknowledgement of its limitations in this emerging area of sociology and social epidemiology and leave room for further social-historical investigations to complement the use of quantitative techniques such as pooled regression.

Political and policy processes (e.g., increasing social security or medical expenditures) are typically considered similar in the countries that are grouped together, but the effect of these processes has the potential to vary across grouped countries because the initial conditions are different in these countries (e.g., degree of social participation, social movements supporting policies). The "sketch" should provide historical explanations of what happens at the aggregate level instead of presenting mere associations among relevant factors. "Carrying out the burden in a causal argument (Freedman 1991)" or account for the "historical proportion" need to be conducted through qualitative case studies or quantitative studies aware of these short comings (Hopkins 1982).

At best, the presentation of a simple summary of associations is insufficient, and, at worst, it will be misleading, as illustrated by Issac and Griffin (1989). These authors claimed that "much conventional quantitative time-series research is 'a historical'…that critical contingencies of social change, understood as the sudden or gradual temporal conditioning of historical-structural relationships (Duncan 1975) are for the most part ignored in quantitative explorations of historical processes (Hernes 1976)." Thus, using the same data and measures as examined in previous studies (Ashenfelter and Pencavel 1969; Edwards 1981; Hannan and Freeman 1988), these researchers conducted a "correlational" variant of the "moving regression" (Brown et al. 1975) or "moving covariance" method (Issac and Griffin 1989) to analyze the relationship between changes in strike frequency and three indicators of union strength for the period from 1882 to 1980. They found sudden structural changes in the relationship, i.e. the change in the direction of the association, in the early 1920s, in the mid- to late-1930s, the mid-1940s and in the mid-1950s, with the most dramatic change in the mid- to late-1930s. These breakpoints correspond to historical changes in labour institutions and regulations and the resulting change in labour militancy or the growth in membership of the American labour movement that had not been identified in previous analyses. These findings, again, point out the need for historical specific analyses in comparative politics and policy studies in sociology and social epidemiology as well. At the same time, the study is a good example of using quantitative analyses to conform to the historical reality. In sum, the alternative to the intrinsic problems of comparative political and policy analysis in sociology and social epidemiology is to incorporate appropriate amendments to existing quantitative methods.

9.5.2 The "Small N" Problem, Statistical Power, Omitted Variables and Sensitivity Analyses

The "small N" problem stems from the fact that the phenomenon we have at hand is a set of complex social processes occurring among a few countries (less than 200) and, usually, much less due to lack of quality datasets in low- and medium-income countries. The number of cases is too small to permit multivariate analyses that include all of the potentially relevant explanatory factors (Kenworthy 2004). Analyses, therefore, run the risk of omitted variable bias. Thus, as it is well known in epidemiology, if a variable that is correlated with both the independent variable of interest and the dependent variable is not included in the regression, the coefficient for the independent variable may overestimate its true effect (Kenworthy 2004).

It is empirically unfeasible to include all explanatory variables, and, even if we could, we would not be able to test their effect in a single model because of multi-collinearity. Therefore, in macro-comparative political and policy analyses, we use various types of sensitivity tests to assess the stability of hypothetical models. First, "extreme bound analysis" can be performed using one explanatory variable and all possible combinations of other variables with less than four explanatory variables (Leamer 1983; Deravi et al. 1990). Also useful is a variety of the "jackknife test," generating a number of bivariate regressions equal to the number of countries by using subsets of datasets. Only seven of the studies reviewed here conducted such sensitivity analyses (Avendano et al. 2009; Chung and Muntaner 2006; Conley and Springer 2001; Bambra et al. 2009; Baum and Lake 2003; Eikemo et al. 2008a; Klomp and de Haan 2009). Political economy of health and welfare regime researchers engaged in comparative population health research would be well served to become acquainted with these analytical methods.

9.6 The Missing Link in Political Epidemiology: Social Class

Social class understood as a power and political relation (as in managerial control, property relations, labour unions, political parties and class based social movements) is absent from social epidemiology. Yet, as suggested by the Whitehall studies (Marmot et al. 1991, 1997) and several other analyses (Muntaner et al. 2010), power relations can be an important social mechanism by which health disparities are generated. The typical pattern of relying on a single ordering of income does not tap into the social mechanisms that explain how individuals arrive at different levels of material resources. Occupational measures cannot account for social inequalities because occupation refers to the technical aspects of work rather than to power relations (such as asset ownership or managerial control). For example, somebody who drives an automobile for a living could be a self-employed owner of a taxicab, a supervisory worker of a taxicab chain, the owner of a taxicab chain, a taxicab driver renting a car or some combination of the above.

Class politics, as opposed to popular research areas such as "globalisation" or "social capital," is absent from social epidemiology (Muntaner 2004). For example, the working classes of low- and middle-income countries may or may not have influence over the international financial institutions that outline developing countries' health policy reforms. Again, without assessing social class power and political relations, we fail to generate mechanisms and explanations to further health disparities research. We can begin to understand the mechanisms that generate differences in income, wealth or credentials if we use social class measures that capture power relations (e.g., property relations, managerial control) (Muntaner and Lynch 1999; Muntaner et al. 2010). We can add even more complexity when class power is mediated (via one's family), is part of a trajectory (e.g., higher education), involves simultaneous positions and is measured at multiple levels or with continuous indicators (e.g., rate of exploitation, value of productive assets owned, number of workers supervised).

We also need to confront the causes of the neglect of power relations in social class research. By focusing on the properties of social positions rather than persons, power relations clash with the lay (middle class) assumption that a person's social class reflects some intrinsic attribute ("will power," "talent," "effort"). For this reason, power relations are simultaneously intriguing and unsettling.

9.7   Bringing Politics Back into Epidemiology

Guided by a political economy of health and welfare state regime framework, our review of 73 studies suggests that there is an association between politics expressed in terms of democracy, globalization, political traditions and welfare states and population health and health inequalities after adjustment for a common range of confounders. The strongest and most consistent associations with improved population health are advanced levels of democracy and egalitarian political traditions, while the health effects of welfare states are inconsistent. This emerging field of study is limited by a dearth of globalization studies, over-reliance on high-income core countries, infrequent use of longitudinal and time-series designs, few sensitivity analyses and limited conceptualizations of politics and power. Research on the association between politics and health has only recently emerged as a body of research, and it is clear that further investigation of this phenomenon is warranted. Informed theory, rigorous methods and conceptual clarity will be needed to reveal how political forces function as a macro-determinant of population health.

Harvard University Professor Richard Lewontin (2001), in his critical analyses of the standards of social sciences, noted that equating the status of experimental sciences and sociology was a self-defeating strategy. Instead, he recommended the use of data simultaneously with explanatory narratives to "fill in" where the data cannot go. The emerging field of the "politics of population health" or the comparative political and policy studies of population health is providing interesting inspirations to sociology and epidemiology and reminds us of the health-defining role of political and other macrosocial factors. However, such cautious warnings as Lewontin has suggested should be applied to this emergent field of sociology and epidemiology as well.

9.8   Conclusions

This chapter has shown that political and welfare state variables are salient determinants of population health and health inequalities and that absolute and relative health differences exist across countries along a range of political variables, including democracy, globalization, welfare states and political tradition. Identifying these associations represents an important first step; however, more work is needed to understand how to apply conflict-based theories to reduce health inequalities.

Conflict-based theories such as political economy of health and welfare regime frameworks emphasize, respectively, how social structures and institutions create, enforce and perpetuate social inequalities in health as well as the extent to which the state, operating as a social system, decommodifies the welfare needs of its citizens to mediate reduce these inequalities. Social epidemiologists are now applying these theories and their associated concepts to yield new important insights and, in the process, are rapidly advancing the sub-field of "political epidemiology" (Gil-González et al. 2009; Muntaner and Chung 2008). Applying political epidemiology to understand population health requires specifying how political and welfare regime variables are proxies for social structural forces that either favour or oppose egalitarian health outcomes and the distribution of proximal social determinants (e.g., socioeconomic resources, affordable housing stock, reliable public transport, green spaces for health recreation or regulation workplace hazards).

To illustrate how health inequalities can be reduced from a political epidemiology perspective, consider the example of political traditions, defined as left-right ideological dimensions, reviewed above. Conceptualizing political traditions as a determinant of population health expands social epidemiology's scope of interest to understand how structural levels of health inequalities are generated, what levels of political jurisdictions are relevant as well as which political forces and ideologies favour egalitarian outcomes. From this viewpoint, reducing health inequalities requires understanding how pro-distributive political parties, social movements, organized labour and other forms of working-class power mobilize to create strong welfare states that institutionalize the equal distribution of social and health-relevant resources. Conversely, to understand how political traditions might contribute to health inequalities, future research can assess the impact of conservative ("right wing") political parties and neo-liberalism in addition to the familiar structural adjustment policies imposed by the World Bank and by the International Monetary Fund on policy arrangements that lead to increased social stratification and class conflict. Advancing these research programs relate well to current work in social epidemiology on the mediating pathways that link social determinants to the health of individuals and populations (Marmot 2000).

Answering this chapter's central question – how does politics influence population health? – offers an important lesson on how future research can be augmented with path-dependent models. Path dependence explains how institutional patterns are created and reproduced from the sequential interplay between historical decisions and contingent events (Mahoney 2000). Applying this logic to the institutional reproduction of health inequalities reveals how historical relations and events influence power mechanisms, institutional characteristics and mechanisms of political change. Thus, achieving health equality is dependent on the path of past political struggles and outcomes in addition to current policies, programs and other factors that mediate population health outcomes. The challenge involves linking health inequalities to a particular set of historical events and demonstrating how these events are themselves contingent upon time and place.

A power-based, path-dependent approach suggests that health inequalities are not inevitable but result from contingent events such as historical transformations (e.g., transition to democratic governance structures); changes in democratic power (e.g., electoral swings between political parties); international relations (e.g., increasing impact of globalization); and social class compromises (e.g., varieties of welfare states). Common to these examples is the inherent conflict between those who are empowered verses those who are powerless through the persistence of political, economic and cultural institutions. The presence of conflict implies that these institutions possess the potential to be influenced, altered and even transformed (Sewell 2009). In this sense, power-based accounts, which integrate political relations and institutional reproduction, offer an intriguing framework for social epidemiology to explain the path-dependent causes of health inequalities as well as their possible reduction. Though political epidemiology remains in its infancy, considerable evidence exists that demonstrates that political factors are as important to population health today as they were during Engels' and Virchow's time.

References

Abbott A (1992) From causes to events: notes on narrative positivism. Sociol Methods Res 20:428–455
Adeyi O, Chellaraj G, Goldstein E et al (1997) Health status during the transition in Central and Eastern Europe: development in reverse? Health Policy Plan 12:132–145
Alvarez-Dardet C, Franco-Giraldo A (2006) Democratisation and health after the fall of the Wall. J Epidemiol Community Health 60:669–671
Aronson RE, Lovelace K, Hatch JW et al (2004) Strengthening communities and the roles of individuals in community life. In: Levy BS, Sidel VW (eds) Social injustice and public health. Oxford University Press, Oxford
Ashenfelter O, Pencavel J (1969) American trade union growth. Q J Econ 83:434–448
Avendano M, Juerges H, Mackenbach JP (2009) Educational level and changes in health across Europe: longitudinal results from SHARE. J Eur Soc Policy 19:301–316
Bambra C (2005) Cash versus services: 'Worlds of welfare' and the decommodification of cash benefits and health care services. J Soc Policy 34:195–213
Bambra C (2006) Health status and the worlds of welfare. Soc Policy Soc 5:53–62
Bambra C, Eikemo TA (2009) Welfare state regimes, unemployment and health: a comparative study of the relationship between unemployment and self-reported health in 23 European countries. J Epidemiol Community Health 63:92–98
Bambra C, Fox D, Scott-Samuel A (2005) Towards a politics of health. Health Promot Int 20:187–193
Bambra C, Pope D, Swami V et al (2009) Gender, health inequalities and welfare state regimes: a cross-national study of 13 European countries. J Epidemiol Community Health 63:38–44
Baum MA, Lake DA (2003) The political economy of growth: democracy and human capital. Am J Polit Sci 47:333–347
Beckfield J, Krieger N (2009) Epi + demos + cracy: linking political systems and priorities to the magnitude of health inequities – evidence, gaps, and a research agenda. Epidemiol Rev 31:152–177
Berkman LF, Kawachi I (2000) Social Epidemiology. Oxford University Press, New York
Besley T, Kudamatsu M (2006) Health and democracy. Am Econ Rev 96:313–318

Borrell C, Espelt A, Rodriguez-Sanz M et al (2009) Analyzing differences in the magnitude of socioeconomic inequalities in self-perceived health by countries of different political tradition in Europe. Int J Health Serv 39:321–341

Brown R, Durbin J, Evans JM (1975) Techniques for testing the constancy of regression relations over time. J Royal Stat Soc 37:149–192

Burnham G, Lafta R, Doocy S et al (2006) Mortality after the 2003 invasion of Iraq: a cross-sectional cluster sample survey. Lancet 368:1421–1428

Burstrom B, Whitehead M, Clayton S et al (2010) Health inequalities between lone and couple mothers and policy under different welfare regimes – the example of Italy, Sweden and Britain. Soc Sci Med 70:912–920

Cereseto S, Waitzkin H (1986) Economic-development, political-economic system, and the physical quality-of-life. Am J Public Health 76:661–666

Chung H, Muntaner C (2006) Political and welfare state determinants of infant and child health indicators: an analysis of wealthy countries. Soc Sci Med 63:829–842

Chung H, Muntaner C (2007) Welfare state matters: a typological multilevel analysis of wealthy countries. Health Policy 80:328–339

Coburn D (2000) Income inequality, social cohesion and the health status of populations: the role of neo-liberalism. Soc Sci Med 51:135–146

Coburn D (2004) Beyond the income inequality hypothesis: class, neo-liberalism, and health inequalities. Soc Sci Med 58:41–56

Cockerham WC (2001) Medical sociology and sociological theory. In: Cockerham WC (ed) The Blackwell companion to medical sociology. Blackwell, Oxford

Commission on Social Determinants of Health (2008) Closing the gap in a generation: health equity through action on the social determinants of health: Final report of the Commission on Social Determinants of Health. World Health Organization, Geneva

Conley D, Springer KW (2001) Welfare state and infant mortality. Am J Sociol 107:768–807

Correa H, Namkoong K (1992) Determinants and effects of health policy. J Policy Model 14:41–63

Côrtes SV (2009) The Unified National Health System: decision-making forums and the political arena in health. Cad Saúd Pública [Portuguese] 25:1626–1633

Dahl E, Fritzell J, Lahelma E et al (2006) Welfare state regimes and health inequalities. In: Siegrist J, Marmot M (eds) Social inequalities in health: new evidence and policy implications. Oxford University Press, Oxford

Deravi MK, Hegji CE, Moberly HD (1990) Government debt and the demand for money: an extreme bound analysis. Econ Inquiry 28:390–401

Duncan O (1975) An introduction to structural equation models. Academic, New York

Edwards P (1981) Strikes in the United States, 1881–1974. St. Martin's Press, New York

Eikemo TA, Bambra C, Judge K et al (2008a) Welfare state regimes and differences in self-perceived health in Europe: a multilevel analysis. Soc Sci Med 66:2281–2295

Eikemo TA, Huisman M, Bambra C et al (2008b) Health inequalities according to educational level in different welfare regimes: a comparison of 23 European countries. Sociol Health Illn 30:565–582

Elola J, Daponte A, Navarro V (1995) Health indicators and the organization of healthcare systems in Western Europe. Am J Public Health 85:1397–1401

Engels F (1958) The condition of the working class in England. Stanford University Press, Stanford

Espelt A, Borrell C, Rodriguez-Sanz M et al (2008) Inequalities in health by social class dimensions in European countries of different political traditions. Int J Epidemiol 37:1095–1105

Espelt A, Borrell C, Rodriguez-Sanz M et al (2010) Answer to the commentary: politics and public health – some conceptual considerations concerning welfare state characteristics and public health outcomes. Int J Epidemiol 39:630–632

Esping-Andersen G (1990) The three worlds of welfare capitalism. Princeton University Press, Princeton

Farfan-Portet M, Popham F, Mitchell R et al (2010) Caring, employment and health among adults of working age: evidence from Britain and Belgium. Eur J Pub Health 20:52–57

Fayissa B (2001) The determinants of infant and child mortality in developing countries: the case of Sub-Sahara Africa. Rev Black Political Econ 29:83–100

Ferrera M (1996) The 'southern' model of welfare in social Europe. J Eur Soc Policy 6:17–37

Finkel SE (1995) Causal analysis with panel data. Sage Publications, Thousand Oaks

Franco A, Alvarez-Dardet C, Ruiz MT (2004) Effect of democracy on health: ecological study. BMJ 329:1421–1423

Freedman D (1991) Statistical models and shoe leather. Sociol Methodol 21:291–313

Frey RS, Al-Roumi A (1999) Political democracy and the physical quality of life: the cross-national evidence. Soc Indic Res 47:73–97

Gauri V, Khaleghian P (2002) Immunization in developing countries: its political and organizational determinants. World Dev 30:2109–2132

Ghobarah HA, Huth P, Russett B (2004) Comparative public health: the political economy of human misery and well-being. Int Stud Q 48:73–94

Gil-González D, Ruiz-Cantero MT, Alvarez-Dardet C (2009) How political epidemiology research can address why the millennium development goals have not been achieved: developing a research agenda. Int Epidemiol Community Health 63:278–280

Gizelis T (2009) Wealth alone does not buy health: political capacity, democracy, and the spread of AIDS. Polit Geogr 28:121–131

Griffin LJ (1992) Temporality, events, and explanation in historical sociology: an introduction. Sociol Methods Res 20:403–427

Grosse Frie K, Eikemo TA, von dem Knesebeck O (2010) Education and self-reported health care seeking behaviour in European welfare regimes: results from the European Social Survey. Int J Public Health 55:217–220

Hall PA (2002) Aligning ontology and methodology in comparative research. In: Mahoney J, Rueschemeyer D (eds) Comparative historical research in the Social Sciences. Cambridge University Press, New York

Hannan MT, Freeman J (1988) The ecology of organizational mortality: American labor unions, 1836–1995. Am J Sociol 94:25–52

Hempel CG (1965) The logic of functional analysis: aspects of scientific explanation. Free Press, New York

Hernes G (1976) Structural change in social process. Am J Sociol 82:513–547

Hopkins TK (1982) The study of the capitalist world-economy: some introductory considerations. In: Hopkins TK, Wallerstein I (eds) World-systems analysis: theories and methodology. Sage Publications, Beverly Hills

Houweling TAJ, Caspar AEK, Looman WN et al (2005) Determinants of under-5 mortality among the poor and the rich: a cross-national analysis of 43 developing countries. Int J Epidemiol 34:1257–1265

Huber E, Stephens JE (2001) Development and crisis of the welfare state: parties and policies in global markets. University of Chicago Press, Chicago

Huber E, Mustillo T, Stephens JD (2008) Politics and social spending in Latin America. J Politics 70:420–436

Idrovo AJ, Ruiz-Rodríguez M, Manzano-Patiño AP (2010) Beyond the income inequality hypothesis and human health: a worldwide exploration. Revista de Saúd Pública 44:695–702

Issac LW, Griffin LJ (1989) A-historicism in time-series analyses of historical process: critique, redirection, and illustrations from U.S. labor history. Am Sociol Rev 54:873–890

Karim SA, Eikemo TA, Bambra C (2010) Welfare state regimes and population health: integrating the East Asian welfare states. Health Policy 94:45–53

Kaufman RR, Segura-Ubiergo A (2001) Globalization, domestic politics and social spending in Latin America: a time-series cross-section analysis, 1973–1997. Dados-Revista De Ciencias Sociais 44:435–479

Kenworthy L (2004) Egalitarian capitalism: jobs, incomes, and growth in affluent countries. Russell Sage, New York

Kick EL, Nasser R, Davis BL et al (1990) Militarization and infant-mortality in the third-world. J Polit Mil Sociol 18:285–305

Klomp J, de Haan J (2008) Effects of governance on health: a cross-national analysis of 101 countries. Kyklos 61:599–614

Klomp J, de Haan J (2009) Is the political system really related to health? Soc Sci Med 69: 36–46

Krieger N (2001) Theories for social epidemiology in the 21st century: an ecosocial perspective. Int J Epidemiol 30:668–677

Labonte R, Schrecker T, Packer C et al (2009) Globalization and health: pathways, evidence and policy. Routledge, New York

Lahelma E, Arber S (1994) Health inequalities among men and women in contrasting welfare states: Britain and three Nordic countries compared. Eur J Public Health 4:213–226

Lake DA, Baum MA (2001) The invisible hand of democracy – political control and the provision of public services. Compara Polit Stud 34:587–621

Lange P, Garrett G (1985) The politics of growth: strategic interaction and economic performance in the advanced industrial democracies, 1974–1980. J Polit 47:792–827

Leamer EE (1983) Let's take the con out of econometrics. Am Econ Rev 73:31–43

Lena HF, London B (1993) The political and economic-determinants of health outcomes – a cross-national analysis. Int J Health Serv 23:585–602

Lewontin RC (2001) It ain't necessarily so: the dream of the human genome and other illusions. New York Review of Books, New York

London B, Williams BA (1990) National politics, international dependency, and basic needs provision – a cross-national analysis. Soc Forces 69:565–584

Lundberg O (2009) Commentary: politics and public health – some conceptual considerations concerning welfare state characteristics and public health outcomes. Int J Epidemiol 37:1105–1108

Lundberg O, Yngwe MA, Stjarne MK et al (2008) The role of welfare state principles and generosity in social policy programmes for public health: an international comparative study. Lancet 372:1633–1640

Mahoney J (2000) Path dependence in historical sociology. Theory Soc 29:507–548

Marmot M (2000) Multilevel approaches to understanding social determinants. In: Berkman LF, Kawachi I (eds) Social epidemiology. Oxford University Press, New York

Marmot MG, Stansfeld S, Patel C et al (1991) Health inequalities among British civil servants: the Whitehall II study. Lancet 337:1387–1393

Marmot MG, Bosma H, Hemingway H et al (1997) Contribution of job control and other risk factors to social variations in coronary heart disease incidence. Lancet 350:235–239

McLean I, McMillan A (2003) Oxford concise dictionary of politics. Oxford University Press, New York

Menon-Johansson MA (2005) Good governance and good health: the role of societal structures in the human immunodeficiency virus pandemic. BMC Int Health Hum Rights 5:4

Moene KO, Wallerstein M (2003) Earnings inequality and welfare spending – a disaggregated analysis. World Polit 55:485–516

Moon BE, Dixon WJ (1985) Politics, the state, and basic human-needs – a cross-national-study. Am J Polit Sci 29:661–694

Moore S, Teixeira AC, Shiell A (2006) The health of nations in a global context: trade, global stratification, and infant mortality rates. Soc Sci Med 63:165–178

Muntaner C (2004) Commentary: social capital, social class, and the slow progress of psychosocial epidemiology. Int J Epidemiol 33:674–680

Muntaner C, Chung H (2008) Commentary: macrosocial determinants, epidemiology, and health policy: should politics and economics be banned from social determinants of health research? J Public Health Policy 29:299–306

Muntaner C, Lynch J (1999) Income inequality, social cohesion, and class relations: a critique of Wilkinson's neo-Durkheimian research program. Int J Health Serv 29:59–81

Muntaner C, Lynch JW, Oates GL (1999) The social class determinants of income inequality and social cohesion. Int J Health Serv 29:699–732

Muntaner C, Lynch JW, Hillemeier M et al (2002) Economic inequality, working-class power, social capital, and cause-specific mortality in wealthy countries. Int J Health Serv 32:629–656

Muntaner C, Borrell C, Kunst A et al (2006) Social class inequalities in health: does welfare state regime matter? In: Raphael D, Bryant T, Rioux MH (eds) Staying alive: critical perspectives on health, illness, and health care. Canadian Scholars Press, Toronto

Muntaner C, Borrell C, Espelt A et al (2009) Politics or policies vs politics and policies: a comment on Lundberg. Int J Epidemiol 39:1396–1397 Epub 2009 Jun 2. PubMed PMID: 19491140

Muntaner C, Borrell C, Varoelen C et al (2010) Employment relations, social class and health: a review and analysis of conceptual and measurement alternatives. Soc Sci Med 71:2130–2140

Navarro V (1989) Why some countries have national health insurance, others have national health service, and the U.S. has neither. Soc Sci Med 28:887–898

Navarro V (1993) Has socialism failed? Health indicators under capitalism and socialism. Sci Soc 57:6–30

Navarro V, Muntaner C (2004) Political and economic determinants of population health and well-being: controversies and development. Baywood Publishing Company, Amityville

Navarro V, Shi LY (2001) The political context of social inequalities and health. Int J Health Serv 31:1–21

Navarro V, Borrell C, Benach J et al (2003) The importance of the political and the social in explaining mortality differentials among the countries of the OECD, 1950–1998. Int J Health Serv 33:419–494

Navarro V, Muntaner C, Borrell C et al (2006) Politics and health outcomes. Lancet 368:1033–1037

Navia P, Zweifel TD (2003) Democracy, dictatorship, and infant mortality revisited. J Democr 14: 90–103

Nordenmark M, Strandh M, Layte R (2006) The impact of unemployment benefit system on the mental well-being of the unemployed in Sweden, Ireland and Great Britain. Eur Soc 8:83–110

Ouweneel P (2002) Social security and well-being of the unemployed in 42 nations. J Happiness Stud 3:167–192

Pillai VK, Gupta R (2006) Cross-national analysis of a model of reproductive health in developing countries. Soc Sci Res 35:210–227

Pope C, Mays N, Popay J (2007) Synthesizing qualitative and quantitative health evidence: a guide to methods. Open University Press, Maidenhead

Ragin CC (1987) The comparative method: moving beyond qualitative and quantitative strategies. University of California Press, Berkeley

Raphael D, Bryant T (2004) The welfare state as a determinant of women's health: support for women's quality of life in Canada and four comparison nations. Health Policy 68:63–79

Rose G (2001) Sick individuals and sick populations. Int J Epidemiol 30:427–432

Ross M (2006) Is democracy good for the poor? Am J Polit Sci 50:860–874

Rostila M (2007) Social capital and health in European welfare regimes: a multilevel approach. J Eur Soc Policy 17:223–239

Rudra N, Haggard S (2005) Globalization, democracy, and effective welfare spending in the developing world. Comp Polit Stud 38:1015–1049

Safaei J (2006) Is democracy good for health? Int J Health Serv 36:767–786

Sanders AE, Slade GD, John MT et al (2009) A cross-national comparison of income gradients in oral health quality of life in four welfare states: application of the Korpi and Palme typology. J Epidemiol Community Health 63:569–574

Sekine M, Chandola T, Martikainen P et al (2009) Socioeconomic inequalities in physical and mental functioning of British, Finnish, and Japanese civil servants: role of job demand, control, and work hours. Soc Sci Med 69:1417–1425

Sen A (1999) Development as freedom. Oxford University Press, Oxford

Sewell WH Jr (2009) From state-centrism to neoliberalism: macro-historical contexts of population health since World War II. In: Hall PA, Lamont M (eds) Successful societies – how institutions and culture affect health. Cambridge University Press, New York

Shalev M (2007) Limits and alternatives to multiple regression in comparative research. Comp Soc Res 24:261–308

Shandra JM, Nobles J, London B et al (2004) Dependency, democracy, and infant mortality: a quantitative, cross national analysis of less developed countries. Soc Sci Med 59:321–333

Shandra JM, Nobles J, London B (2010) Do non-governmental organizations impact health? A cross-national analysis of infant mortality. Int J Comp Sociol 51:137–164

Shen C, Williamson JB (1997) Child mortality, women's status, economic dependency, and state strength: a cross-national study of less developed countries. Soc Forces 76:667–700

Shen C, Williamson JB (2001) Accounting for cross-national differences in infant mortality decline (1965–1991) among less developed countries: effects of women's status, economic dependency, and state strength. Soc Indic Res 53:257–288

Stroup MD (2007) Economic freedom, democracy, and the quality of life. World Dev 35:52–66

Tapia Granados JA (2010) Politics and health in eight European countries: a comparative study of mortality decline under social democracies and right-wing governments. Soc Sci Med 71:841–850

Tsai MC (2006) Does political democracy enhance human development in developing countries? A cross-national analysis. Am J Eco Sociol 65:233–268

Veenhoven R (2000) Well-being in the welfare state. J Comp Policy Anal 2:91–125

Veenhoven R, Ouweneel P (1995) Livability of the welfare-state appreciation-of-life and length-of-life in nations varying in state-welfare-effort. Soc Indic Res 36:1–48

Verba S (1967) Some dilemmas in comparative research. World Polit 20:111–127

Virchow RLK (1985) Report on the typhus epidemic in Upper Silesia. In: Rather LJ (ed) Rudolph Virchow: collected essays on public health and epidemiology. Science History Publications, Canton

Wejnert B (2008) Effect of global democracy on women's reproductive health: 1970–2005, cross-world analysis. Marriage Fam Rev 3(4):14–37

Whitehead M, Burstrom B, Diderichsen F (2000) Social policies and the pathways to inequalities in health: a comparative analysis of lone mothers in Britain and Sweden. Soc Sci Med 50:255–270

Wilkinson RG, Pickett K (2010) The spirit level: why more equal societies almost always do better. Allen Lane, London

Zambon A, Boyce W, Cois E et al (2006) Do welfare regimes mediate the effect of socioeconomic position on health in adolescence? A cross-national comparison in Europe, North America, and Israel. Int J Health Serv 36:309–329

Zweifel TD, Navia P (2000) Democracy, dictatorship, and infant mortality. J Democr 11:99–114

Part III
Research Tools in Action

Chapter 10

Structural Violence and Structural Vulnerability Within the Risk Environment: Theoretical and Methodological Perspectives for a Social Epidemiology of HIV Risk Among Injection Drug Users and Sex Workers

Tim Rhodes, Karla Wagner, Steffanie A. Strathdee, Kate Shannon, Peter Davidson, and Philippe Bourgois

Contents

10.1	Introduction	206
10.2	From the Individual to the Social	207
10.3	Methodological Challenges	210
10.4	Four Case Studies	211
	10.4.1 Case Study One: Policing and the "Structuration" of HIV Vulnerability Through Fear	212
	10.4.2 Case Study Two: Gendered Power Relations and HCV Seroconversion Among Street-Based Youth IDUs	215
	10.4.3 Case Study Three: Structural Violence, Power and HIV Prevention Among Female and Transgendered Sex Workers in an Urban Setting	218
	10.4.4 Case Study Four: HIV Risk in the Context of Deportation: The Modifying Role of Gender	221
10.5	Discussion	222
	10.5.1 Structural Vulnerability	223
	10.5.2 Mixing Method and Theory	225
10.6	Conclusions	226
References		227

T. Rhodes (✉)
London School of Tropical Medicine and Hygiene, 15-17 Tavistock Place,
London WC1H 9SH, UK
e-mail: Tim.Rhodes@lshtm.ac.uk

K. Wagner • S.A. Strathdee • P. Davidson
Division of Global Public Health, Department of Medicine, UC San Diego, California, USA

K. Shannon
Department of Medicine, University of British Columbia
and BC Centre for Excellence in HIV/AIDS

P. Bourgois
Department of Anthropology, University of Pennsylvania

P. O'Campo and J.R. Dunn (eds.), *Rethinking Social Epidemiology:
Towards a Science of Change*, DOI 10.1007/978-94-007-2138-8_10,
© Springer Science+Business Media B.V. 2012

Abstract The transmission of HIV is shaped by individual-environment interactions. Social epidemiologic approaches thus seek to capture the dynamic and reciprocal relationships of individual-environment interactions in the production and reduction of risk. This presents considerable methodological, theoretical and disciplinary challenges. Drawing upon four research case studies, we consider how methods and concepts in the social and epidemiologic sciences might be brought together towards understanding HIV risk as an effect of social, cultural and political condition. The case studies draw upon different combinations of methods (qualitative, ethnographic and quantitative) and disciplines (sociology, anthropology and epidemiology) in different social contexts of HIV vulnerability (street settings in Russia, Serbia and North America and a cross-border setting in Mexico) among a range of marginalised high-risk populations (injection drug users and female and transvestite sex workers). These case studies illustrate the relevance of the social science concepts of "structural violence" and "structural vulnerability" for a social epidemiology of HIV risk. They also explore how social epidemiologic work can benefit from the mixing of social science methods and theories. We contend that social epidemiology cannot advance in its understanding of structural vulnerability without embracing and relying upon ethnographic and qualitative approaches. We put forward the linked concepts of "structural violence," "structural vulnerability" and "risk environment" as building blocks for a theory-informed social epidemiology of HIV risk among marginalised populations.

Abbreviations

GIS   Geographic Information Systems
HCV   Hepatitis C virus
IDU   injection drug user
SRO   single room occupancy

10.1   Introduction

HIV transmission is influenced by an interaction between biological, individual and environmental factors. Social epidemiologic approaches thus seek to delineate how the distribution of HIV in populations is shaped by the "risk environment," that is, by determinants that extend beyond "proximal" individual-level factors and their behavioural mediators (Farmer 2009; Krieger 2008; Rhodes 2002). This presents considerable methodological, theoretical and disciplinary challenges. In this chapter, we consider how methods and concepts in the social and epidemiologic sciences might be brought together towards understanding HIV risk as an effect of social, cultural and political condition. Our interest is in mapping how social, political and economic structures generate and reproduce vulnerability to HIV, especially among socially marginalised populations, including injection drug users (IDUs) and sex workers. This brings into focus how multiple interacting social factors create a context of vulnerability to HIV risk across multiple marginalised populations. We, therefore, outline a case for a "social epidemiology of structural vulnerability" applied to HIV. In doing so, we emphasise the critical role of qualitative methods and social science theory in capturing and representing the "lived experience" of embodied structural vulnerability inside a mixed-method and cross-disciplinary approach. We suggest that social epidemiology cannot advance in its practical understanding of structural vulnerability without embracing and relying on ethnographic and qualitative approaches. Our aim is not merely to outline a case for a social epidemiology of structural vulnerability but also to reflect upon some of the limits, opportunities and challenges likely to be created through such cross-methodological and disciplinary work.

10.2 From the Individual to the Social

The field of public health, and in HIV specifically, has increasingly moved towards an understanding that health is an outcome of social and structural conditions and, in particular, sociocultural, economic and political inequalities (Farmer 1999; Navarro and Mutaner 2004). Accompanying this understanding is a growing critique of biomedical approaches to health research, which tend to emphasize individual-level factors over environmental or structural ones and which fail to adequately capture the social structural production of risk or the facilitators of change. In the case of HIV, however, the interplay between health and social marginalisation is, or should be, so visible as to be unavoidable (Farmer et al. 1996). This critique identifies a tendency in public health and the behavioural sciences to operationalize risk as primarily resulting from individual action and responsibility and, in doing so, cautions against an over reliance upon individual-level models of rational choice decision making. Behavioural interventions alone have been shown to only account for a modest reduction in HIV incidence in the absence of social and structural interventions and policies (Copenhaver et al. 2006). This critique also cautions against the "victim blaming" tendency of individual-level models, which give sole or primary emphasis to individual choice and agency as determinants of risk and risk behaviour. In contrast, social epidemiologic approaches seek to situate risk and risk responsibility as something shared between individuals, communities and environments – especially among the social and political-economic institutions that have a key role in risk production. While epidemiologic research has shown that physical, social, economic and policy environment factors are independently associated with HIV infection among vulnerable groups such as drug users, few studies have fully operationalized a social epidemiologic approach from the outset (Strathdee et al. 2010). Here we advocate for a shift "from the individual to the social" in public health, which emphasises, first, that the health of individuals and communities is an *embodiment of their social condition* and, second, that health improvement requires *social and structural change*.

One overarching heuristic for guiding research and intervention on HIV risk as an effect of social condition is the "risk environment" framework (Rhodes 2002, 2009; Rhodes et al. 2005; Strathdee et al. 2010). This has been defined as the space, whether social or physical, in which a variety of environmental factors interact to increase the chances of risk occurring (Rhodes 2002; Rhodes et al. 2003). The risk environment is conceptualised as comprising *types of environment* (physical, social, economic and policy) interacting with *levels of environmental influence* (micro and macro). This same logic implies an "enabling environment" framework of social and structural change (Table 10.1). This heuristic has given impetus to a number of studies investigating the primacy of social context in HIV and other risks related to injection drug use and sex work (Strathdee et al. 2010, 2008b; Rhodes et al. 2005; Moore 2004; Small et al. 2006; Shannon et al. 2008a, b; Cooper et al. 2009; Green et al. 2009). Within an overarching framework of risk environment, there are a number of overlapping (and to some extent competing) concepts in social science that have provided the conceptual foundations for social epidemiologic work, including in the field of HIV and drug use. These concepts include "political economy" and "structural violence." Social epidemiologic approaches have long drawn attention to an overlap with *political economy* (Krieger 2001, 2008; Doyle 1979). For Krieger (2008), health "cannot be divorced from considerations of political economy and political ecology." This reflects parallel assertions in the social sciences that the HIV risks of drug use or sex work are "virtually meaningless outside their sociocultural as well as political economic contexts" (Bourgois 2003) and that drug use is "the epiphenomenal expression of deeper, structural dilemmas" (Bourgois 1995). Crucially, political-economic perspectives posit social conditions as rendering *particular* sectors of the population vulnerable to harm. This "structuration of risk" is illustrated through the incarceration and enforcement-based policies that disproportionately affect those using drugs and working in the sex industry as well as those already suffering intense and systematic discrimination, including racial discrimination (Jurgens et al. 2010).

A related concept informing social epidemiologic work to date is *structural violence*. Structural violence is distinct from personal or direct violence in that it is embedded in social structures whereby "unequal power" shapes "unequal life chances" (Galtung 1990). Poverty, racism and gender inequalities provide examples (Farmer et al. 1996; Walter et al. 2004). Each of these may perpetuate constraints in agency, leading to unequal opportunity and disproportionate social suffering for the marginalised (Farmer 2010). Crucially, the institutionalisation and everyday internalization of structural violence can render it invisible or unnoticeable (Scheper-Hughes 1996). The embodied effects of structural violence may be understood as "oppression illness," which is the "product of the impact of suffering from social mistreatment," a type of "stress disorder," where the source of stress is "being the object of widespread and enduring social discrimination, degradation, structural violence and abusive derision," whether overt or hidden (Singer 2004). Drug use, itself, can be seen as a form of "self-medication" for oppression illness, providing "pain intolerance," "chemical intervention" and a "solution" (Singer 2004). The internalization of social suffering (Kleinman et al. 1997) reproduces a cycle of

Table 10.1 The risk and enabling environment: selected examples related to HIV, drug injecting and sex work

		Micro-environment	Macro-environment
Physical	Risk	Drug using, injecting and sex work locations Drug injecting in public spaces Prisons and detention centres	Drug trafficking and distribution routes Trade routes and population mobility Geographical population shifts and population mixing
	Intervention	Creating safer drug using sites (e.g., sharps disposal, lighting) Developing supervised injecting facilities Prison-based harm reduction interventions and alternatives to prison	Changes to trafficking interdiction policies Interventions at truck stops and train stations Cross-border interventions Changes to immigration laws and routine enforcement practices
Social	Risk	Social and peer group "risk" norms and intimate partner violence Local policing practices and "crackdowns" Community health and welfare service access and delivery	Gender inequalities and gendered risk Stigmatisation and marginalisation of drug users Weak civil society and community advocacy
	Intervention	Social network and peer-based interventions Shelters for homeless and for battered partners Police partnership and training projects Developing low threshold accessible services for drug users	Fostering collective actions and political mobilization for social and human rights in combination with policy changes Mass media and social marketing of harm reduction Strengthening civil society infrastructure and self-help
Economic	Risk	Cost of living and cost of health treatments Cost of prevention materials Lack of income generation and employment	Lack of health service revenue and spending Growth of informal economies Uncertain economic transition
	Intervention	Subsidised and free treatment Distribution of free prevention materials Micro-economic enterprise and employment schemes	Increase investment in harm reduction relative to enforcement National health insurance schemes Laws governing employment rights
Policy	Risk	Availability and coverage of clean needles and syringes Program-level policies governing distribution of materials Access to low-threshold and social housing	Public health policy governing harm reduction and drug treatment Laws governing possession of drugs Laws governing protection of human and health rights
	Intervention	Scaling-up pharmacy-based syringe provision Secondary syringe distribution programmes Hostel-based and housing neighbourhood development	Legal reform enabling the scaling-up of harm reduction Legal reform enabling the protection of drug user rights National policy changes regarding public health strategy

Source: Rhodes (2009)

risk production in which those marginalised can become complicit, including unconsciously, in their ongoing structural subordination (Bourdieu 2000).

Critiques of political economy perspectives and the ways in which structural violence informs social epidemiologic work emphasise that they tend to be "over deterministic," underplaying the role of agency, subjectification and non-material forces in the reciprocal processes of individual-environment interactions (Bourgois and Schonberg 2009; Duff 2007; Giddens 1984; Biehl et al. 2007; Butler 1997; Foucault 1995; Pine 2008). It is critical that social epidemiologic approaches capture the dynamism of agency-structure transformations, in which environments constrain as well as enable agency, and are thus also produced and reproduced by participant practices. We take up these points below in the case study descriptions and discussion of the "structural vulnerability" of HIV risk.

10.3 Methodological Challenges

Rather than relying on reductionist models that hypothesize direct, linear associations between "risk factors" and "outcomes," a shift towards a social understanding of HIV vulnerability can "scale up" an understanding of risk to embrace the dynamic, reciprocal associations amongst individuals and their social, physical and political-economic environments. Attention to the multilevel, complex systems that influence health outcomes, however, is not without its methodological challenges. In fact, developing research methods that can delineate causal and theoretical pathways in the social determinants of HIV is a critical step to informing social and structural interventions for reducing HIV risk (Strathdee et al. 2010; Rhodes 2009).

Researching causal pathways to HIV transmission demands a shift from binary epidemiologic models of simple "cause and effect" to "multilevel" models, which emphasise HIV as an outcome of multiple contributing factors at once interacting together (Galea and Vlahov 2002). Social determinants that derive from the risk environment perspective are often "non-linear" and "indirect" in their effects, and this presents considerable challenges to delineating causative relationships (Krieger 1994). Measuring the effects of structural violence, for example, is not as simple as assessing phenomena such as the direct experience of physical violence or economic dislocation; structural violence extends beyond the individual to the social structures that perpetuate poverty, racism, gender inequalities and other forms of systemic marginalisation, which ultimately shape HIV risk. HIV is thus an outcome of a "complex system" of interactions occurring within and between individuals and their environments, with the challenge being to better capture the dynamism of these reciprocal relations through mixed-methods research.

Understanding these complex systems requires an iterative and multidisciplinary approach in which qualitative evidence and social science theory help to map conceptions of "risk environment" and related risk pathways. Although there is a rich theoretical and empirical tradition in the social sciences of investigating health as an effect of social inequality and condition (Engels 1892), public health has not dialogued systematically with social science theory and methods. In a research environment increasingly characterized by transdisciplinary and mixed-methods approaches, both social science and traditional epidemiologic approaches can benefit from the strategic integration of the other's theoretical approaches and research methods (Mason 2006). Such a synthesis has the potential to increase the public health impact of both fields by generating grounded conceptual frameworks with testable causal pathways contributing to intervention development on the one hand and by providing socially-situated interpretations of epidemiologic data on the other.

10.4   Four Case Studies

We will draw upon four short case studies to illustrate the relevance of the concepts of structural violence and structural vulnerability in social epidemiology studies of the HIV risk environment. Our four case studies explore relationships between viral harms (HIV and hepatitis C virus) and social condition. Case Study One explores the "structuration" of HIV risk through the everyday internalization of fear induced by policing practices among injection drug users in Russia and sex workers in Serbia. Case Study Two explores the legitimization of violence against young female IDUs in San Francisco leading to heightened vulnerability to hepatitis C (HCV). Case Study Three focuses on police-enforced displacement of female sex workers in Vancouver to remote, violent neighbourhoods that heighten their risk of violence and limit their capacity to negotiate condom use. Case Study Four explores gendered patterns of international migration and deportation associated with the risk of HIV infection in the United States/Mexico border region.

Each case study employs a different design and, taken as a group, show the strategic advantage of integrating multiple methodological approaches. Case Study One emphasises the critical role of ethnographic and qualitative research in capturing and representing the "lived experience" of embodied structural vulnerability, including as a means of informing subsequent epidemiologic study. Case Study Two demonstrates how the simultaneous use of ethnographic participant observation and epidemiologic survey research can both inform and refine research questions when ethnography uncovers associations that may be difficult to detect using quantitative measures. Case Study Three uses a participatory research approach to incorporate quantitative questionnaire data, social mapping and in-depth qualitative interviews in an iterative design that explicitly accounts for the complex physical and social environment in which HIV risk behaviour occurs. Case Study Four shows how counterintuitive findings from a classically-designed epidemiologic cohort study can be contextualized and interpreted through the use of supplemental qualitative research informed by social science theory. Our aim is not only to make a case for a social epidemiology of structural vulnerability (as applied to HIV) but also to highlight some of the methodological and theoretical challenges facing cross-disciplinary public health research.

10.4.1   Case Study One: Policing and the "Structuration" of HIV Vulnerability Through Fear

Data were drawn from qualitative studies among injecting drug users in Russia, in 2003, and sex workers in Serbia, in 2005, to capture the lived effects of HIV risk environment in which policing practices played a key role (Sarang et al. 2010; Rhodes et al. 2008).

One of the most visible structural mechanisms perpetuating social suffering and HIV risk among vulnerable populations of IDUs and sex workers is the criminal justice system, especially policing practices. International evidence links policies emphasizing repressiveness through law enforcement with higher levels of risk for health and HIV, and a growing epidemiologic literature points towards policing practices and fear of the criminal justice system as important factors (Strathdee et al. 2010; Rhodes 2009; Cooper et al. 2009; Friedman et al. 2006; Pollini et al. 2008).

Russia provides an acute example (as do other parts of Eastern Europe witnessing massive outbreaks of HIV among drug injectors). The enactment of criminal and administrative codes relating to drugs possession combine with aggressive police surveillance, resulting in the mass incarceration of drug users and other minority groups and a prison system linked to HIV outbreaks (Bobrik et al. 2005; Sarang et al. 2006). Intense police surveillance fosters reluctance to seek help or carry sterile needles for fear of arrest, caution, fine or detention (Rhodes et al. 2003). Police contact, from arrest to assault, is associated with increased risk of syringe sharing (Strathdee et al. 2010; Sarang et al. 2010; Pollini et al. 2008; Rhodes et al. 2004).

Qualitative research among 209 IDUs in three Russian cities (Moscow, Volgograd and Barnaul) illustrates the "structural violence" of drug policies emphasizing criminalization (Sarang et al. 2010). Everyday policing practices, and especially *extrajudicial practices*, generated a pervasive sense among drug injectors of *being at risk*, in turn reinforcing a sense of stigma, powerlessness and, importantly, a *fatalistic acceptance of harm and suffering*. Through the internalization of the effects of policing practices, we see the *embodiment* of social conditions into everyday risk perceptions and practices. Of key importance is the *fear* of policing practices and how this acted as an indirect force of structural violence affecting capacity for HIV risk avoidance.

First, drug injectors felt under inescapable surveillance ("You cannot hide from them" and "They know everything about us"). While the sense of being under pervasive surveillance was presented as normative, it is what police might do with such surveillance opportunity that drug users feared. The power of the police was ubiquitously perceived among drug injectors as *limitless* (captured by the Russian term *bespredel*).

The extortion of money and the planting of evidence were, for example, presented as common practices, with the latter also resulting in unjust incarceration. Yet extortion was seen as mundane. Drug users were participants in, and complicit with, extortion. It had an immediate function, for money was exchanged for freedom. This was seen as a risk management strategy.

But police physical violence and assault was perceived entirely differently. Physical violence by the police was experienced as an extreme act of moral indignation, aggression and subordination. It was police brutality that induced most fear: "I'm very afraid;" "I was so shit scared;" and "Fear, fear, that is the main thing." Fear acts as both an effect and a force of structural violence. Here, Sergei (aged 27), an occasional injector from Volgograd, tells a story of how police violence produces fear:

> We were just standing, talking, with my girlfriend. So a policeman comes by and asks to show my passport, as they always do. I didn't have them. ...So he takes me out into his booth. ...After they searched me and couldn't find anything, they just started to call someone, peek into my eyes, and say like I'm high or something. And they just start to get to me. Then my girl comes in. They searched her too, and found the pack of Russian cigarettes [where the cannabis was]. And that was it. Now we're 100% junkies, and things are off and rolling. He locks us both on to these bars. There were maybe five other people in there. And he just starts to bully my girl. He says, "Your girl is a bitch, she's a toad, a turd, I can see it in her eyes." And he starts to wind me up. And when I start reacting, he just tears me out of there and starts to beat me, methodically on my belly, legs, and other parts so as not to bruise me too much. Then when he got tired, he just stretched me out on the floor, put handcuffs behind my back, pulled my legs through my arms and just left me there. I don't know how long I just laid there, or why they bullied me, even though I didn't even have anything. No reason. I don't know what to call that. This is just scary. ...I don't know. I'm still in a trance from all this horror.

The physical suffering narrated by Sergei has human rights and public health implications. It also has *practical consequences*, as the internalization of fear exacerbates structural vulnerability to HIV and other health risk. A state of fear heightens concerns to evade detection, resulting in rushed injections, short-cuts in needle hygiene, injecting in "hidden" locations (such as at dealers' houses) and sharing needles and syringes to reduce the risk of arrest for carrying injecting equipment: "Fear. This is the main reason [for syringe sharing]. ...You just try and inject quick, quick, quick, and you don't give a damn whether it's clean" and "I am afraid, and so I hide. And so everything [drug injecting] takes place [on the street] in filth." Fear can also lead to avoiding pharmacies and other needle and syringe outlets in an attempt to avoid arrest should the police be present. More subtly, all state representatives, including helping agencies, become feared as a source of risk: "Although the pharmacy was two houses away from me, always, always, the police stood there" and "Why I haven't gone to the exchange? Well, shit, I'm scared, that's why. It's dangerous. Who knows who is there."

It can be seen here how political processes of everyday violence cross over from public space to traumatize personal space and then cross back as collective experience (Kleinman 1991). Policing practices feature inside a broader complex of multiple interacting social and material inequalities, which over time become *institutionalized* and *normalized*. When internalized, the effects of such structural violence may be expressed as individual deficits, as psychological harm, powerlessness, and fatalism to risk.

A second example of qualitative research, focusing on the policing of female and transvestite sex workers in Serbia (Rhodes et al. 2008), illustrates further how policing practices targeting the vulnerable are best seen not in social isolation but as institutionalized expressions of a wider complex of normative social and moral regulation. Among street-based sex workers in Belgrade and nearby Pančevo, violence, especially police violence, was a primary concern. While client violence was not uncommon, police violence was perceived as the greater threat and as less open to risk management: "You can manage your clients somehow, but to be honest, the greatest threat to us is the police." Sexual services were provided to police without payment as well as secured by them through deception and coercion, often involving violence or the threat of it: "And at the end of the job he shows me his badge, and says like 'Give me my money back now'. That's what he does" and "They want blowjobs, fucks. I work for free, just so they don't take me in." Attempts to resist such demands could also incite violence: "He wants me to blow him for free. I don't want to. Later, when he gets me on my shift, he beats me silly. Beats me silly" and "He beats me up with a baton. And several times I had to be [have sex] with him. I really had to. I was forced."

Being coerced into providing sex to police in this setting was described as an *exchange for freedom* (from detainment, arrest or fine) enforced by a pervasive risk, sometimes realized, of physical violence (Rhodes et al. 2008). Again, we see fear induced by policing practices acting as an indirect force of structural violence. Embodied fear produced fatalist risk acceptance to the inevitability of violence ("I can't fight destiny") and an internalized sense of police "rights" to victimize ("They have a right to beat us because we do this prostitution thing").

This study shows that while serving to protect state and public interests, policing practices can reproduce underlying societal injustices, fears and inequalities, including regarding gender, sexuality, drug use and ethnicity. Enforced sexual acts and payments to police were experienced as a form of governmentality, as if for moral wrong doing, to "bring sex workers to their senses." Significantly, police "moral punishments" for selling sex were inextricably linked inside a broader complex of social discrimination, especially towards Roma and transvestites. In Serbia, Roma are a minority ethnic group subjected to immense social discrimination and Roma sex workers, most of whom were Kosovo refugees and all of whom were working as transvestites, were subjected to extreme acts of police violence:

> They [police] kicked, kicked, kicked the hell out of us. Just transvestites. They took me to the woods, down by the bridge. They stripped everything off me. Flashlight in the eyes. I said a million times "Take me away. Did you come to arrest me? Arrest me then, but do not beat me up". That makes it worse: "Shut up, motherfucker, shut up!"
> They [police] started going wild, only on us transvestites. They let the girls go. They just pick us up, and go to the woods, and go wild on us. …First, they beat us in the woods, and then they take us to the station. And then, they tell us at the station "Hey, freshen up", and they beat us up in the bathroom.
> I didn't know where the blows were coming from. …They just have this hate. Whether it's towards prostitutes or specifically trannnies. But it's terrible.

We see in these examples how qualitative research documents the everyday lived effects of the risk environment, shaping risk identities. Mapping pathways between individual risk actions and their structural contexts is inherently complex because these effects are *reciprocal* as well as often *indirect* and *non-linear*. They shape values and patterns of subjectivities that can promote risk-taking practices. In this case example, *fear* and *discrimination* have direct as well as indirect effects on individual and collective capacity to reduce risk. Fear and discrimination are vectors of structural violence that can promote HIV risk. It is unlikely we could have uncovered their importance through traditional epidemiologic methodologies.

10.4.2   Case Study Two: Gendered Power Relations and HCV Seroconversion Among Street-Based Youth IDUs

Data were drawn from a prospective cohort study of young out-of-treatment IDUs in San Francisco (2000–2002) that included the simultaneous coordinated collection of epidemiologic survey research and anthropological participant observation.

In coordination with a prospective epidemiologic study of HCV and HIV transmission among out-of-treatment youth injectors, we simultaneously collected classic anthropological participant observation data among participants involved in an epidemiologic study. The epidemiologic study screened young (< 30 years old) IDUs for HCV and HIV and enrolled HCV-negative individuals into a prospective cohort. Participants were re-tested for HCV and HIV and quantitatively interviewed on a quarterly basis. A central aim was to explore behavioural differences between those who seroconverted for HCV and those who did not. The primary ethnographer was a young woman (approximately the same age as the average age of the youth injectors) and also a former outreach worker and epidemiologic questionnaire administrator for the project. She befriended and accompanied members of a series of extended social networks of neighbourhood-based youth injectors in their natural environment on the street. This involved frequenting street corners, parks, single room occupancy (SRO) hotels, hidden injection locales, homeless encampments, jails, hospitals, clinics, social service waiting rooms and needle exchange sites. She also accompanied the youth injectors in their daily search for drugs and income (primarily through panhandling, shoplifting, street-based sex work and retail drug sales). Ethnographic participants were initially selected through a classic opportunistic snowball sample of young women and men. Over time participants were then more strategically selected through the infrastructure of the epidemiologic project to develop causal explanations for social processes that might explain or contradict the emerging findings on risky practices and seroconversion.

Almost immediately, because of the positionality of the ethnographer, the subject of intimate partner violence within romantic relationships emerged as the primary theme organizing the lives of the young women surviving on the street in these social networks. The ethnographer was able to triangulate observational and self-report data on how romantic sexual relationships affected the details of heroin and methamphetamine injection practices as well as income generating strategies.

The ethnographic data revealed that newly arrived young women – especially those under 18 – entering this adolescent drug scene developed romantic relationships with older, more experienced men who had violent reputations and who displayed jealous dispositions. These relationships protected them from harassment and rape by other men and also initially provided them with abundant access to drugs and advice on how to be street smart. Because of their number of years on the street, almost all of these "successful" domineering male street injectors were HCV infected. Some women were self-consciously aware of the protective benefits of selecting a partner with a "macho" and violent reputation. Most, however, understood their choice of partner in romantic terms. Many interpreted violent male love as inevitable and even desirable: "The more he hits you the more he loves you."

The male partners generally attempted to oblige the women to conduct all their drug consumption exclusively with them. They often insisted on maintaining physical control over needle use and administered injections to the women. This allowed them to consume more than half of all the drugs they consumed together. It also reduced the opportunities for the women to meet other men and form alternative romantic relationships. Almost all the women eventually gravitated towards sex work to raise money for drugs, both for themselves and for their romantic partner. Over time, they would become the primary income generators within the relationship.

The ability to explore and document the details of the social logics for gendered violence was informed by social science theories of gender power relations with an emphasis on the concept of structural violence and the normalization of everyday interpersonal violence. The ethnographer's findings about the prevalence of violence against women among street youth injectors and the romantic discourse surrounding it was also consistent with Bourgois and colleagues' (2004, 2009) simultaneous documentation of violence against women in other street-based drug use scenes.

Regular monthly meetings with the epidemiologic team allowed the project to compare the emerging qualitative and quantitative findings and to redefine priorities for both qualitative data collection and for statistical analyses. The primary epidemiologic outcome measure for statistical analysis was seroincidence. At first there was no detectable association between HCV seroincidence and gender, despite the fact that the ethnographic findings strongly suggested that gender and violence were primary factors driving risk for bloodborne pathogen infection. The epidemiologists worried that the qualitative findings were driven by an ideological bias towards feminist theory and had "no basis in the science." Unfortunately, there were no questions in the epidemiologic survey that assessed the factors uncovered in the ethnographic research – particularly with respect to exposure to violence and the details and influence of romantic relationships. New questions were drafted, but the field staff responsible for quantitative interviewing expressed concerns that asking sensitive questions about intimate partner violence and related issues might be potentially traumatic for respondents. The field staff felt that asking such questions might be considered unethical, given their lack of psychological therapeutic training and dearth of services available. A number of the investigative team concurred, and the proposed questions were never added. In contrast, using ethnographic methods to discuss intimate violence was not ethically problematic. The research participants actively sought the company of the ethnographer to discuss their personal concerns over violence in their lives. This occurred in the context of warm, long-term friendship relationships in their natural environment. It sometimes led to improved self-protective behaviours on the part of the women.

By the end of the second year, the epidemiologic project documented an elevated rate of seroconversion among women compared to men (34.4% versus 23.4%), but this association did not reach statistical significance, possibly due to the inadequate number of seroconverters (approximately 27 seroconversions per year). We searched the epidemiologic survey for proxy variables for the social dynamics that were being documented ethnographically. One factor we were able to document was an age differential in sexual partnerships (i.e., men older than women). Also documented was a biologically implausible predictor of HCV seroconversion in the survey data, i.e. having a sexual partner who is an injection drug user, despite the current understanding that hepatitis C is very rarely sexually transmitted. This same biologically implausible association has also been reported in the literature on other large epidemiologic studies of HCV seroconversion (Miller et al. 2002). We were able to draw on our qualitative data to identify this finding as being a proxy variable reflecting gender power dynamics in romantic or sexually active dyadic relationships generally permeated by violence, jealousy and control.

This case study highlights one of the multiple challenges of integrating theory and methods into a social epidemiology of risk. The association between being a woman and HCV risk was tenuous and difficult to document through the quantitative data, despite the overwhelming qualitative evidence of the young women being at consistently more elevated risk then young men immediately upon entering the street scene. How can this lack of concordance between the two approaches be explained? One explanation is that variables that measure significant social power categories (such as gender and race/ethnicity) are highly correlated with many other variables and behaviours; therefore, it is difficult to disentangle them from other closely related variables. This is further complicated by the fact that significant power categories often have contradictory effects on risk. In certain contexts they can be protective and in others risk-enhancing. As an example, a woman in a relationship with an older, violent, highly controlling male who forbids her to inject with others may be both protected by the power relationship (in that the size of the pool of people she injects with shrinks) and put at risk by that same violent power relationship (if the male partner is infected with hepatitis C and controls all aspects of injecting). The complexity of overlapping disjunctive risks and vectors propelled by social dynamics may explain the often contradictory findings across studies and within studies around the category of gender and sexuality in the United States (e.g., Bourgois 2002; Bourgois et al. 2004; Collier et al. 1998; Strathdee et al. 2001; Hahn et al. 2001). These inconsistent quantitative findings illustrate the utility of introducing the social science concept of "social structural plausibility" in conjunction with that of biological plausibility and statistical association (Auerbach 2009).

A second explanation for the lack of concordance rests in the differing aims and methodological foci of the epidemiologic and ethnographic components of the research. The stated aims of the quantitative research were to find behavioural differences between those active injectors who became infected with hepatitis C and those who did not. Within this framework, an ideal outcome would have been to discover a significant association between seroconversion and a specific injecting practice, leading to an individualized behavioural intervention that would assist individual injectors to avoid infection. By contrast, the ethnographic research was inherently more oriented toward exploring and describing structural risks – in this case, the complex interplay between gender power roles and the normalization of romantic violence and seroconversion described above. It is, therefore, perhaps unsurprising that the micro-practice-oriented quantitative data did not speak well to the broader structural issues emerging from the qualitative data.

Large-scale epidemiologic projects also have what might be termed a "logistic inertia." Statistical methods usually hinge on testing specified hypotheses, which, in turn, tend to require large sample sizes to produce statistically significant outcomes. As such, re-purposing a quantitative study in midstream to respond to emerging findings requires a fundamental re-design of the study. In anticipation of this logistical inertia, the co-investigators and project directors of the ethnographic arms of the study held discussions during the grant writing phase before beginning the study to develop one neutral, quantifiable question about whether respondents had "pooled money with others to buy drugs to inject." This question tested an anthropological hypothesis about the risk imposed by the reciprocal obligations for paraphernalia sharing imposed by the "moral economy" of drug exchanges (Bourgois 1998). This variable had no biological meaning, in that pooling money in itself cannot result in the transmission of a bloodborne virus, but it did have clear connections to the social contexts in which paraphernalia sharing can occur. Interestingly, this variable was one of only four variables independently associated with HCV seroconversion in multivariate analysis (Hahn et al. 2002).

The overarching pragmatic lesson from this collaborative study was that planning for mixed-methods studies must go beyond the boilerplate text now often used to justify such collaborations on grant proposals and must assume from the beginning of the study that both qualitative and quantitative processes *will* generate observations that can be tested or explored by the other. As such, thought needs to be given to *how* this will be carried out, for instance, through regular meetings, circulation of fieldwork notes and preliminary statistical analyses, development of proxy variables, additional targeted sampling and so on.

10.4.3 Case Study Three: Structural Violence, Power and HIV Prevention Among Female and Transgendered Sex Workers in an Urban Setting

Data were drawn from a multi-methods, community-based research study (2005–2008) in partnership with a local sex work agency in Vancouver, Canada.

This study was developed as a community-based research partnership between an academic institution and a local sex work agency to examine the factors shaping HIV prevention among street-based sex workers over a 2-year period (Shannon et al. 2007). The study was conceived as a multi-methods study using a participatory action research approach, including an open prospective cohort (interview-administered research questionnaire and HIV screening at baseline and semi-annual follow-up visits over a 2-year period), social mapping completed alongside each questionnaire study visit and purposive sampling for qualitative in-depth interviews with a subset of the study sample (street-based sex workers). The study was purposefully designed to integrate a team of current and former sex workers as "peer researchers." This team of peer researchers served as both key informants or experts and research facilitators. They were involved in content and questionnaire development and facilitation and interpretation of results, together with the academic research team. Their lived experience as sex workers and sometimes inconsistent consumers of public health messages provided critical "insider" insight into the complexities and dynamics shaping HIV prevention in the street-based sex industry.

Within Vancouver, Canada, as in many other international settings, the buying and selling of sex is legal, and yet criminal sanctions exist around most aspects of sex work (such as communicating and soliciting in public spaces, operating a brothel and living off the avails of prostitution). This study contributes to the growing literature on how enforcement of criminal sanctions facilitates the exacerbation of "risk." Specifically, despite substantial program availability of HIV prevention resources in the inner city community of Vancouver (an area known as the Downtown Eastside), this study's findings collectively revealed how structural violence mediates individual agency, reducing the capacity of sex workers to access resources and negotiate risk reduction (Shannon et al. 2008a). Our analyses of narratives drew on the risk environment framework (Rhodes 2002) and theoretical constructs of violence and power that emphasize the interconnectedness of interpersonal (Scheper-Hughes 1996; Bourgois et al. 2004), structural (Farmer 2004) and symbolic (Epele 2002; Bourdieu 2001) violence. We drew on a broad understanding of power and agency, building on earlier ethnographic studies (Bourgois 1998; Wojcicki 2002; Wojcicki and Malala 2001), which explored ways in which sex workers' decision making and interpersonal risk negotiations might be rational, economic coping strategies in the face of social and structural violence. This relational understanding of power is developed in post-structural feminist critiques of institutionalized forms of social control and the discursive production and regulation of sexuality (Foucault 1981; Nencel 2001; Weedon 1987). At the micro level, the ubiquitous "everyday violence" of "bad dates" (i.e., violent clients) intersected with a discourse of disposal of symbolic violence and a lack of legal recourse to violence at a macro level in forcing sex workers to prioritize the immediate threat of violence over the negotiation of condom use with clients. At the meso level, local policing and enforcement of criminal sanctions (such as legal restrictions on working indoors) affected sex workers' control over dates and their ability to negotiate HIV risk reduction, both directly through the threat of police violence, harassment and coercion and indirectly through displacement to isolated public spaces and lack of access to safer indoor spaces to service clients.

This study's qualitative work was conducted by the same team members in parallel with social mapping and baseline quantitative data collection and helped inform questionnaire development and subsequent social epidemiologic constructs, theory and analyses that provided empirical confirmation of the qualitative findings. For example, social epidemiologic analyses using mapping and questionnaire data revealed a geographic correlation between physical areas of avoidance due to violence and police harassment and the health access core (i.e., the area with the highest concentration of services and resources for vulnerable populations), which resulted in displacement of sex workers to outlying, isolated areas away from health and harm reduction resources (Shannon et al. 2008a). The use of mixed methods allowed us to elucidate the social meanings ascribed to place among sex workers that initially emerged from the qualitative interviews and to explore and map the empirical associations with HIV risk. For example, analyses of mapping data using geographic information systems (GIS) combined with questionnaire responses identified geographic clustering (or "hotspots") of coercive, unprotected sex by clients among sex workers working in isolated public spaces compared to main streets and commercial areas (Shannon et al. 2009b). In multivariate analyses, adjusting for potential confounding effects of individual and interpersonal factors, structural factors, including enforced displacement, servicing clients in cars or public spaces and client-perpetrated violence, were independently associated with reduced ability to negotiate condom use among sex workers (Shannon et al. 2009a, b). The construct of structural police violence identified in qualitative studies by ourselves and others (Rhodes et al. 2008) emerged as being directly related to elevated likelihood of rape and client-perpetrated violence among sex workers (Shannon et al. 2009a, b). This study moved forward the importance of analysing the relational and gendered negotiation of condom use in HIV prevention studies with sex workers rather than relying on an overly simplistic construct of "unprotected sex" coded as a binary variable at the individual level in traditional epidemiologic analyses. This study also underlined the importance of upstream contextual factors in the casual pathway to gendered condom negotiation and subsequent risk for HIV transmission.

These results document how structural and everyday violence mediate the negotiation process of condom use and other risk reduction practices among sex workers, resulting in a heightened risk of HIV transmission. At the same time, the lived experiences of sex workers documented from the qualitative research articulate how certain risky sexual and drug use practices are rational coping strategies in the face of large scale social and structural violence and, as such, highlight the importance of active inclusion of sex workers' experiences in redefining prevention policies and programmes. For example, sex workers describe how informal self-regulation mechanisms (e.g., prices charged for dates) can help promote a work culture of condom use, underscoring the importance of enhanced structural support for sex work collectives (e.g., networks, unions) in regulating safer industry practices. This initial work is now being tested through social cohesion measures in follow-up questionnaires. Adopting a social epidemiologic approach that combines qualitative, mapping and quantitative data sources helped us to capture the complexity of the daily lived experiences of sex workers in informing a re-conceptualized HIV prevention response and move beyond individual-level strategies. These results point to a critical need for safer environment interventions (e.g., managed sex work zones and safer indoor work spaces) and structural policy support (e.g., legal reforms, sex work collectivism and empowerment) in stemming violence and, in turn, facilitating an "enabling environment" for condom negotiation in the sex industry.

10.4.4 Case Study Four: HIV Risk in the Context of Deportation: The Modifying Role of Gender

These data were drawn from a prospective epidemiologic study of injection drug users in Tijuana, Mexico (2006–2008) that employed quantitative survey data supplemented by subsequent in-depth qualitative interviews.

The initial study was a classically designed, epidemiologic study examining HIV risks among male and female IDUs in Tijuana, Mexico. Baseline data from this study were examined in a logistic regression model to identify correlates of HIV infection, through which a significant association was found between HIV risk and years spent living in Tijuana (Strathdee et al. 2008b). Further exploration showed that this association was modified by gender (Strathdee et al. 2008a). Females who had lived in Tijuana longer had higher HIV risk; whereas, among males, the converse was true (shorter time periods lived in Tijuana were associated with greater HIV risk). Since this finding was counterintuitive, additional descriptive analyses were conducted to study the motivations for moving to Tijuana by gender. This revealed that most females moved to Tijuana voluntarily, primarily for reasons associated with employment or family. In contrast, males were primarily involuntary migrants, with the most common reason for living in Tijuana being deportation from the United States (i.e., 55% of male migrants were deportees). Indeed, further logistic regression models revealed that deportation explained the association between shorter time span lived in Tijuana for males and higher HIV risk. From an epidemiologic perspective, the question remained: how does deportation create an elevated risk for HIV among males? Is it a marker for a high-risk subset of male migrants who became HIV-infected in the United States prior to deportation? Or is deportation a true risk factor for HIV infection, representing a destabilizing force that disrupts social networks and creating economic and social vulnerabilities? In either case, research strategies employing a strictly epidemiologic perspective had reached their limit in terms of being able to identify how these sociopolitical forces were influencing HIV risk either directly or indirectly.

To explore these questions in more depth, subsequent studies were undertaken that drew from a social science perspective, both methodologically and theoretically, to "scale up" our understanding of the observed statistical association between deportation and HIV risk among men to consider the sociopolitical context in which HIV risk is produced. Methodologically, the studies were qualitative in nature, employing in-depth interviews to help "unpack" deportation as a construct among male drug injectors (Ojeda et al. 2010). In-depth interviews among male deportees explored themes of social isolation, stigma, unemployment, limited access to health and social services and cultural identity. Pre-deportation influences included social factors (e.g., friends and/or family and post-migration stressors) and environmental factors (e.g., drug availability) that were perceived to contribute to substance use initiation in the United States. Post-deportation experiences pointed to the role of shame and loss of familial, social and economic support that exacerbated drug use and led to a sense of hopelessness and despair. From a theoretical perspective, the research identified deportation and United States-Mexico relations as a form of structural violence – a macro-level change in the risk environment that arises as a result of sociopolitical and cultural forces. This research provides a rich context for understanding the interplay between deportation and HIV risk in a manner that moves beyond the identification of statistical associations signifying individual-level "risk factors" into a depiction of the structural and environmental context in which bi-national politics, economic opportunity (or lack thereof) and sociocultural factors produce a system of structural violence that elevates HIV risk for certain individuals. Through the integration of epidemiologic and social science methods into a "social epidemiology of deportation," this research also suggests multilevel targets for intervention. At a micro level, it suggests the need to implement supportive services for deportees. At a macro level, it points to the need to examine factors such as the United States' health and immigration policies and whether they are working at odds.

10.5   Discussion

Conventional public health interventions and research primarily target individuals by promoting behaviour change through imparting knowledge, skills, motivation and/or empowerment using a cognitive model of rational choice theory in medical decision making. There is a growing recognition in the fields of public health and medicine, however, of the ways social inequality imposes risk on vulnerable population groups. This recognition is informed by an acknowledgement that a larger "risk environment" precedes and influences individual decision making (Rhodes 2002, 2009). In the case studies presented above, we have highlighted how a behavioural science perspective focused solely on individual-level constructs often fails to recognize the broader sociocultural and structural political economic framework in which risk behaviour occurs. A failure to incorporate an appreciation for socioeconomic and cultural context in public health research often also fails to uncover causal pathways. Moreover, it tends towards the design of primarily individual-level interventions that, at best, have limited impact and, at worst, result in victim blaming or further harm to already vulnerable individuals. These case studies advocate for the use of an approach that integrates social science and epidemiologic methods to enable a focus on social inequality at the local level while avoiding the tendency to individualize risk. It also offers a way to understand the *reciprocal relationships* between political-economic structures and the internalization and embodiment of vulnerability and harm. Social science concepts emerging as especially useful in the development of social epidemiologic approaches include: the Marxist structural violence framework (Farmer 2010); theories of "structuration" (Giddens 1984), including the "logics of everyday practice" (Bourdieu 1977, 1990); the destructive effects of "symbolic violence" (whereby socially vulnerable populations come to accept their location in an oppressive social hierarchy that imposes risky practices on them for which they blame themselves) (Bourdieu 2000, 2001); and Foucault's (1995) approach to discursive power and subjectification.

10.5.1   Structural Vulnerability

We propose that a "social epidemiology of HIV risk vulnerability" can elucidate the ways *structural violence* (Scheper-Hughes 1996; Farmer 2004; Galtung 1969) and *structural vulnerability* (Quesada et al. 2011) within the *risk environment* (Rhodes 2002, 2009) affect the health of individuals within distinctly patterned population groups and social contexts. The term "vulnerability" refers to a location in a social structure that makes an individual of a particular group prone to suffering from the effects of structural violence. It opens a linear, structural political economy analysis to broader theoretical domains to address the individual embodiment of the cultural, psychodynamic, symbolic and discursive dimensions of power. This is especially important in our contemporary historical moment because it counteracts the rhetoric of blame that creeps inadvertently into individualized approaches to behaviour change. A critical theoretical analysis of how larger structural and/or cultural forces shape intimate ways of being in the world also de-legitimizes punitive approaches targeted towards stigmatized populations, such as drug users and sex workers. Structural vulnerability thus draws attention to the larger upstream forces and processes that place specific population groups at a disadvantage for health and well-being by highlighting the biological and embodied effects of economic, social, gender and racial discriminations. It draws attention to how the embodied suffering of particular population groups is not only historically located but also reproduced through every day cultural practices interacting with the repressive effects of state policies.

One critique of political economy perspectives is that they *underplay* agency, positioning individuals as largely passive in their complicity to "structural determinants." The relationship between individuals and their environments is ongoing and reciprocal. Risk environments constrain how agency is enabled, but they are at once also a product and adaptation of agency. It is critical that social epidemiologic approaches capture the dynamism of the reciprocity of individual-environmental interactions. Risk environments thus feature in a process of what Giddens has termed *structuration* (Giddens 1984). Structuration posits that structure is not "external" to individuals, for the "constitution of agents and structures are not two independently given sets of phenomena, a dualism, but represent a duality" (Giddens 1984). This means that "social systems are both medium and outcome of the practices they recursively organise" and that structure is "not to be equated with constraint but is always both constraining and enabling" (Giddens 1984). Foucault

(1981) would refer to this as the "positive" effects of power and would identify them as processes of "subjectification." Bourdieu (2000) might identify this dynamic as a process of "habitus formation." We, therefore, caution against models of risk environment that perpetuate dichotomous models of "structure" and "agency." We see risk environments as capacitating individuals to act according to particular kinds of *habitus*, wherein socially acquired practices and habits are reproduced iteratively, and often unconsciously, through every day practices (Bourdieu 1977, 1990) that also incorporate processes of governmentality and the positive effects of power (Foucault 1981). Risk environments, then, are embodied through *participation*, through ways of being in the world and of understanding the ethics of self-formation or subjectivity.

The concept of vulnerability implicates social conditions and is intended to transcend the conceptualization of "at risk populations" (as the Vancouver case study emphasizes with respect to condom negotiations by vulnerable sex workers) in which individuals engage in risky practices with an accompanying connotation of individual guilt (e.g., Quesada et al. 2011; Hernandez-Rosete et al. 2005; Rocha 2006). As Bronfman et al. (2002) note, "while risk points to a probability and evokes an individual behaviour, vulnerability is an indicator of inequity and social inequality and demands responses in the sphere of the social and political structure. It is considered that vulnerability determines the differential risks and should therefore be what is acted upon." Vulnerability is produced as the outcome of position in a hierarchical social order and a network of power relationships that constrain agency. Structural positioning influences personal decision making, limits life options and frames choices. It also determines how vulnerable populations make sense of their ailments and afflictions. Structural vulnerability is both a "space of vulnerability" (Rocha 2006) and an "embodiment of social hierarchy;" it is a "space that configure(s) a specific set of conditions in which people live, and sets constraints on how these conditions are perceived, how goals are prioritized, what sorts of actions and responses might seem appropriate, and which ones are possible" (Bronfman et al. 2002 as cited in Quesada et al. 2011). As an embodiment of social hierarchy, risk taking can be understood as the result of forms of violence enacted through cultural rationales and managed through modes of governmentality, often in a social milieu and political context of marked indifference to those afflicted (Watts and Bohle 1993).

Our case studies dealt with the gendering of risk as one, often core, way of exploring the structuration of vulnerability to HIV and related infectious diseases. They also examined the ways embodied distress at the individual level is shaped by criminalization and law enforcement, in this instance, through everyday street-level policing practices in Vancouver, Russia and Serbia that may, themselves, structure risk differentially by gender. Gender is particularly interesting because of the multiple and complex ways it articulates, with distinct material forces, cultural values, individual practices and political policies (including immigration and law enforcement), and it becomes a primary vector for structural violence. The Tijuana case is illuminative because it suggests that males and females are differentially propelled across the United States/Mexico border by subsistence crisis as well as by immigration and/or deportation law enforcement, resulting in HIV risk taking across gender divides. The San Francisco case demonstrates the gendered, dissonant patterns to subjectification effects of normalized romantic violence against women. The Russia and Serbia case study highlights how day-to-day policing practices targeting the vulnerable induce an internalized state of oppression illness characterized by a subjectivity of fear that not only limits HIV prevention capacity but that reproduces and reinforces wider social, gender and racial inequalities in these societies.

10.5.2 Mixing Method and Theory

Our case studies employed different approaches to the use of mixed methods for documenting and analyzing complex social structural dynamics. Thus, in addition to the heightened understanding engendered by the integration of theoretical approaches, these case studies also illustrate both the challenges and added benefit of integrating the methodological approaches that are hallmarks of the disciplines. For example, the San Francisco case study illustrates the limitations of using probabilistic statistical analysis based on quantifiable individual-level variables to measure higher order social and cultural dynamics because variables that reflect social structural power relations, by definition, interface with multiple confounding and risky practices. The same gendered logics that normalize violence against women can sometimes prevent them from taking risks with other infected injectors. The jealous dyadic relationships that isolate them socially can be protective or toxic depending on the serostatus of the dominating partner. Simply describing a statistical association between HCV incidence and gender in San Francisco failed to describe the complicated structural and social processes that influenced this association. It was through the added contribution of in-depth ethnographic work that we were able to unpack the mechanisms behind the observed statistical pattern. In the Tijuana case, the initially counterintuitive statistical associations served as an inspiration for both additional quantitative analyses and a new qualitative component to the study that was designed to explore and contextualize the findings. In the Vancouver case, simultaneous implementation of geographic mapping, quantitative and qualitative data collection capitalized on local knowledge of study participants to explain the relationships between HIV vulnerability, social meanings and the built environment.

It is important to note that the San Francisco, Vancouver and Tijuana case studies each used a different mix of cross methodological dialogue, revealing the flexibilities of mixing methods. As the field of public health research increasingly adopts mixed-methods designs in order to capitalize on their ability to broaden and contextualize our understanding of complex multilevel influences on health, more researchers will face the challenge of successfully synthesizing data derived from multiple sources and methods. While integration of data from various sources is often stated as a goal of mixed-methods designs, both epistemological and methodological barriers to such integration have been identified (Bourgois 2002; Moss 2003; Bryman

2007). Synthesis and integration, however, does not require absolute agreement between data generated through different methods; the integration of mixed-methods results may, in fact, provide a sum that is greater than the individual qualitative and quantitative parts (Mason 2006; Bryman 2007). In the case studies presented here, we have demonstrated how ethnographic and qualitative methods can be used to develop and refine epidemiologic research questions in order to quantify associations that were observed in the field (Case Study Two) or to begin to understand the mechanisms behind counterintuitive associations detected through quantitative analyses (Case Study Four). A particular challenge facing mixed-methods design is the difficulty inherent in distilling broad social or cultural constructs down into variables that can be measured using epidemiologic approaches. A second challenge is to make the shift from deterministic, linear models to a greater emphasis on the dynamic systems in which individuals are embedded. Systems thinking requires an attention to the interactions, processes and, often contradictory, feedback loops inherent in complex social and environmental systems (Strathdee et al. 2010).

10.6 Conclusions

Bringing the concepts of structural violence, structural vulnerability and risk environment into the basic lexicon of social epidemiology would revitalize our subdiscipline's distinguished mid-nineteenth century historical roots. As Rudolf Virchow, one of the discipline's founders (who was trained as a physician, an anthropologist and as a pathologist) wrote about his experience with the typhus epidemic of 1847–1848 in Upper Silesia: "Medical statistics will be our standard of measurement: we will weigh life for life and see where the dead line thicker among the workers or among the privileged" (Taylor and Rieger 1984). The very real consequences of structural vulnerability are shorter lives subject to a disproportionate load of suffering. Recognizing the analytical terms structural violence and structural vulnerability within the risk environment is only a first step for the challenge of a critical social epidemiology that moves beyond the classroom, the laboratory and the clinic to develop upstream interventions that impact larger populations who are systematically subject to risk taking because of their subordinated status in society.

Already many public health and medical schools have instituted curricula to address "socially vulnerable populations" (King and Wheeler 2007). The paradigm of structural violence and structural vulnerability within a concrete risk environment extends this focus by linking health, political economy, culture and subjectivity to re-conceive risk as a structural outcome. Methodologically, it draws upon "thick" qualitative descriptions and critical analysis of the quantifiable relationship between risk taking and specific relations of power (Doyle 1979; Bourgois et al. 2004; Singer 2001). Despite the danger of reification inherent in any diagnostic tool, we envision that a clinical or public health outreach translation of structural vulnerability might take the form of administering screening protocols in clinics and on the street or in social service or carceral settings (Quesada et al. 2011). The goal would be to widen the public health gaze towards an awareness of the embodied effects of social positioning in order to legitimize the allocation of increased resources (medical, social service and political) to the disenfranchised in the name of public health and to improve the quality of outreach services and care for the poor in the name of "best medical practices," "public health efficacy" and "evidence-based practice." It is not only a matter of training and sensitizing individual researchers and outreach workers to "see" risky individuals as structurally vulnerable but also a question of establishing viable institutional practices for health practitioners. Insisting that both health practitioners and the systems they work within include structural vulnerability as an etiological agent promoting risk taking pushes public health and medicine to extend their purview towards becoming more fully social as well as towards recognizing health as a fundamental human right.

References

Auerbach J (2009) Transforming social structures and environments to help in HIV prevention. Health Aff (Millwood) 28:1655–1665

Biehl JG, Good B, Kleinman A (2007) Subjectivity: ethnographic investigations. University of California Press, Berkeley

Bobrik A, Danishevski K, Eroshina K et al (2005) Prison health in Russia: the larger picture. J Public Health Policy 26:30–59

Bourdieu P (1977) Outline of a theory of practice. Cambridge University Press, Cambridge

Bourdieu P (1990) The logic of practice. Stanford University Press, Stanford

Bourdieu P (2000) Pascalian meditations. Stanford University Press, Stanford

Bourdieu P (2001) Masculine domination. Stanford University Press, Stanford

Bourgois P (1995) In search of respect: selling crack in El Barrio. Cambridge University Press, Cambridge

Bourgois P (1998) The moral economies of homeless heroin addicts: confronting ethnography, HIV risk, and everyday violence in San Francisco shooting encampments. Subst Use Misuse 33:2323–2351

Bourgois P (2002) Anthropology and epidemiology on drugs: the challenges of cross-methodological and theoretical dialogue. Int J Drug Policy 13:259–269

Bourgois P (2003) Crack and the political economy of suffering. Addict Res Theory 11:31–37

Bourgois P, Schonberg J (2009) Righteous dopefiend. University of California Press, Berkeley

Bourgois P, Prince B, Moss A (2004) Everyday violence and the gender of hepatitis C among homeless drug-injecting youth in San Francisco. Hum Organ 63:253–264

Bronfman MN, Leyva R, Negroni MJ et al (2002) Mobile populations and HIV/AIDS in Central America and Mexico: research for action. AIDS 16(Suppl 3):S42–S49

Bryman A (2007) Barriers to integrating quantitative and qualitative research. J Mix Methods Res 1:8–22

Butler J (1997) The psychic life of power: theories in subjection. Stanford University Press, Stanford

Collier K, Kotranski L, Semaan S et al (1998) Correlates of HIV seropositivity and HIV testing among out-of-treatment drug users. Am J Drug Alcohol Abuse 24:377–393

Cooper HL, Bossak B, Tempalski B et al (2009) Geographic approaches to quantifying the risk environment: drug-related law enforcement and access to syringe exchange programmes. Int J Drug Policy 20:217–226

Copenhaver MM, Johnson BT, Lee IC et al (2006) Behavioral HIV risk reduction among people who inject drugs: meta-analytic evidence of efficacy. J Subst Abuse Treat 31:163–171

Doyle L (1979) The political economy of health. Pluto Press, London

Duff C (2007) Towards a theory of drug use contexts: space, embodiment and practice. Addict Res Theory 15:503–519

Engels F (1892) The condition of the working-class in England 1844. Swan Sonnenschein, London

Epele ME (2002) Gender, violence and HIV: women's survival in the streets. Cult Med Psychiatry 26:33–54

Farmer P (1999) Infections and inequalities: the modern plagues. University of California Press, Berkeley

Farmer P (2004) An anthropology of structural violence. Curr Anthropol 45:305–325

Farmer P (2009) "Landmine boy" and the tomorrow of violence. In: Rylko-Bauer B, Whiteford L, Farmer P (eds) Global health in times of violence: school for Advanced Research Advanced Seminar Series. School for Advanced Research Press, Santa Fe

Farmer P (2010) Partner to the poor: a Paul Farmer reader. University of California Press, Berkeley

Farmer P, Connors M, Simmons J (1996) Women, poverty, and AIDS: sex, drugs, and structural violence. Common Courage Press, Monroe

Foucault M (1981) Power/knowledge: selected interviews and other writings, 1972–1977. Pantheon/Random House, New York

Foucault M (1995) Discipline and punish: the birth of the prison. Vintage Books, New York

Friedman SR, Cooper HL, Tempalski B et al (2006) Relationships of deterrence and law enforcement to drug-related harms among drug injectors in US metropolitan areas. AIDS 20:93–99

Galea S, Vlahov D (2002) Social determinants and the health of drug users: socioeconomic status, homelessness, and incarceration. Public Health Rep 117(Suppl 1):S135–S145

Galtung J (1969) Violence, peace, and peace research. J Peace Res 6:167–191

Galtung J (1990) Cultural violence. J Peace Res 27:291–305

Giddens A (1984) The constitution of society: outline of the theory of structuration. University of California Press, Berkeley

Green TC, Grau LE, Blinnikova KN et al (2009) Social and structural aspects of the overdose risk environment in St. Petersburg, Russia. Int J Drug Policy 20:270–276

Hahn JA, Page-Shafer K, Lum P et al (2001) Hepatitis C virus infection and needle exchange use among young injection drug users in San Francisco. Hepatology 34:180–187

Hahn JA, Page-Shafer K, Lum PJ et al (2002) Hepatitis C virus seroconversion among young injection drug users: relationships and risks. J Infect Dis 186:1558–1564

Jurgens R, Csete J, Amon JJ et al (2010) People who use drugs, HIV, and human rights. Lancet 376:475–485

King T, Wheeler B (2007) Medical management of vulnerable and underserved patients: principles, practice, and populations. McGraw-Hill, New York

Kleinman AJK (1991) Suffering and its professional transformation. Cult Med Psychiatry 15:275–301

Kleinman A, Das V, Lock MM (1997) Social suffering. University of California Press, Berkeley

Krieger N (1994) Epidemiology and the web of causation – has anyone seen the spider? Soc Sci Med 39:887–903

Krieger N (2001) Theories for social epidemiology in the 21st century: an ecosocial perspective. Int J Epidemiol 30:668–677

Krieger N (2008) Proximal, distal, and the politics of causation: what's level got to do with it? Am J Public Health 98:221

Martinez H-R D, Hernandez GS, Villafuerte BP et al (2005) Del riesgo a la vulnerabilidad. Bases metodológicas para comprender la relación entre violencia sexual e infección por VIH/ITS en migrantes clandestinos. Salud Ment 28:20–26, Spanish

Mason J (2006) Six strategies for mixing methods and integrating data in social science research. University of Manchester, Manchester

Miller CL, Johnston C, Spittal PM et al (2002) Opportunities for prevention: hepatitis C prevalence and incidence in a cohort of young injection drug users. Hepatology 36:737–742

Moore D (2004) Governing street-based injecting drug users: a critique of heroin overdose prevention in Australia. Soc Sci Med 59:1547

Moss A (2003) Put down that shield and war rattle: response to Philippe Bourgois. Int J Drug Policy 14:105–109

Navarro V, Mutaner C (2004) Political and economic determinants of population health and well-being: controversies and developments. Baywood Publishing Company, Amityville

Nencel L (2001) Ethnography and prostitution in Peru. Pluto Press, London

Ojeda VD, Robertson AM, Hiller SP et al (2010) A qualitative view of drug use behaviors of Mexican male injection drug users deported from the United States. J Urban Health 88:104–117

Pine A (2008) Working hard, drinking hard: on violence and survival in Honduras. University of California Press, Berkeley

Pollini RA, Brouwer KC, Lozada RM et al (2008) Syringe possession arrests are associated with receptive syringe sharing in two Mexico-US border cities. Addiction 103:101–108

Quesada J, Hart L, Bourgois P (2011) Structural vulnerability and the health of Latino migrant laborers. Med Anthropol 30:339–362

Rhodes T (2002) The 'risk environment': a framework for understanding and reducing drug-related harm. Int J Drug Policy 13:85–94

Rhodes T (2009) Risk environments and drug harms: a social science for harm reduction approach. Int J Drug Policy 20:193–201

Rhodes T, Mikhailova L, Sarang A et al (2003) Situational factors influencing drug injecting, risk reduction and syringe exchange in Togliatti City, Russian Federation: a qualitative study of micro risk environment. Soc Sci Med 57:39–54

Rhodes T, Judd A, Mikhailova L et al (2004) Injecting equipment sharing among injecting drug users in Togliatti City, Russian Federation: maximizing the protective effects of syringe distribution. J Acquir Immune Defic Syndr 35:293–300

Rhodes T, Singer M, Bourgois P et al (2005) The social structural production of HIV risk among injecting drug users. Soc Sci Med 61:1026–1044

Rhodes T, Simic M, Baros S et al (2008) Police violence and sexual risk among female and transvestite sex workers in Serbia: qualitative study. BMJ 337:a908

Rocha JL (2006) AIDS and migrants: a perverse association. Revista Envio 303

Sarang A, Rhodes T, Platt L et al (2006) Drug injecting and syringe use in the HIV risk environment of Russian penitentiary institutions: qualitative study. Addiction 101:1787–1796

Sarang A, Rhodes T, Sheon N et al (2010) Policing drug users in Russia: risk, fear, and structural violence. Subst Use Misuse 45:813–864

Scheper-Hughes N (1996) Small wars and invisible genocides. Soc Sci Med 43:889–900

Shannon K, Bright V, Allinott S et al (2007) Community-based HIV prevention research among substance-using women in survival sex work: the Maka Project Partnership. Harm Reduct J 4:20

Shannon K, Kerr T, Allinott S et al (2008a) Social and structural violence and power relations in mitigating HIV risk of drug-using women in survival sex work. Soc Sci Med 66:911–921

Shannon K, Rusch M, Shoveller J et al (2008b) Mapping violence and policing as an environmental-structural barrier to health service and syringe availability among substance-using women in street-level sex work. Int J Drug Policy 19:140–147

Shannon K, Kerr T, Strathdee SA et al (2009a) Prevalence and structural correlates of gender based violence among a prospective cohort of female sex workers. BMJ 339:b2939

Shannon K, Strathdee SA, Shoveller J et al (2009b) Structural and environmental barriers to condom use negotiation with clients among female sex workers: implications for HIV-prevention strategies and policy. Am J Public Health 99:659–665

Singer M (2001) Toward a bio-cultural and political economic integration of alcohol, tobacco and drug studies in the coming century. Soc Sci Med 53:199–213

Singer M (2004) The social origins and expressions of illness. Br Med Bull 69:9–16

Small W, Kerr T, Charette J et al (2006) Impacts of intensified police activity on injection drug users: evidence from an ethnographic investigation. Int J Drug Policy 17:85–95

Strathdee S, Galai N, Safaiean M et al (2001) Sex differences in risk factors for HIV seroconversion among injection drug users: a 10-year perspective. Arch Intern Med 161:1281–1288

Strathdee SA, Lozada R, Ojeda VD et al (2008a) Differential effects of migration and deportation on HIV infection among male and female injection drug users in Tijuana, Mexico. PLoS One 3:e2690

Strathdee SA, Lozada R, Pollini RA et al (2008b) Individual, social, and environmental influences associated with HIV infection among injection drug users in Tijuana, Mexico. J Acquir Immune Defic Syndr 47:369–376

Strathdee SA, Hallett TB, Bobrova N et al (2010) HIV and risk environment for injecting drug users: the past, present, and future. Lancet 376:268–284

Taylor R, Rieger A (1984) Rudolf Virchow on the typhus epidemic in Upper Silesia. Sociol Health Illn 6:201–217

Walter N, Bourgois P, Loinaz M (2004) Masculinity and undocumented labor migration: injured Latino day laborers in San Francisco. Soc Sci Med 59:1159–1168

Watts M, Bohle HG (1993) The Space of vulnerability: the causal structure of hunger and famine. Prog Hum Geogr 17:67

Weedon C (1987) Feminist practice and poststructural theory. Blackwell Publishers, Oxford

Wojcicki JM (2002) Commercial sex work or ukuphanda? Sex-for-money exchange in Soweto and Hammanskraal Area, South Africa. Cult Med Psychiatry 26:339–370

Wojcicki JM, Malala J (2001) Condom use, power and HIV/AIDS risk: sex-workers bargain for survival in Hillbrow/Joubert Park/Berea, Johannesburg. Soc Sci Med 53:99–121

Chapter 11
Realist Review Methods for Complex Health Problems

Maritt Kirst and Patricia O'Campo

Contents

11.1 Introduction 232
11.2 A "Realist" Approach to Systematic Review 233
11.3 A Realist Systematic Review of Intimate Partner Violence
Screening Programs 236
11.4 The Utility of Realist Review: A Comparison of Review
Findings on Intimate Partner Violence Screening Programs 239
11.5 Challenges in Conducting Realist Review 241
11.6 Discussion and Conclusion 242
References 243

Abstract Social epidemiologists are undertaking research to understand an increasingly complex set of social factors and processes given the complicated health problems encountered today. Systematic reviews are powerful tools to assess the effectiveness of interventions by utilizing a transparent and rigorous method for summarizing and synthesizing the existing research literature. In light of the increasing complexity of health problems and interventions to address these problems, their subsequent evaluation must not only explore the magnitude of the interventions' impact but must also include an examination of underlying intervention theory in order to fully assess effectiveness. Drawing on an example from our work synthesizing evidence on intimate partner violence screening programs, we argue in

M. Kirst (✉)
Ontario Tobacco Research Unit, Dalla Lana School of Public Health, University of Toronto,
155 College Street, 5th floor, Toronto, ON M5T 3M7, Canada
e-mail: maritt.kirst@utoronto.ca

P. O'Campo
Centre for Research on Inner City Health, St. Michael's Hospital, 30 Bond Street,
Toronto, ON M5B 1W8, Canada
e-mail: O'CampoP@smh.ca

P. O'Campo and J.R. Dunn (eds.), *Rethinking Social Epidemiology:*
Towards a Science of Change, DOI 10.1007/978-94-007-2138-8_11,
© Springer Science+Business Media B.V. 2012

this chapter for greater adoption of systematic review methods informed by realist philosophy in the field of social epidemiology. Such research methods are important tools for the identification of key intervention mechanisms and contextual effects in the comprehensive evaluation of interventions that will inform the development of solutions to complex health problems.

Abbreviations

IPV   Intimate partner violence
RCT   Randomized controlled trial

11.1   Introduction

Social epidemiologists are undertaking research to understand an increasingly complex set of social factors and processes given the level of complexity of health problems encountered today (Kaplan 2004). This complexity relates to health as affected by a variety of social, political and economic factors simultaneously. Health interventions that try to address these determinants are by necessity complex, constituting a variety of interconnected program components that render them difficult to evaluate (Egan et al. 2009; Gamble 2008; Paterson et al. 2009). To generate evidence about the success of these interventions, social epidemiologists need to expand the tools that are available to them to accurately assess this complexity; thus, new approaches to evaluate, systematically review and synthesize evidence are required (Egan et al. 2009; Gamble 2008).

Systematic reviews are powerful tools to assess the effectiveness of interventions by utilizing a transparent, rigorous method for summarizing and synthesizing the existing research literature. Such reviews are undertaken to inform clinical decision making and the development of effective health policies and interventions (Bambra 2011; Bambra et al. 2010). Often, systematic reviews focus upon determining the magnitude of change or health improvement related to an intervention and rely on statistical techniques (e.g., pooled estimates of effectiveness or meta-analyses). However, qualitative or narrative syntheses can also be conducted to describe success across interventions (Mays et al. 2005; Popay et al. 2006). While determining the magnitude of intervention impact is important, it is equally, if not more, important to determine *how* and *why* interventions fail or succeed (Donaldson 2007; Pawson 2006). For this reason, the focus of evaluations, as well as systematic reviews, must include an examination of underlying theories of change in health interventions.

To date systematic reviews have been most useful when the interventions are straightforward and external factors can be controlled in implementation (e.g., through randomized controlled trial (RCT) design) (Petticrew and Roberts 2006). In situations when the intervention is less complex (e.g., evaluation of a pharmaceutical intervention for the treatment of a specific disease outcome), the intervention is typically implemented according to a standardized protocol, making it easier for systematic reviewers to isolate intervention components and assess their effectiveness. However, Conventional systematic review methods are typically not well suited to interventions that address structural determinants of health, as these determinants inherently add complexity to interventions and their implementation. Conventional systematic review methods also do not typically account for the effects of external or contextual factors. For example, with complex interventions that may have multiple components or uncertain outcomes (Gamble 2008; Rogers 2008), it is more difficult for systematic reviewers to identify all relevant components of the intervention, such as whether the implementation adhered to a protocol, whether there were synergistic effects of intervention components and whether there were contextual effects that could have led to the confounding of outcomes (Egan et al. 2009). If evaluation strategies are to isolate mechanisms and synergies that lead to the success or failure of interventions for complex health problems, new systematic review tools need to be developed that pay careful attention to the influence of social and related contextual factors which cannot be controlled for during intervention implementation (Gamble 2008; Pawson and Tilley 1997; Westley et al. 2006).

In this chapter, we argue for greater adoption of realist review methods within the field of social epidemiology that seek to identify key intervention mechanisms and account for contextual effects in order to more comprehensively evaluate complex interventions and inform solutions to complex health problems.

11.2   A "Realist" Approach to Systematic Review

The realist approach to systematic review acknowledges that the effects of interventions such as programs and policies are crucially dependent on context and implementation. This approach to systematic review is based on realism, a philosophy that holds that social systems are "open" and complex, making the study of these social systems and determination of causality extremely difficult using the traditional methods of the natural sciences due to a lack of control over social factors and contextual influences (Pawson 2006) (see Chapter 2 for an in-depth discussion of realism and critical realism). The realist approach is aligned with a generative model of causality in the sense that it seeks to identify causal explanation of regularities *and* irregularities in social phenomena (Pawson 2006). In systematic review, the realist approach seeks to identify the underlying theory or mechanism of an intervention that leads to success. This approach also seeks to learn from failure in order to best discern "what works for whom, in what circumstances, in what respects and how" (Pawson et al. 2004).

While there are many similarities to conventional systematic reviews, realist reviews are best suited for the examination of complex interventions, as they focus on the inclusion of diverse evidence in an attempt to learn and explain how interventions work. In this sense, realist reviews do not adhere to a strict hierarchy of evidence where RCTs are automatically considered the best type of study upon which to draw inferences. Rather evidence of multiple types can be used to inform "what works" and to generate a theoretical explanation of why programs succeed or fail. Realist review seeks to learn from (rather than control) real world phenomena such as diversity, change, idiosyncrasy, adaptation, cross-contamination and program failure (Pawson 2006). As a result, the realist review approach is useful for not just identifying whether a program works but more importantly *how* and *why* it works. This approach is consistent with more solution-focused research by identifying key mechanisms and contextual factors that facilitate program success or failure, and thus it provides important information with which to improve existing programs and to facilitate the replication and implementation of programs. Realist reviews have recently been conducted to evaluate complex health-related interventions including community-based programming for homeless individuals experiencing concurrent mental health and substance use disorders, intimate partner violence screening programs, housing interventions, smoking cessation programs, and school feeding programs (Greenhalgh et al. 2007; Jackson et al. 2009; Kaneko 1999; O'Campo et al. 2011, 2009).

Similar to conventional systematic reviews, key stages in the realist review process include: (1) defining the topic and scope of the review; (2) identifying and collecting the evidence; (3) appraising the evidence and extracting data; (4) synthesizing the evidence; and (5) disseminating findings to stakeholders (Pawson 2006). Yet, unlike a conventional review, these steps happen in a non-linear and overlapping manner. For example, while in conventional reviews, one often sets the topic, keywords and identifies the databases to search before embarking on the review (e.g., Higgins and Green 2008), realist reviews move back and forth between the different stages and allow for revisions of these aspects at any time in the review. To be clear, such revisions in realist reviews should be documented and the process should be replicable, but not all aspects of the review have to be fixed before the review begins.

While many of the stages of the realist review resemble those that would be followed in a conventional systematic review, there are a number of other differences between these two approaches. Table 11.1 compares the differences in approach and outcomes for realist versus conventional systematic reviews.

One of the most fundamental differences between realist and conventional systematic reviews relates to the research question. The focus of a realist review is to explain *how* and *why* an intervention works; whereas, a conventional systematic review is focused on determining *whether* a specific intervention works or, sometimes when there are a selection of programs, *which* program works best. Furthermore, in the process of trying to isolate program mechanisms and contextual factors, realist reviews include a wide range of types of evidence, such as quantitative and qualitative research, theoretical research, grey literature,

Table 11.1 Comparison between realist and conventional systematic review approaches

	Realist review	Conventional systematic review
Type of intervention	Complex	Straightforward; discrete
Focus	Explanatory: *How* and *why* does "x" work to improve well-being	Judgemental: By how much does "x" improve well-being
Relevant types of evidence	Includes a wide range of research (i.e., both quantitative and qualitative)	Mostly quantitative research on effectiveness
Evidence source	Peer reviewed literature, policy reviews, stakeholder consultations, focus groups, grey literature (e.g., reports, conference proceedings)	Mostly peer reviewed quantitative research on effectiveness
Method	Theory-driven synthesis: Deconstructs intervention into component theories; contextual data retained and basic theory is refined concerning applicability in context	Statistical synthesis/ Meta-analysis: Data from individual studies are combined statistically and then summarized
Results	Identification of mechanisms and underlying theory that facilitates program success	Statistic of program effectiveness

interactions with program designers or staff, and other program-related information that is evaluative as well as more descriptive; whereas, conventional systematic reviews include primarily quantitative, experimental studies that have been peer reviewed (Bambra 2011). Both types of reviews can incorporate quality appraisal, but the assessment criteria are different. A realist review does not just focus on power and quality of study design, but, similar to narrative reviews, also assesses the amount of descriptive information or extent of information on intervention theory provided by the study that is helpful for identifying mechanisms and context.

The realist review uses conventional systematic review steps as a guiding framework, but incorporates more sub-stages than a conventional review. It also incorporates theory-driven synthesis, whereby the underlying theory or explanatory mechanism is sought, and the impact of contextual factors on intervention workings is considered. This is contrary to the more statistical synthesis of the meta-analytic approach that dominates more conventional systematic reviews. Furthermore, as mentioned earlier, steps are not sequential but are overlapping and iterative in the realist review approach.

The process of conducting realist reviews is best highlighted through the use of an example, as very few examples exist and methods are sparsely described in most published realist reviews. The discussion will now focus on a realist review of evidence conducted by the authors and their colleagues on intimate partner violence screening programs in health care settings. This section of the chapter is adapted from an article originally published in *Social Science and Medicine* in 2011 (see O'Campo et al. 2011).

11.3   A Realist Review of Intimate Partner Violence Screening Programs

Intimate partner violence (IPV) is a growing public health problem. High morbidity, mortality and health care utilization among victims result from IPV (Bonomi et al. 2009; Campbell 2002; Campbell et al. 2002; O'Campo et al. 2009). Because of these adverse consequences, professional organizations have been calling for screening and intervention for IPV in health care settings since the 1990s (U.S. Preventive Services Task Force 2004; Wathen and MacMillan 2003b; American Academy of Family Physicians 2005; American Medical Association 2000; Cherniak et al. 2005). Yet, despite the serious health consequences and widespread calls for screening in health care settings, gaps exist in knowledge with respect to screening. In the past 10 years, a number of systematic reviews have been conducted to determine whether health care-based IPV screening programs are effective (Nelson et al. 2004; Ramsay et al. 2002; Wathen and MacMillan 2003a, b). These studies have concluded that insufficient evidence exists to show effectiveness of these programs in reducing partner violence, and, as a result, controversy exists concerning their implementation.

In light of this debate, we undertook a realist review of evidence on universal IPV screening programs in health care settings to synthesize the published grey- and peer-review literature, in order to examine *how* and *why* these programs work (or do not work) and identify mechanisms related to program success or failure. Unlike previous systematic reviews of IPV screening programs, which have reviewed evidence on different types of IPV screening programs (e.g., universal[1] and case-finding[2] screening approaches) within the same review (Nelson et al. 2004; Ramsay et al. 2002), we chose to focus our review on universal IPV screening programs in order to ensure that information about common program mechanisms could be extracted and compared. Another key difference between this review and previous syntheses was that most previous evaluations and reviews have focused on the reduction or elimination of IPV as the primary outcome. Instead, we focused our review on a more proximal outcome to IPV screening, namely the rate of IPV disclosure and detection. As shown in Fig. 11.1, the success of screening should not be determined by whether changes have occurred in IPV prevalence given the multiple intervening steps (e.g., disclosure, referral and access to services) that must occur between IPV screening and reduction or elimination. Moreover, this pathway is influenced by interpersonal or relationship factors at multiple points. For example, whether a victim accesses services for IPV resolution may be dependent upon factors, such as the relationship involved, fear of violence and economic considerations, which are out of the control of the health care

---

[1] An intimate partner violence screening approach in which all women are screened regardless of illness or high-risk presentations.

[2] An intimate partner violence screening approach in which only women who are suspected to be victims are screened.

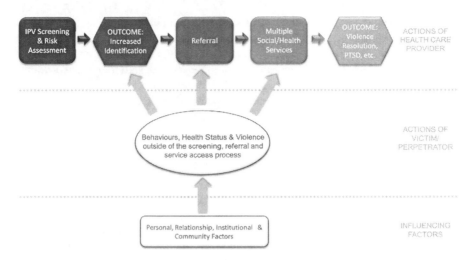

Fig. 11.1 Pathway between IPV screening and changes or reduction of IPV

provider and setting in which screening occurs. This framework supports the idea that the reduction of IPV prevalence is an inappropriate outcome for the evaluation of IPV screening programs.

The first step in our review process was to search the literature. Our search yielded 5,046 scholarly articles on IPV screening programs. During the initial review process, we applied inclusion criteria to studies containing evaluative data on programs in health care settings that implemented universal IPV screening. The studies reviewed included information about screening outcomes including rates of IPV screening, disclosure and identification or detection.

During the synthesis process, we sought to determine mechanisms related to successful program outcomes such as increased rates of screening, disclosure and identification, and, in so doing, identified common components of programs that were successful as well as those that experienced failure. Over the course of this process, we determined that IPV programs that included numerous components at multiple levels were more successful at achieving increased screening outcomes. For this reason, we classified each of the programs as having a "comprehensive" or "non-comprehensive" approach to IPV screening implementation. Programs were considered to be "comprehensive" if they incorporated numerous program components and included institutional support for IPV screening.

Six programs were classified as comprehensive and incorporated a combination of the following program components at multiple systems levels (i.e., in multiple sites and settings and/or involving various types of health care staff), which were linked to program success: (1) institutional support for IPV interventions; (2) immediate access and referral to onsite or offsite support services; (3) thorough initial and ongoing training; and (4) use of effective and detailed screening protocols.

All of the comprehensive programs had strong institutional support that facilitated their ability to operate at a systems level. Strong *institutional support* involved the investment, approval and support for the integration or institutionalization of all aspects of the program at high levels within the health care setting or institution. Its presence in these programs meant that knowledge of the importance and the nature of the screening program was communicated to health care staff across departments and sites, including frontline nurses and other providers and health care administrators, which led to raised awareness and support for the programs to address IPV (McCaw et al. 2001; McColgan et al. 2010; Short et al. 2002; Spangaro 2007; Ulbrich and Stockdale 2002).

Successful screening programs provided identified victims with *immediate access to support services*, such as mental health services, safe shelters or transitional housing, health care and legal services, either immediately through an onsite case manager or social worker or by rapidly referring victims to offsite services (McCaw et al. 2001; McColgan et al. 2010; Short et al. 2002). Those programs that did not have onsite services and referred victims offsite emphasized the importance of maintaining ongoing communication and linkages with community service providers in order to facilitate a smooth and timely referral process (Ulbrich and Stockdale 2002).

Many of the successful programs incorporated *thorough initial and ongoing training* for health care providers on how to screen and how to appropriately respond when a victim discloses violence. Several of the studies of the programs offering thorough, ongoing training noted increased provider self-efficacy, comfort and confidence with screening, which was subsequently related to increased screening rates (McCaw 2001; Short 2002; Ulbrich and Stockdale 2002; Spangaro 2007; Wills et al. 2008).

The use of *effective screening protocols* was another component of many of the successful screening programs reviewed. These screening protocols were detailed and clearly outlined for providers when and how to screen and clarified how to ask sensitive screening questions (e.g., through the use of standardized questions), how to assess patient safety and how to refer patients to support services (Hadley et al. 1995; McCaw et al. 2001; Spangaro 2007; Ulbrich and Stockdale 2002).

Eleven universal IPV screening programs were considered to be non-comprehensive, as they consisted of few screening program components and/or lacked the key component of institutional support. For example, some of these programs introduced screening questions with limited supports to staff, conducted staff training over short periods of time and/or lost institutional support to sustain programming (Coyer et al. 2006; Gadomski et al. 2001; Grunfeld et al. 1994; Lo Vecchio et al. 1998; Ramsden and Bonner 2002). These programs tended to yield only limited increases in IPV screening outcomes that were not statistically significant or sustained post-intervention. These findings highlighted the importance of the ongoing implementation of several program components as opposed to implementing just one or two on a short-term basis.

Our realist-informed review highlighted that comprehensive, multi-component universal IPV screening programs were the most successful at yielding increased screening outcomes. The literature consulted suggested that screening efforts were more successful when providers: (1) accepted the responsibility of screening for

IPV; (2) were comfortable with the screening process; and (3) have the resources and time to assess and assist the victim (e.g., Short et al. 2002; Wills et al. 2008). Many of the comprehensive programs have shown that implementation of multiple program components can serve to increase provider self-efficacy and comfort with screening and subsequently promote screening behaviour. The relation between self-efficacy, behaviour change and the influence of contextual and interpersonal factors has been supported extensively in the literature by the social cognitive theory of behaviour change (Bandura 1988). The social cognitive theory for behaviour and behaviour change focuses on changes resulting from the interaction among behaviours (i.e., the desired behaviour or, in this case, IPV screening behaviour), personal factors (i.e., the person's beliefs and cognitive competencies) and the environment (i.e., social influences and structures within the environment, e.g., the health care setting). The theory explains *how* and *why* these components are necessary to achieve effective IPV screening. The relationship between the availability of multiple IPV screening program components within the health care environment and provider self-efficacy and comfort with screening reflects the underlying program theory or mechanism of change that results in increased IPV screening outcomes, as seen in Fig. 11.2.

11.4 The Utility of Realist Review: A Comparison of Review Findings on Intimate Partner Violence Screening Programs

The IPV intervention process is complex in that there are a number of steps that need to take place in various contexts, that is by individual victims, within health care settings and within the community, before IPV can be reduced (Fig. 11.1). Previous reviews of IPV programs have used a broader focus by examining effectiveness of both universal (i.e., every patient is screened) and case-finding (i.e., only those suspected of abuse are screened) screening programs as well as non-health care setting programs or efforts to improve IPV-related referrals within the same review (Nelson et al. 2004; Ramsay et al. 2002; Wathen and MacMillan 2003a). Previous reviews have examined a wide variety of screening outcomes, especially changes in IPV prevalence, and have not facilitated an in-depth look at program mechanisms related to any particular outcome. As a result, we felt that the realist review approach was well suited to explain how IPV screening programs work for a more proximal outcome of the IPV intervention process, namely IPV screening and detection of victims. Furthermore, previous reviews of IPV programs have typically taken a conventional systematic review approach and were focused on assessing *whether* these programs work. In the process, these reviews only considered quantitative evaluative evidence and did not review other program materials that may have provided more in-depth, descriptive information about program workings. As a result, they did not address *how* or *why* these programs work, or do not work.

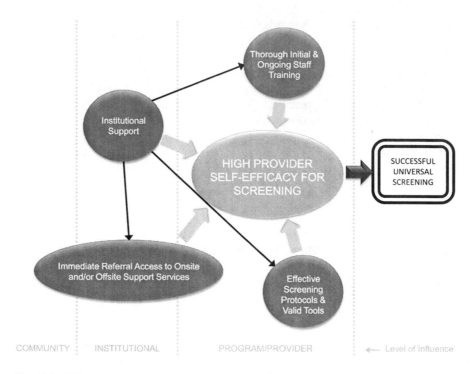

Fig. 11.2 IPV screening in health care settings: what works

The methodological weaknesses of prior reviews and the overwhelming conclusion that there is insufficient evidence to support IPV screening in health care settings has had negative practical consequences in these settings. For example, one review deemed that "implementation of screening programmes in health care settings is not justified by current evidence" due to lack of program information and methodological flaws in existing studies (Ramsay 2002). This conclusion was made despite significant increases in IPV detection in six out of the ten screening-related studies reviewed. Based on prior reviews, there has likely been lack of mobilization and action regarding the implementation of IPV screening and detection in many health care settings, creating a missed opportunity to help IPV victims along the complex continuum of assistance and support towards a reduction in violence (Fig. 11.1), as well as a missed chance to better evaluate these programs.

Similar to previous reviews, we also encountered problems with the quantity and quality of evaluative evidence provided on universal IPV screening programs in this review. The evaluation of such a complex social problem as IPV is extremely difficult given the relative complexity of such interventions and the ethical constraints with respect to study design (e.g., ethical limitations to conducting a true RCT of an IPV screening intervention that would involve withholding services to victims who had disclosed) (Spangaro et al. 2009). Nevertheless, our realist-informed review on universal screening programs for IPV contributes to knowledge on the effectiveness of screening programs to address IPV and further advances the methods of systematic review for complex health interventions. It does so by considering information from various types of program evidence (qualitative and descriptive and pre- and post-designs) in order to facilitate greater understanding of how programs function. The review isolated a program theory of *how* and *why* screening programs for IPV can be successful in increasing IPV detection in health care settings. While it is not clear from the review which program components are the most important to program success, the program components identified herein and the systems-level approach can be tailored to almost any health care department or setting. Better evidence regarding the effectiveness of universal IPV screening programs is certainly needed through continued, strong evaluation design. However, it is still possible to learn from existing evidence and programming in order to identify promising practices and increase understanding of how to implement better interventions to address this serious public health problem (Spangaro et al. 2009).

11.5 Challenges in Conducting Realist Reviews

We now turn to a discussion of challenges to conducting realist reviews of complex health and social interventions in order to present a balanced argument as well as to present some suggestions for advancing this methodological approach.

The process of conducting a realist review is time consuming given its iterative nature and the various types of evidence that need to be sourced. To which problems and programs a realist review is best applied is ambiguous and certain technical details of the approach, for example the quality appraisal of various types of evidence, are still under-developed given the few published examples available from which to draw. In order to address the latter challenge, we have turned to and have adapted quality appraisal techniques and tools from the narrative synthesis literature (Dixon-Woods et al. 2005; Mays et al. 2005; Popay et al. 2006) to appropriately assess the methodological rigour and quality of evidence but remain inclusive of all types of information (e.g., quantitative, qualitative, scholarly and grey literature) that may carry important details of program mechanism.

Similar to conventional systematic reviews, realist reviewers are constrained by the state of the evidence on the topic being reviewed. In general, if evaluation studies are poorly designed and have limited power, then reviewers are limited in the conclusions that they may draw with respect to program effectiveness. In realist reviews, these limitations are further compounded by a dearth of detailed information about program implementation and contextual factors that may assist in elucidating program mechanisms. This issue is most problematic with evidence published in academic journals due to manuscript page limits and perhaps a lack of awareness by evaluators of the importance of reporting such information for purposes of systematic review. Furthermore, we found that evaluators were generally unwilling to provide more information when contacted, typically a long time after their evaluation has been completed, to ask their impressions regarding success or failure of the programs. In order for appropriate information regarding program mechanism and context to be gleaned, it is perhaps necessary for academic journals to increase their page limits for evaluation research of complex health and social programs and to raise awareness among evaluators of the need to report detailed information on program implementation and context (O'Campo et al. 2009). It may also be necessary to include key informant interviews with evaluators as a key step in realist review methodology in order to learn enough about program mechanisms and the impact of context on outcomes.

While not unique to realist reviews, the process of review can become even more time consuming if a multi- or transdisciplinary team is involved due to challenges with integrating and collaborating in the context of differing disciplines, types of knowledge and research agendas. Many of our reviews have taken a cross-disciplinary approach, but more methodological inquiry into cross-disciplinary realist review is needed. Cross-disciplinary research collaboration is important when addressing complex health problems, and may be facilitated through the use of "terms of reference" that outline governance guidelines for respectful collaboration, intellectual property and data usage (Kirst et al. 2011).

11.6   Discussion and Conclusion

In this chapter, we present a new synthesis tool that could be a complement to existing review approaches being used in social epidemiology. It should be emphasized that this new tool needs further refinement, which can be easily remedied by increased application of realist review along with careful documentation and publication of the approaches undertaken with each new application. To further support realist reviews of all types, whether they are in social epidemiology or in other fields, published program evaluations need to be more explicit in several areas including underlying program theory and discussion of why programs were successful or why they failed.

The example provided herein represents a first step in implementing this new tool. As well, in this particular instance, the gap between the knowledge generated by a realist approach on *how* successful IPV screening programs work versus the failure of past conventional systematic reviews to support IPV screening programs is noteworthy. Despite the high prevalence of lifetime IPV and the widespread calls by professional organizations for the implementation of universal screening programs, the evidence generated by prior reviews has precluded the extensive implementation of such programs. For those programs that have been implemented, past syntheses provided little guidance as to critical program components related to program success. The focus on the theory of realist review has addressed this problem for the case of IPV screening. Not only did this realist-informed review provide stronger support for the implementation of IPV screening, but this type of synthesis also revealed critical ingredients and how they work to support strong IPV screening programs. A logical next step in this story is to begin to implement and evaluate programs that are consistent with "comprehensive" IPV program components. A further advantage of the realist approach taken was the identification of the conceptual underpinnings of successful programs that may or may not be limited to the health care context. Thus, while the evidence synthesized in this review was specific to health care settings, it is reasonable to consider implementing such programs outside of the health care setting and to document whether the model is more widely applicable.

As noted in multiple chapters throughout this book (see Chapters 1 and 10) as well as by authors elsewhere (Navarro 2009; Putnam and Galea 2008), social epidemiology must expand its focus toward more structural determinants of health to identify the critical causes of adverse population well-being. Furthermore, to accelerate the generation of solution-focused research to address pressing problems such as the growing social inequities in health globally, systematic reviews are an important tool to determine whether and how structural and social interventions improve well-being. Given the multiple levels at which structural interventions typically operate and the mismatch between complexity and conventional systematic reviews, social epidemiologists should adopt and improve methods of realist review as an additional approach to generate knowledge to support social change.

References

American Academy of Family Physicians (2005) Violence (position paper): AAFP policy and advocacy statement. http://www aafporg/online/ en/home/policy/ policies/v/violencepositionpaper.html. Accessed 7 Mar 2011

American Medical Association (2000) AMA data on violence between intimates. In: 2000 interim meeting of the American Medical Association. Report of the council on scientific affairs. http://www.ama-assn.org/ama1/pub/upload/mm/443/csai-00.pdf. Accessed 7 Mar 2011

Bambra C (2011) Real world reviews: a beginner's guide to undertaking systematic reviews of public health policy interventions. J Epidemiol Community Health 65:14–19

Bambra C, Gibson M, Sowden A et al (2010) Tackling the wider social determinants of health and health inequalities: evidence from systematic reviews. J Epidemiol Community Health 64:284–291

Bandura A (1988) Social cognitive theory and social referencing. In: Feinman S (ed) Social referencing and social construction of reality. Plenum, New York

Bonomi A, Anderson M, Reid R et al (2009) Medical and psychosocial diagnoses in women with a history of intimate partner violence. Arch Intern Med 169:1692–1697

Campbell J (2002) The health consequences of intimate partner violence. Lancet 359:1509–1514

Campbell J, Snow-Jones A, Dienemann J (2002) Intimate partner violence and physical health consequences. Arch Intern Med 162:1157–1163

Cherniak D, Grant L, Mason R et al (2005) Intimate partner violence consensus statement. J Obstet Gynaecol Can 27:365–418

Coyer S, Plonczynski D, Baldwin K et al (2006) Screening for violence against women in a rural health care clinic. J Rural Nurse Health Care 6:47

Dixon-Woods M, Agarwal S, Jones D et al (2005) Synthesising qualitative and quantitative evidence: a review of possible methods. J Health Serv Res Policy 10:45–53

Donaldson S (2007) Program theory-driven evaluation science: strategies and applications. Lawrence Erlbaum, New York

Egan M, Bambra C, Petticrew M et al (2009) Reviewing evidence on complex social interventions: appraising implementation in systematic reviews of the health effects of organizational-level workplace interventions. J Epidemiol Community Health 63:4–11

Gadomski A, Wolff D, Tripp M et al (2001) Changes in health care providers' knowledge, attitudes, beliefs and behaviors regarding domestic violence, following a multifaceted intervention. Acad Med 76:1045

Gamble J (2008) Developmental evaluation primer. JW McConnell Family Foundation, Montreal

Greenhalgh T, Kristjansson E, Robinson V (2007) Realist review to understand the efficacy of school feeding programmes. BMJ 335:858–861

Grunfeld AF, Ritmiller S, Mackay K et al (1994) Detecting domestic violence against women in the emergency department: a nursing triage model. J Emerg Nurs 20:271–274

Hadley SM, Short LM, Lezin N (1995) WomanKind: an innovative model of health care response to domestic abuse. Womens Health Issues 5:189–198

Higgins JPT, Green S (2008) Cochrane handbook for systematic reviews of interventions. http://www.cochrane-handbook.org/. Accessed June 2008

Jackson L, Langille L, Lyons R et al (2009) Does moving from a high-poverty to lower-poverty neighborhood improve mental health? A realist review of "Moving to Opportunity". Health & Place 15:961–970

Kaneko M (1999) A methodological inquiry into the evaluation of smoking cessation programmes. Health Educ Res 14:433–441

Kaplan GA (2004) What's wrong with social epidemiology, and how can we make it better? Epidemiol Rev 26:124–135

Kirst MJ, Schaefer-McDaniel N, Hwang S et al (2011) Moving Forward: The Future of Transdisciplinary Health Research. In Kirst M, Schaefer-McDaniel N, Hwang S & O'Campo P (eds) pp 161–167. Converging disciplines: a transdisciplinary research approach to urban health problems. Springer, New York

Lo Vecchio F, Bhatia A, Sciallo D (1998) Screening for domestic violence in the emergency department. Eur J Emerg Med 5:441–444

Mays N, Pope C, Popay J (2005) Systematically reviewing qualitative and quantitative evidence to inform management and policy making in the health field. J Health Serv Res Policy 10:S6–S20

McCaw B, Berman WH, Syme SL et al (2001) Beyond screening for domestic violence: a systems model approach in a managed care setting. Am J Prev Med 21:170–176

McColgan M, Cruz M, McKee J et al (2010) Results of a multifaceted intimate partner violence training program for pediatric residents. Child Abuse Negl 34:275–283

Navarro V (2009) What we mean by social determinants of health. Int J Health Serv 39:423–441

Nelson HD, Nygren P, McInerney Y et al (2004) Screening women and elderly adults for family and intimate partner violence: a review of the evidence for the U.S. Preventive Services Task Force. Ann Intern Med 140:387–396

O'Campo P, Kirst M, Schaefer-McDaniel N et al (2009) Community-based services for homeless adults experiencing concurrent mental health and substance use disorders: a realist approach to synthesizing evidence. J Urban Health 86:965–989

O'Campo P, Kirst M, Tsamis C et al (2011) Implementing successful IPV screening programs in health care settings: evidence generated from a realist systematic review. Soc Sci Med 72: 855–866

Paterson C, Baarts C, Launso L et al (2009) Evaluating complex health interventions: a critical analysis of the 'outcomes' concept. BMC Complement Altern Med 9:18

Pawson R (2006) Evidence-based policy: a realist perspective. Sage Publications, London

Pawson R, Tilley N (1997) Realistic evaluation. Sage Publications, London

Pawson R, Greenhalgh T, Harvey G et al (2004) Realist synthesis: an introduction. In: ESRC research methods programme: RMP methods paper series. University of Manchester, Manchester

Petticrew M, Roberts H (2006) Systematic reviews in the social sciences: a practical guide. Blackwell Publishing, Oxford

Popay J, Roberts H, Sowden A et al (2006) Guidance on the conduct of narrative synthesis in systematic reviews: a product from the ESRC methods programme. Lancaster, Institute for Health Research

Putnam S, Galea S (2008) Epidemiology and the macrosocial determinants of health. J Public Health Policy 29:275–289

Ramsay J, Richardson J, Carter YH et al (2002) Should health professionals screen women for domestic violence? Systematic review. BMJ 325:314

Ramsden C, Bonner M (2002) A realistic view of domestic violence screening in an emergency department. Accid Emerg Nurs 10:31–39

Rogers PJ (2008) Using programme theory to evaluate complicated and complex aspects of interventions. Evaluation 14:2948

Short LM, Hadley SM, Bates B (2002) Assessing the success of the WomanKind program: an integrated model of 24-hour health care response to domestic violence. Women Health 35:101–119

Spangaro JM (2007) The NSW Health routine screening for domestic violence program. N S W Public Health Bull 18:8689

Spangaro J, Zwi A, Poulos R (2009) The elusive search for definitive evidence on routine screening for intimate partner violence. Trauma Violence Abuse 10:55–68

U.S. Preventive Services Task Force (2004) Recommendation statement: screening for family and intimate partner violence. Ann Intern Med 140:382–386

Ulbrich PM, Stockdale J (2002) Making family planning clinics an empowerment zone for rural battered women. Women Health 35:83–100

Wathen CN, MacMillan HL (2003a) Interventions for violence against women: scientific review. JAMA 289:589–600

Wathen CN, MacMillan HL (2003b) Prevention of violence against women: recommendation statement from the Canadian Task Force on Preventive Health Care. CMAJ 169:582–584

Westley F, Quinn Patton M, Zimmerman B (2006) Getting to maybe: how the world is changed. Vintage Canada, Toronto

Wills R, Ritchie M, Wilson M (2008) Improving detection and quality of assessment of child abuse and partner abuse is achievable with a formal organisational change approach. J Paediatr Child Health 44:92–98

Chapter 12
Addressing Health Equities in Social Epidemiology: Learning from Evaluation(s)

Sanjeev Sridharan, James R. Dunn, and April Nakaima

Contents

12.1 Introduction 248
12.2 Why Should Social Epidemiologists Bother with Evaluations? 250
12.3 The Complexities of Conceptualizing Health Inequities 251
12.4 Moving Beyond Programs: The Ecology of Health 253
12.5 Intersectoral Responses to Health Inequities: Background 254
12.6 A Realist Approach to Evaluating Complex Interventions 255
    12.6.1 The Key Components of the Complex Intervention 257
    12.6.2 The Program Theory of the Complex Interventions 257
    12.6.3 Learning from the Evidence Base 258
    12.6.4 The Anticipated Timeline of Impact 258
    12.6.5 Learning Framework for the Evaluation 258
    12.6.6 The Pathways of Influence of an Evaluation 259
    12.6.7 Assessing the Impact of the Health Intervention 259
    12.6.8 Learning About the Pathways of Impact of the Complex
          Intervention over Time 260
    12.6.9 Spreading Learning from an Evaluation 260
    12.6.10 Reflections on Sustainability 261
12.7 Conclusions 261
References 262

S. Sridharan (✉)
The Evaluation Centre for Complex Health Interventions, St. Michael's Hospital,
30 Bond Street, Toronto, ON M5B 1W8, Canada
e-mail: SridharanS@smh.ca

J.R. Dunn
Department of Health, Aging and Society, McMaster University, Kenneth Taylor Hall 226,
1280 Main Street West, Hamilton, ON L8S 4L8, Canada
e-mail: jim.dunn@mcmaster.ca

A. Nakaima
Independent Consultant

P. O'Campo and J.R. Dunn (eds.), *Rethinking Social Epidemiology:*
Towards a Science of Change, DOI 10.1007/978-94-007-2138-8_12,
© Springer Science+Business Media B.V. 2012

Abstract This chapter examines how evaluations and evaluative thinking can help in the social epidemiologic study of *complex interventions*. There is increasing interest within the field of social epidemiology in studying interventions, as well as increasing pressure from funders and decision makers to make research more relevant for addressing social problems. Within the field of evaluation, there is a parallel move towards embracing the study of complex interventions – the very kinds of interventions that will almost invariably be the focus of social epidemiology. Using the example of interventions that seek to address health inequities in urban settings, we introduce a framework of steps through which evaluations can impact such health inequities. Rather than discussing a series of tools and methods, we use these steps to describe the importance of thinking evaluatively in addressing complex social problems. Specifically, we highlight a realist approach to evaluation. This approach focuses not only on *whether* an intervention works, but also on *how* it works, *for whom* and *under what conditions* (Pawson and Tilley 1997). This perspective marks a significant departure from traditions of other branches of epidemiology, such as clinical epidemiology, where the *whether* question is paramount and the *how* question is less important, often because of the uniformity and simplicity of interventions (e.g., administration of a drug). Research within epidemiology on social interventions has been relatively uncommon to date, and this chapter seeks to provide some guidance to expanding the literature on the health effects social interventions by engaging with cutting-edge theory on thinking evaluatively.

Abbreviations

RCT   randomized controlled trial
SES   socioeconomic status

12.1   Introduction

This chapter examines how evaluations and evaluative thinking can help in the social epidemiologic study of *complex interventions*. There is increasing interest within the field of social epidemiology in studying interventions, as well as increasing pressure from funders and decision makers to make research more relevant for addressing social problems. Within the field of evaluation, there is a parallel move towards embracing the study of complex interventions – the very kinds of interventions that will almost invariably be the focus of social epidemiology. We use the example of interventions that seek to address health inequities in urban settings in this paper. We introduce a framework of steps by which evaluations can make a difference to such health inequities. Rather than discussing a series of tools and methods, we use these steps to describe the importance of thinking evaluatively in addressing complex social problems.

In this chapter, we highlight a realist approach to evaluation. This approach focuses not only on *whether* an intervention works, but also on *how* it works, *for whom* and *under what conditions* (Pawson and Tilley 1997). As noted earlier (see Chap. 2), the defining feature of the realist approach is its heavy emphasis on understanding the contexts and mechanisms needed for interventions to work in addressing problems like health inequities. In so doing, the realist approach also problematizes the dynamics of an intervention as they play out over time, for instance, eschewing, to some extent, a strict notion of "fidelity." This perspective is a significant departure from traditions of other branches of epidemiology, such as clinical epidemiology, where the *whether* question is paramount and the *how* question is less important, often because of the uniformity and simplicity of interventions (e.g., administration of a drug). Yet while social epidemiologists naturally draw methodological guidance from epidemiology, we argue that the lessons learned about investigating complex interventions within evaluations research are an equally important source of guidance. In this chapter, the term *intervention* is used broadly and includes preventative, curative, behavioural and intersectoral macrosocial interventions that may simultaneously focus on multiple sectors (e.g., water, health services and education) and on routine health services, such as primary health care.

Research within epidemiology on social interventions has been relatively uncommon to date (Berkman 2004). Phenomena like income, education, race, *et cetera*, are attributes and characteristics of individuals and communities and are not immediately amenable to interventions that would change them in the same way that one would, for example, try to redress a vitamin deficiency with a supplement. Although there are examples of social epidemiologic interventions, they tend to focus on redressing the *effects* of low socioeconomic status (SES) or vulnerability, either by using interventions that: (1) are targeted at high-risk groups (e.g., smoking cessation aimed at low-income individuals); or (2) attempt to change the conditions in which people of low SES live that may affect their health (e.g., putting affordable, nutritious foods in convenience stores in low SES neighbourhoods). These two types of interventions address not only the *mechanisms* by which low SES translates into poor health, but also the ways in which *context* is involved in the causal chain between low SES and poor health. In other branches of epidemiology from which social epidemiology draws much of its logic and methods it is relatively unimportant *how* or *why* an effect is seen (e.g., drug trials), nor is it considered part of the problem to analyze *under what conditions* and *for whom* the intervention works. Indeed, the logic of the randomized controlled trial (RCT) attempts to exclude such questions from explicit consideration. In these ways, the parent discipline of social epidemiology and many of its siblings explicitly avoid complexity in favour of simplicity and reductionism through control of a variety of confounders, either by design or by analysis. We suggest that these phenomena, mechanisms and contexts, the cornerstones of a realist approach to interventions, are critical to thinking evaluatively about social epidemiologic research on complex interventions.

Interventions focussed on health inequities are complex in multiple ways. Surprisingly little research on the evaluations of complex health interventions focuses on the sources and nature of complexity (Riley et al. 2008). In our experience, interventions focussed on long-term outcomes such as health inequities need to address at least three different kinds of complexity. First, there is complexity due to the multiple, interacting components that are involved in complex health interventions. A second source of complexity is the dynamic nature of programs, which has implications for both program theory and evaluation design. A third source of complexity is due to contextualization. Public health programs are located in specific settings, and the act of translating an initiative into a specific setting requires adaptation to local conditions (see Chap. 15). The absence of a clear *a priori* theory implies that complex health interventions rarely have a blueprint at the outset for how their suspected mechanisms will operate in the specific interventional context. Intervention adaptation (i.e., adaptation of subjects in the target population to the intervention) provides another source of complexity that is usually ignored in most evaluation and social epidemiologic research on interventions. Each of these sources of complexity has multiple interacting components, and both dynamic complexity and contextualized complexity have implications for theory and design.

Realism is one of the very few evaluation and social science approaches that attempts to address complexity of interventions. The realist-based approach has many strengths, but most of all it shifts the focus of social epidemiologic research from "does a program work?" to "what is it about a program that makes it work?"

12.2   Why Should Social Epidemiologists Bother with Evaluations?

Evaluation can be defined both as a means of assessing performance and as a means of identifying alternative ways to deliver services. For example, the new Canadian federal policy on evaluation defines evaluation as "the systematic collection and analysis of evidence on the outcomes of programs to make judgments about their relevance, performance and alternative ways to deliver them or to achieve the same results" (Treasury Board of Canada Secretariat 2009).

Evaluations have multiple purposes and ways of responding to health inequities. As described in Table 12.1, evaluation of health interventions can determine not only if a given program or policy makes a difference in impacting health inequities, it can also begin to elucidate the theory about and causal mechanisms of social processes and their impacts on health inequities. In this sense, engaging in evaluations research can assist social epidemiologists in informing solutions to growing social problems and can move the field of social epidemiology towards more solution-focused research (see Chap. 1). Furthermore, social epidemiologists should consider conducting evaluations research as a means of engaging in policy approaches to epidemiology, in which methods are applied to specific problems defined by end users of knowledge (e.g., decision makers within organizations or at varying levels of government). Conducting evaluations research is also a means of engaging in public approaches to epistemology, in which research is undertaken with and for those who are affected by the issues under study.

Table 12.1 Multiple purposes of evaluations

Purposes of evaluations	Description
Assessment of merit and worth	"...the development of warranted judgments about the effects and other value characteristics of a project or policy" (Mark et al. 2000). In the context of urban health inequities, the question posed is: Did the intervention make a difference in impacting urban health inequities? This purpose of evaluation is most closely aligned with the experimental/ trials view of evaluation
Program and organizational improvement	"...efforts are made to provide timely feedback designed to modify and enhance project operations" (Mark et al. 2000). Given the complex nature of intersectoral approaches to health inequities, program and organizational improvement might be very critical to programs and systems that attempt to impact health inequities
Oversight and compliance	"...estimate the extent to which a project meets specified expectations such as the directives of statutes, regulations, or other mandates, including requirements to reach specified levels of performance" (Mark et al. 2000). This purpose of evaluation can also connect with the "fidelity" of the implementation of intervention: Is the intervention being implemented as planned?
Knowledge development	"...refers to efforts to discover and test general theories and propositions about social processes and mechanisms as they occur in the context of social policies and projects" (Mark et al. 2000). This is an especially important purpose of evaluations of interventions that target health inequities. Given the complexity of intersectoral approaches to addressing inequities, there is quite often a lack of clarity on the theory (and the causal mechanisms) that informs the development of the interventions at the outset of the intervention. *One of the important purposes of evaluation is to develop clarity on the intervention theory over time*

12.3   The Complexities of Conceptualizing Health Inequities

We start with a model that explicates the evaluative challenges of addressing health inequities (Sridharan et al. 2009). For simplicity, this model illustrates the limitations of typical approaches to redressing inequities (i.e., remedial, service-oriented, unisectoral approaches), as opposed to suggesting structural change to address the root causes of inequity (see Chaps. 1, 6, 9 and 10). This model also does not consider the multiple complexities involved in intersectoral approaches to addressing health inequities, which we look at elsewhere in this chapter.

The model outlined in Fig. 12.1 describes three levels. The first level is that of the individuals (e.g., residents of a city or a community) whose downstream health needs are being met by multiple providers and sectors. At the second level, there are upstream and downstream systems of delivery (e.g., community providers, hospitals, short-term interventions, etc.). Finally, at the third level, there is a

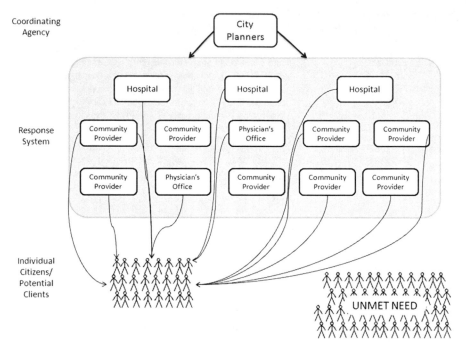

Fig. 12.1 A multilevel model of health needs

coordinating body (e.g., health department or city planner) – in reality, multiple coordinating bodies at different levels of government. Such entities are responsible for ensuring that the health system and related sectors are meeting the heterogeneous needs of the population, that the various health care providers' and services' responses to health inequities are coordinated and that the system does not systematically disadvantage some individuals or groups of individuals. Furthermore, these coordinating bodies must avoid the problem of fragmentation in which entities focus and act on the parts of a system "without adequately appreciating their relation to the evolving whole," as such fragmentation can function to increase social inequities (Stange 2009).

Whitehead (1992) defines health inequities as "differences in *health* that are avoidable, unfair and unjust" (emphasis added) and systematically related to social inequality and disadvantage. Whitehead further emphasizes reducing these systematic differences (see related discussions in Sen 2002 and Culyer 2007). This definition raises a number of questions that are relevant to social epidemiologists: How can an intervention that is often uncoordinated with the other aspects of the health system or other sectors help enhance health outcomes? What role can an intervention play in equalizing the outcomes for individuals whose needs are not being met? How can social epidemiologic research address the root causes of health disparities that lie in the broader social and economic systems far beyond the health sector?

Despite oversimplifying, the model for understanding health needs presented in Fig. 12.1 makes three points:

1. Any intervention of either a policy or program is part of the ecology of a complex system, part of a social determinants approach to health with both upstream and downstream needs, such that a number of individuals' needs are being met through a range of interventions.
2. For some individuals, there will need to be coordination between multiple providers.
3. There are a large number of individuals whose needs are *not* being met by upstream or downstream interventions. It is highly likely that there are a large number of individuals with complex disadvantages who might not have their needs met through a single provider or through the primary care system.

These points highlight the challenges for social epidemiologists when engaged in evaluations research. When conducting an evaluation, social epidemiologists need sufficiently detailed data to understand the *context* of the complex system in which the intervention is located. Furthermore, they need to explicate the *mechanisms* by which the interventions can make a difference (e.g., coordination between multiple providers), and also highlight the *dynamic processes* that may be responsible for the generation of the health inequities (e.g., dynamics of unmet need). They require knowledge of what service interventions and program mixes work for whom and under what contexts. Simply stated, t*he challenge of evaluations research within the field of social epidemiology is to locate the intervention being evaluated within the context of the processes that generate health inequities in the first place.*

Social epidemiologists must also recognize the role of data not just for measurement and operationalization but also for planning an actionable response to addressing health inequities (see Chap. 4). This is a difficult challenge, as often there is "a paucity of data to inform decisions about which individual or contextual interventions (i.e., interventions that address the environment or that are most equitably available to people regardless of their SES or behaviour) will contribute the most to reducing disparities and improving health" (Gerberding 2005). However, data may not be enough. Social epidemiologists must also leverage knowledge of past patterns of participation and engagement with social interventions and the health system to develop a strategic response to health inequities.

12.4 Moving Beyond Programs: The Ecology of Health

While the earlier discussion described a singular intervention, it is important when conducting evaluations research to also consider the broader health system (Watt et al. 2011). The need to move beyond a focus on individual programs is also driven by an increased understanding of the social determinants of health, which calls for intersectoral approaches to addressing health inequities. Intersectoral actions imply a move away from piecemeal, fragmented solutions towards thinking more broadly about a network of solutions.

In order to move beyond a singular focus on programs, social epidemiologists must learn more about the ecology of health. In other words, social epidemiologists must understand who engages and does not engage with the regular health system. The big question for addressing health inequities is not simply "does intervention 'A' work?" but rather "how best does the 'ecology of services' work as a whole to make a difference to an individual's unmet needs and quality of services?" An intersectoral systems approach offers the advantage of focusing on such connections: "it is a paradigm or perspective that considers connections among different components, plans for the implications of their interaction, and requires transdisciplinary thinking as well as active engagement of those who have a stake in the outcome to govern the course of change" (Leischow and Milstein 2006).

12.5   Intersectoral Responses to Health Inequities: Background

Developing intersectoral approaches to addressing health inequities will require a theoretical framework that describes how "collaborative problem-solving capacity" can be developed (Sridharan and Gillespie 2004). Moreover, there needs to be greater focus on how evaluation frameworks can help with the development of such intersectoral approaches (Fox 1996). There is limited evidence on good models for developing intersectoral partnerships (Babiak 2009; Shapira et al. 1997), and there are relatively few examples of collaborations between upstream and downstream organizations or any evidence that such collaborations matter in addressing health inequities. Furthermore, while the challenges of developing intersectoral responses are big at the programmatic level, the challenges are even greater if one seeks to create synergies between policies. Social epidemiologists engaged in evaluations research can help to promote coordination between policies by determining for policy makers the most effective ways to integrate public programs and policies such that the coordinated system has synergistic effects (Smith and Spenlehauer 1994).

In addition to planning and initiating intersectoral partnerships, work is required to sustain these partnerships once formed (Bourdages et al. 2003; Sridharan et al. 2006). At the programmatic level, the factors that predict sustainability of cross-program collaborations include "having a history of collaboration, a diverse and broad coalition, a clear vision and operation guidelines and diversified and sufficient funding" (Rog et al. 2004). Of course, cross-sectoral approaches, as valuable as they may be, do not often address broader structural causes of inequities. Despite strong potential, there is also a dearth of research on the health impacts of such interventions (e.g., changes in income support, unemployment insurance and other programs and policies) (Berkman 2004). Where such studies have been done, the complexity is seldom fully addressed, limiting the knowledge that can be drawn from the research. Even then, the traditional simplistic approaches to understanding the nature of the intervention are insufficient. This chapter discusses how evaluation methods, approaches and designs can help address some of these challenges.

12.6 A Realist Approach to Evaluating Complex Interventions

Pawson et al. (2004) describe seven characteristics of complex interventions. Table 12.2 describes the seven characteristics that might emerge in planning an evaluation from a realist approach. Programs are dynamic (i.e., change over time),

Table 12.2 Pawson et al.'s (2004) features of complex interventions

Features of complex interventions	Examples of evaluation questions
The intervention is a theory of theories	What are the stakeholders' theories of the intervention? Do different stakeholders have different theories of how the intervention will impact health inequities?
The intervention involves the actions of people	How do key stakeholders co-construct the intervention? What are the active ingredients of each of the interventions? Is the actual "journey" of the intervention different from the planned "journey"? Is there buy-in from the stakeholders for the theory of the intervention?
The intervention consists of a chain of steps	What are the implications of a complex chain of program activities for impacting long-term outcomes such as health inequities? How do upstream and downstream interventions connect with the causal chain implicit in the intervention?
These chains of steps or processes are often not linear, and involve negotiation and feedback at each stage	How does user involvement change the planned intervention over time?
Interventions are embedded in social systems and how they work is shaped by this context	How did the context of the intervention influence the planning and implementation of the intervention? What role did the organizational context play in shaping the eventual intervention?
Interventions are leaky and prone to be borrowed	How and why did the intervention change over time? Did the program theory change over time?
Interventions are open systems and change through learning as stakeholders come to understand them	How did the experience of implementing a complex intervention change program staff's perceptions of the mechanisms involved in impacting long-term outcomes? What are the implications of such learning for future interventions?

Adapted from (Pawson et al. 2004)

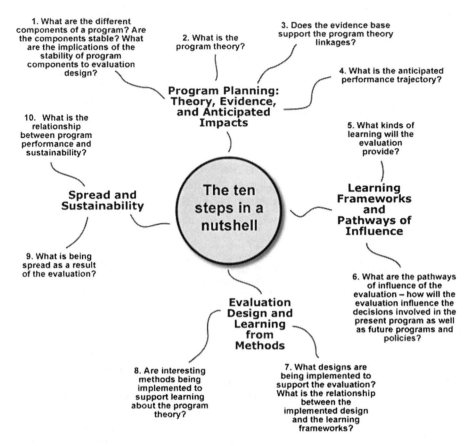

Fig. 12.2 Key issues in valuating complex health interventions (Reprinted from Sridharan and Nakaima 2011, © 2010. With permission from Elsevier)

depend critically on the context in which they are implemented and change as a result of stakeholder reasoning. One of the implications of a realist view to complex programs is a recognition that program implementers need help to align complex programming with long-term goals (such as health equity).

Based on the above discussions, we propose the following four-part framework for evaluating health inequities:

- Intervention planning, implementation and theory
- Structure of evaluation influence
- Design, data and methods
- Spread and sustainability

The following subsections each consider one of ten questions that need to be addressed as part of the framework of evaluation (Fig. 12.2). Each subsection describes the question in detail. Taken as a whole, these subsections address some basic "how to" issues that need to be considered in the evaluation of complex health interventions. Many of these issues are described in greater detail in a recent publication (Sridharan and Nakaima 2011).

12.6.1 The Key Components of the Complex Intervention

One of the surprising aspects of the evaluation literature is that there is little reflection on the implications of the complexity of the intervention for the evaluation, a weakness it shares with social epidemiologic research on the health (equity) impacts of interventions. Will the evaluation for a simple aspirin-type intervention follow the same approach as designing an evaluation system or a complex community initiative focused on health inequities? There is often a haste to rush into the evaluation without a thorough understanding of the intervention, which has consequences that have been described above. But since interventions are "complex systems thrust upon complex settings" (Pawson et al. 2004), the work of carefully describing all components of the intervention and its context is critical. Complexity has implications for both the stability and the dynamic nature of the components of an intervention. A complex health intervention with very many components that change over time may need a very different evaluation design than a simple intervention that is stable over time (Morell 2010; Patton 2010).

12.6.2 The Program Theory of the Complex Interventions

Fundamental to the evaluation of a complex intervention is developing some initial ideas of how the intervention (or, from a strategic perspective, a complex set of interventions) is likely to work. Specifically, how will an intervention address health equity outcomes? What is the relationship between the processes that constitute the complex intervention and its short- and long-term outcomes? Under what contextual conditions is the complex intervention likely to work (Mayne 2001; Pawson and Tilley 1997; Pawson 2006; Pawson and Sridharan 2009)? What mechanisms are needed for the intervention to thrive? And, quite fundamental to health equities: is the intervention likely to have very heterogeneous impacts for different groups in various contexts? A proliferation of questions surfaces on developing the initial program theory. Given both the complexity of the intervention and the incomplete knowledge that initially exists in understanding how to address health inequities, part of the focus of the evaluation needs to be sensitive to the development of an emergent theory of change for the intervention over the course of the evaluation (Sridharan and Nakaima 2011). *In our experience with evaluations of interventions that target health inequities, a program theory is often not at all explicit.* Although the development of the program theory is not necessarily going to become core to the discipline of social epidemiology, if epidemiologists are going to have an impact in research on interventions, it is an activity they should be promoting and participating in.

12.6.3   Learning from the Evidence Base

Although an intervention may be new, the reality is that there often exists an evidence base of how similar interventions have done in other fields and in other contexts. The program theory can be further strengthened by conducting an evidence synthesis for each of the linkages of the program theory. This is the approach adopted by a recent method of synthesis called realist synthesis (Pawson et al. 2004; Pawson 2006). The focus of this method of synthesis is on understanding the mechanisms and contexts in which each of the key linkages in the program theory is likely to fire. Rather than focusing on average-level effects of complex interventions, realist synthesis zeroes in on the underlying mechanisms of change and on whether a mechanism operates differently in differing contexts (see Chap. 11). Moreover, there may be invaluable information on the mechanisms of interest that are used in health programs from completely different substantive areas (e.g., crime and delinquency), and such information may also be valuable.

12.6.4   The Anticipated Timeline of Impact

A complex intervention might take time to impact health outcomes. It is important that the evaluation help develop knowledge about the anticipated timeline of impact of complex health interventions. According to Berkman (2004), one of the reasons that many very promising social interventions studied in RCTs have failed to show a sizeable impact on health is that not enough time was allowed. The state of knowledge of social science theory is such that information on anticipated timelines of impact for complex health interventions is often missing. One approach that we have used successfully in prior evaluations is to engage stakeholders who have been involved in prior interventions to help explicate such an anticipated timeline of impact (Cook 2000; Sridharan et al. 2006). Understanding what outcomes are likely to be impacted by the complex health intervention and when is important to the evaluation design and in moderating expectations among researchers, decision makers and community partners.

12.6.5   Learning Framework for the Evaluation

There needs to be clarity on the types of learning that an evaluation of a complex health intervention can provide. Multiple types of learning about a complex intervention might be possible from an evaluation. These "learnings" include: learning about the impacts of the complex health intervention, learning about the dynamic processes that might be critical for the complex intervention to work and learning about the organizational context that might be necessary for the complex intervention to flourish. All evaluations should be guided by the types of information that are needed by stakeholders and the timing of such needs (i.e., when will the information be useful?). This focus on utilization may not be as obvious as it might sound – far too many decisions about evaluations are based on abstract notions of rigour that sometimes do not correspond to generating information in a timely manner that stakeholders will find useful.

12.6.6   The Pathways of Influence of an Evaluation

Just as there is need for clarity about the pathways by which a complex intervention can impact outcomes, there is a similar need to be clear about the pathways by which the evaluation can influence future and present innovations. Recent evaluation literature (Mark and Henry 2004; Henry and Mark 2003) describes the multiple individual, interpersonal and collective processes by which evaluations can bring about influence. While there has been some research on knowledge translation of research based on interventions in social epidemiology (Petticrew et al. 2011), such thinking needs to be incorporated into the development of the evaluation of health innovations. Ultimately, an evaluation is an investment that can come at the expense of other programming resources, so there needs to be clarity on the pathways of influence by which the evaluation itself can make a difference.

12.6.7   Assessing the Impact of the Health Intervention

A fundamental step in evaluation is developing a design that includes methods and measures to understand if the complex intervention is working. This implies: (1) understanding what a successful impact is defined as for the intervention; (2) having clarity on the timeline of impact; (3) developing clear measures that can be used to study the impact of the intervention; (4) that measures to study the impact be informed by the theory of change of the complex intervention; (5) that the measurement system should include measures of the dynamic contexts and mechanisms that might be necessary for the complex intervention to work; and (6) an evaluation design that can help rule out alternative explanations for changes in key outcomes. A good evaluation design also needs to shed light on the actual program's mechanism of change or, alternatively, test the hypothesized mechanism of change. It is crucial to have measures of the impact on aspects of the program theory in all circumstances, but particularly if the intervention does not meet expectations on the endpoint outcomes. In such cases, knowledge about the impact on markers of the program theory or on intermediate outcomes is essential (Berkman 2004). Knowledge about the impact on program theory elements might also be extremely critical in assessing the generalizability of the program in order to make decisions about replicating or adapting a program to a new setting. A good design should shed light on the contexts needed and the mechanisms by which programs work.

A number of evaluation theorists argue for the need for a counterfactual (i.e., a comparison or control group to study what would happen in the absence of the intervention), and this is also the case in social epidemiology (Berkman 2004; Kaufman and Poole 2000). While such designs have strengths, depending on the complexity of the intervention, they might not be practical because there may be lack of clarity of what constitutes the intervention at the start of implementation. The intervention might evolve over time and might depend heavily on local context for the positive impacts to accrue. An experimental design might not pay as clear attention to contextual factors that might be very critical in the success of an intervention (Pawson and Tilley 1997). For many interventions, in other words, the study design must adapt to the intervention in order to maximize what can be learned from it, rather than the other way around, which is more common.

12.6.8   Learning About the Pathways of Impact of the Complex Intervention over Time

One key step in the evaluation of a complex intervention is to learn about a theory of change of the complex intervention over the course of its implementation. Given the nonlinear nature of some complex interventions (Patton 2010), there are likely to be many "surprises" (Morell 2010) in the processes by which a complex intervention can impact outcomes. An emergent theory of change needs to reflect on the processes by which complex interventions can impact outcomes over time. Some of the points to consider in developing such an emergent theory of change include the following: (1) pay close attention to the unintended consequences of a complex intervention (Morell 2010; Patton 2010); (2) focus on both the "macro" social processes and the "micro" individual-level contexts that are essential for the impacts of the intervention; (3) if possible, explore the systems dynamics underlying the process of change of the intervention; and (4) pay attention to both the networks and the key events in the course of the implementation of the intervention that are important for the impact of the intervention. A wide variety of methodologies are available to explicate such emergent theories of change (Patton 2010; Sridharan and Nakaima 2011).

12.6.9   Spreading Learning from an Evaluation

A key purpose of the evaluation is also to reflect on what the types of learning need to be spread as a result of the evaluation (Massoud et al. 2006). A complex intervention typically might consist of many components; an evaluation needs to reflect on the parts of the intervention that are worth replicating in other settings. Is it all of the components? Are there only certain components of the complex intervention that need to be replicated widely? Or is the focus on more specific learning, like knowledge about the context and mechanisms that enhance the success of the intervention?

12.6.10   *Reflections on Sustainability*

Evaluations also provide enormous opportunities to help decide whether interventions need to be sustained. There is often an implicit claim that evaluations help make decisions about sustaining innovations. Yet the relationship between performance and sustainability in the evaluation literature continues to be very limited. Issues of sustainability and performance are especially relevant for complex interventions because often the timelines of impact of complex interventions might be very unclear. Sometimes an intervention might not produce tangible benefits for many years before it results in huge impacts. Understanding such anticipated timelines of impact becomes especially critical given the potential nonlinear patterns of change that might be part of the impact processes of complex interventions.

Should an innovation be discontinued if it does not meet performance targets? As discussed in Sridharan and Nakaima (2011), this is a difficult question, and especially for some complex health interventions, because the trajectory of impact of even a successful intervention can be quite nonlinear, as previously stated. Some performance outcomes might get worse before they get better. Additionally, there is no reason for the trajectory of the performance outcomes to be linear or monotonic over time. Key ideas related to sustainability include:

1. Decisions to sustain the intervention should be guided by a theory that can help inform the drivers of performance of the intervention. Without a clear program theory it is hard to tell whether the intervention needs more investment or less.
2. There is a need to pay attention to the process by which performance targets are set. Milstein et al. (2007) make the point strongly about the lack of rigour and quality by which performance targets are set.
3. There is a need to pay attention to the systems dynamics involved in the process of implementing social interventions. The nature of the impacts of the social interventions might be such that they take a while to accrue.

12.7   Conclusions

In this chapter, we have attempted to draw upon evaluations research and, notably, new innovations in the realist approach to evaluation to offer concepts that could be helpful in rethinking the role of social epidemiology in its examinations of interventions that may affect health and health equity. In so doing, we have illustrated what can be learned from evaluations research as a field of study, and we have also expanded upon traditional notions of what can and should be learned from evaluations. We have not been prescriptive in our approach; social epidemiologists who are engaged in research on interventions and their impact on health equity are best placed to rethink the subdiscipline. Of course, one question that we have sidestepped is whether a social epidemiologist is still a social epidemiologist if they take all of the suggestions from realist evaluation. We think that social epidemiology has many unique contributions to offer the study of the health (equity) impacts of interventions and that learning from evaluations represents an opportunity, not a threat. That opportunity is to give social epidemiologists more potential tools and concepts to bring to their engagement with the problem of reducing health inequities.

References

Babiak KM (2009) Criteria of effectiveness in multiple cross-sectoral interorganizational relationships. Eval Program Plann 32:1–12

Berkman L (2004) Introduction: seeing the forest and the trees – from observation to experiments in social epidemiology. Epidemiol Rev 26:2–6

Bourdages J, Sauvageau L, Lepage C (2003) Factors in creating sustainable intersectoral community mobilization for prevention of heart and lung disease. Health Promot Int 18:135–144

Cook TD (2000) The false choice between theory-based evaluation and experimentation. New Dir Eval 87:27–34

Culyer AJ (2007) Equity of what in health care? Why the traditional answers don't help policy – and what to do in the future. Healthc Pap 8:12–26

Fox J (1996) Promoting independent assessments of MDB anti-poverty investments: bringing civil society in. IDR Rep 12:1–9

Gerberding JL (2005) Protecting health: the new research imperative. JAMA 294:1403–1406

Henry GT, Mark MM (2003) Beyond use: understanding evaluation's influence on attitudes and actions. Am J Eval 24:293–314

Kaufman JS, Poole C (2000) Looking back on "Causal Thinking in the Health Sciences.". Annu Rev Public Health 21:101–119

Leischow SJ, Milstein B (2006) Systems thinking and modeling for public health practice. Am J Public Health 96:403–405

Mark MM, Henry GT (2004) The mechanisms and outcomes of evaluation influence. Evaluation 10:35–57

Mark MM, Henry GT, Julnes G (2000) Evaluation: an integrated framework for understanding, guiding, and improving policies and programs. Jossey Bass, San Francisco

Massoud MR, Nielsen GA, Nolan K et al (2006) A framework for spread: from local improvements to system-wide change. IHI Innovation Series white paper. Institute for Healthcare Improvement, Cambridge

Mayne J (2001) Addressing attribution through contribution analysis: using performance measures sensibly. Can J Program Eval 16:1–24

Milstein B, Jones A, Homer JB et al (2007) Charting plausible futures for diabetes prevalence in the United States: a role for system dynamics simulation modeling. Prev Chronic Dis 4:A52

Morell JA (2010) Evaluation in the face of uncertainty: anticipating surprise and responding to the inevitable. Guilford Press, New York

Patton MQ (2010) Developmental evaluation: applying complexity concepts to enhance innovation and use. Guilford Press, New York

Pawson R (2006) Evidence-based policy: a realist perspective. Sage Publications, London

Pawson R, Sridharan S (2009) Theory-driven evaluation of public health programmes. In: Killoran A, Kelly M (eds) Evidence-based public health: effectiveness and efficiency. Oxford University Press, Oxford

Pawson R, Tilley N (1997) An introduction to scientific realist evaluations. In: Chelimsky E, Shadish WR (eds) Evaluation for the 21st century: a handbook. Sage Publications, Thousand Oaks

Pawson R, Greenhalgh T, Harvey G et al (2004) Realist synthesis: an introduction. In: ESRC research methods programme: RMP methods paper series. University of Manchester, Manchester

Petticrew MP, Chalabi Z, Jones D (2011) To RCT or not to RCT: deciding when more evidence is needed for public health policy and practice. J Epidemiol Community Health. J Epidemiol Community Health. Published online on 7 April 2011. http://jech.bmj.com/content/early/2011/06/07/jech.2010.116483.short

Riley BL, MacDonald J, Mansi O et al (2008) Is reporting on interventions a weak link in understanding how and why they work? A preliminary exploration using community heart health exemplars. Implemen Sci 3:27

Rog D, Boback N, Barton-Villagrana H et al (2004) Sustaining collaboratives: a cross-site analysis of The National Funding Collaborative on Violence Prevention. Eval Program Plann 27: 249–261

Sen A (2002) Why health equity? Health Econ 11:659–666

Shapira P, Kingsley G, Youtie J (1997) Manufacturing partnerships: evaluation in the context of government reform. Eval Program Plann 20:103–112

Smith A, Spenlehauer V (1994) Policy evaluation meets harsh reality: instrument of integration or preserver of disintegration? Eval Program Plann 17:277–287

Sridharan S, Gillespie D (2004) Sustaining problem-solving capacity in collaborative networks. Criminol Public Policy 3:221–250

Sridharan S, Nakaima A (2011) Ten steps to making evaluations matter. Eval Program Plann 34(2):135–146

Sridharan S, Campbell B, Zinzow H (2006) Developing a stakeholder-driven timeline of change for evaluations of social programs. Am J Eval 27:148–162

Sridharan S, Gardner B, Nakaima A (2009) Steps towards incorporating health inequities into a performance measurement and management framework: analysis of the hospital health equity plans. Toronto Central Local Health Integration Network, Toronto. http://www.torontoevaluation.ca/tclhin/PDF/LHIN%20final%20October%2015%20send.pdf. Accessed 11 Apr 2011

Stange KC (2009) The problem of fragmentation and the need for integrative solutions. Ann Fam Med 7:100–103

Treasury Board of Canada Secretariat (2009) Archived [2009-03-31] – policy on evaluation. http://www.tbs-sct.gc.ca/pol/doc-eng.aspx?id=12309. Accessed 11 Apr 2011

Watt G, O'Donnell C, Sridharan S (2011) Building on Julian Tudor Hart's example of anticipatory care. Prim Health Care Res Dev 12:3–10

Whitehead M (1992) The concepts and principles of equity and health. Int J Health Serv 22: 429–445

Part IV
Making a Difference

Chapter 13
Knowledge Translation and Social Epidemiology: Taking Power, Politics and Values Seriously

Kelly Murphy and Patrick Fafard

Contents

13.1	Introduction	268
13.2	Starting Assumptions About Social Epidemiology	269
13.3	Making Research Relevant: A Cursory Look at the Emergence of Knowledge Translation in the Health Sciences	270
13.4	The Tension Between Conventional KT and Social Epidemiology	272
	13.4.1 KT Understands Policy Change in Terms of Problems, Not Processes	272
	13.4.2 Conventional KT Is Concerned with Individual, Not Collective, Action	274
	13.4.3 Conventional KT Assumes Shared, Not Contested, Definitions of Problems	275
	13.4.4 Conventional KT Leaves Little Room for Advocacy	276
13.5	KT and Knowledge Constitutive Interests	278
13.6	Taking Politics, Power and Values Seriously in KT	279
13.7	Conclusions	281
References		281

Abstract Although demand for evidence-based policies and programs to reduce population health inequities is intensifying, the influence of social epidemiology on public policy remains limited. In clinical and health services research domains, *knowledge translation* strategies have been developed to increase the impact of research evidence in policy making and practice. We review the applicability of these strategies for increasing the practical impact of social epidemiology research,

K. Murphy (✉)
Centre for Research on Inner City Health, St. Michael's Hospital, 30 Bond Street, Toronto, ON M5B 1W8, Canada
e-mail: MurphyKe@smh.ca

P. Fafard
Graduate School of Public and International Affairs, University of Ottawa, 55 Laurier Avenue East, Desmarais Building, Room 11105, Ottawa ON, K1N 6N5, Canada
e-mail: Patrick.Fafard@uottawa.ca

P. O'Campo and J.R. Dunn (eds.), *Rethinking Social Epidemiology:
Towards a Science of Change*, DOI 10.1007/978-94-007-2138-8_13,
© Springer Science+Business Media B.V. 2012

drawing on the *knowledge constitutive interests* framework developed by Jürgen Habermas. We find that conventional knowledge translation characterizes policy change and the role of research in technical-instrumental terms that do not reflect the complex social, political and values-based dimensions of policy change and research use that come into play in relation to the reduction of health inequities. While conventional knowledge translation approaches may work in some cases, for social epidemiology to play a significant role in advancing social change, knowledge translation strategies that acknowledge and respond to the intersections of power, politics, values and science also need to be developed.

Abbreviations

CIHR   Canadian Institutes of Health Research
KT   knowledge translation
MMR   measles, mumps and rubella

13.1 Introduction

The World Health Organization Commission on Social Determinants of Health (2008) called action on the determinants of health an "ethical imperative." Social epidemiologists should have important roles to play in the Commission's call to action. Social epidemiology has identified a number of important relationships between socioeconomic inequality and population health. Moreover, the measurement tools and conceptual constructs developed by social epidemiologists can be used to evaluate health outcomes associated with policy and program interventions both inside and outside of the health care system (Oakes and Kaufman 2006; Berkman and Kawachi 2000; Braveman 2006). This research evidence should be particularly valuable for guiding policy initiatives to reduce health inequities (Graham 2004). However, the influence of social epidemiology on current public policy making in North America remains relatively hard to see (Raphael 2003; Asthana and Halliday 2006). In this chapter we ask, why doesn't health equity research in particular, and social epidemiology in general, have a bigger role to play in promoting social and political change? Simply put, in this chapter, we argue that the answer lies in the fact that the tools available, which we designate here as "conventional" knowledge translation, assume that research knowledge is to be used for solving problems; whereas, social epidemiology, at its core, often emphasizes deeper and quite distinct goals of explanation and, ultimately, social change.

There are many ways to explain the limited policy impact of social epidemiology, several of which are explored in other chapters in this book (see Chaps. 1, 3 and 15). Our approach is to look at the tools and techniques that are offered to health researchers in the rapidly expanding *research utilization* or, what is more frequently referred to as, *knowledge translation* (KT), literature. These tools are intended help *make health research relevant* and to *move health research into practice and policy*. In what follows we ask, first, "What were these tools designed to do?" and, second, "Are these tools suited to health equity research and the goals of social epidemiologists?"

This chapter proceeds as follows. First, we outline our assumptions about some of the defining characteristics of social epidemiology. These assumptions inform all of our observations that follow; therefore, we feel it is important to state them at the outset. Next, we briefly introduce conventional KT, as it has emerged and gained prominence in health research communities in Canada and elsewhere. With this foundation, we identify four core premises underpinning conventional KT and critically assess the relevance of these premises for social epidemiology and policy challenges related to health inequities. As an alternative, and drawing on the work of Jürgen Habermas, we suggest that conventional KT, which was designed to advance the practical impact of clinical and health services research, emphasizes an *instrumental* (problem-solving) role for research knowledge in society. In contrast, social epidemiology is characterized by *hermeneutical* (explanatory) and *emancipatory* (equity-seeking) goals (Habermas 1971). These are fundamentally different approaches to knowledge use, and, we will argue, they give rise to different approaches for bridging the gap between research and practice. Consequently, conventional KT tools and techniques will often be ill-suited and inadequate for advancing the impact of social determinants of health research. We conclude with an outline of an alternative KT framework that may be more appropriate for social epidemiology to increase its impact on social policy. Simply put, it encourages social epidemiologists to either align themselves more closely with the instrumental approach to KT in clinical and health services research and move from problem-focused to solution-focused research or move to a form of engaged scholarship. The latter involves researchers becoming more active and engaged as true public intellectuals or, more simply, by actively engage with the media, speaking out on issues that contribute to the health of marginalized populations and becoming active members of advocacy coalitions and other forms of collective action to reform health and social policy. This latter framework takes power, politics and values seriously in strategies to promote social change through research. In other words, social epidemiology is a heterogeneous enterprise and social epidemiologists need to find the KT approach that fits their needs.

13.2 Starting Assumptions About Social Epidemiology

Neither of us is a social epidemiologist, but our arguments in this chapter rest on some core assumptions that we have made about social epidemiology (particularly, health equity research) as a knowledge project. First, we understand social epidemiology as a project that explicitly investigates social, economic and political determinants of health, disease and wellbeing in populations (Krieger 2001).

Second, most social epidemiology research is scrupulously positivist, aiming to produce falsifiable, empirical measures of these relationships. Third, we are assuming that researchers in social epidemiology and related disciplines face increasing pressure from research funding agencies and others to increase the practical impact of their scientific activity even if this practical orientation is in tension with the very nature of the discipline.

Thus, we are also assuming that, unlike almost all other health science disciplines, social epidemiology has, implicitly if not explicitly, a strong normative dimension, one that emphasizes social critique. Social epidemiology illuminates harmful effects of social conditions on health so that (eventually) the relevant social conditions can be targeted and modified and so that population health can be improved (Berkman and Kawachi 2000; Wilkinson and Pickett 2009; Chernomas and Hudson 2009). Finally, precisely because social epidemiology has the potential to inform radical change, we assume that social epidemiologists are genuinely interested in contributing to practical population health improvement but that they may also feel constrained by what they, and others, see as their roles as scientists.

13.3   Making Research Relevant: A Cursory Look at the Emergence of Knowledge Translation in the Health Sciences

The last two decades have been marked by the demand for research, in fields as varied as international development, energy and environmental science and even the social sciences and humanities, to demonstrate practical value and *return on investment* (Murphy and Topple 2003; Buxton et al. 2004). Perhaps nowhere has this demand been expressed as urgently as it has been in relation to health services and health research. Concern for health research to show practical impact is due, in part, to unprecedented cost pressures from health care experienced in most Western countries over this period and a universal need for strategies to contain expenses while also making people healthier (Limoges et al. 1994).

While the role of research in practice and policy making has received longstanding attention in some scholarly disciplines (e.g., science and technology studies, sociology and political science) (Bernal 1939; Merton 1973; Rose and Rose 1970), research utilization is a relatively new focus of attention in the health sciences. Since the late 1990s, Canadians – who pioneered the evidence-based medicine movement (Evidence-Based Medicine Working Group 1992; Sackett et al. 2000) and who have also been leaders in advancing the argument for health research utilization (Lemieux-Charles and Champagne 2004) – have bundled these ideas under the concept of *knowledge translation* or KT (Straus et al. 2009a, b). Canada's premier federal health research funding agency, the Canadian Institutes of Health Research (CIHR), has adopted KT as a core mandate and defines it as "the exchange, synthesis and ethically-sound application of knowledge – within a

Table 13.1 Increasing research impact: traditional scientific dissemination versus knowledge translation

	Traditional dissemination	Knowledge translation
Who is the intended audience?	• Other researchers	• Decision makers
To do what?	• Increase awareness • Increase understanding • Foster further research	• Take action: guide policy making, programming, or practices
By what means?	• Publish in scientific journals	• Explain key messages from research results in accessible, plain language • Synthesize research results from multiple studies • Align research inquiry and funding with decision maker priorities • Involve decision makers in the research process, i.e. integrated KT (Tibelius and Stirling 2007), in accessible plain language • Synthesize research findings to address decision maker questions • Target research funds to address strategic problems (Lomas et al. 2003)

complex system of interactions among researchers and users – to accelerate the capture of the benefits of research for Canadians through improved health, more effective services and products, and a strengthened health care system" (Tibelius and Stirling 2007). Other allied terms used to describe this concept may be more familiar to some readers, such as knowledge transfer, knowledge mobilization, linkage and exchange, research transfer, implementation and dissemination or research uptake. Implementation science is a newer term, describing evaluative research to assess the effectiveness of KT strategies (BiomedCentral 2010). Because KT is an expression that is widely gaining ground in other countries (Pablos-Mendez and Shademani 2006), and other disciplinary domains (Carden 2009), it is the term that we will use throughout this chapter.

KT frameworks for health are premised on perceived structural and/or cultural gaps between the individuals and organizations responsible for health care delivery and those responsible for conducting research. However, KT assumes that scientific publication in peer-reviewed journals is too passive a dissemination practice for there to be a real impact of research on policy, programs and practice.

As outlined in Table 13.1, knowledge translation is different from traditional scientific dissemination in at least three important aspects: (1) the intended audience for research extends far beyond academe to include practitioners and decision makers; (2) the goal is not only to inform but to have an effect on decisions and problems; and (3) the method of knowledge sharing involves active outreach on the part of the research community (Graham and Tetroe 2007).

Explicit and implicit assumptions about the nature of the research/decision-making divide and the proper role of scientific knowledge in policy development have given rise to different recommendations for KT activities; however, all approaches tend toward agreement that "tailor and target" approaches are the best strategies for enhancing the practical influence of research evidence. From these directives we can derive a set of boilerplate KT principles to guide health researchers:

- Understand the decision maker's problem from the decision maker's point of view;
- Interact closely with that decision-making individual or organization to ensure the research project explores aspects of the problem and potential solutions that matter to the decision maker; and
- Explain the research results to the decision maker in terms that are meaningful and actionable and that help the decision maker to solve the problem.

The question then becomes whether and to what extent these core KT principles are an effective guide for social epidemiology. In our view the answer is often "*no*" because of tensions (if not a fundamental disconnect) between some of the core assumptions that underlie conventional approaches to KT and at least parts of the project that is social epidemiology.

13.4   The Tension Between Conventional KT and Social Epidemiology

In our view, conventional KT may not be particularly useful for increasing the impact of social epidemiology on policy, program and practice choices. We want to show how conventional KT is not always relevant or effective for social epidemiology for three reasons: first, because KT understands in terms of problems, not processes; second, because KT targets individual rather than collective action; third, because it assumes shared, rather than contested definitions of policy problems; and fourth and finally, because conventional KT leaves little room for advocacy.

13.4.1   KT Understands Policy Change in Terms of Problems, Not Processes

First, as KT moves from clinical settings to the policy process, it retains a framework that emphasizes problem-solving, characterized in terms of discrete *decision events* that are closely linked to, if not elided with, *implementation* of evidence-based *solutions*. For example, in clinical settings the theory is that effective KT will make it more likely that clinicians will follow clinical practice guidelines. As a result, one of the metrics for evaluating conventional KT more generally is whether or not problems get solved and decisions are made to bring relevant rules and procedures into line with the best available evidence. While the impact of conventional

KT on clinical decision making has been mixed, the complex implications for policy and program change that may be generated through social epidemiology defy the reduction of evidence to *decision support* and the reduction of policy making to *problem solving*.

For a government to respond to the implications, for example, of a report on correlations between housing affordability and health status in a given jurisdiction (Dunn 2002), it would likely require negotiation and coordination across multiple departments, agencies and levels of government and would operate over a number of years (Leone and Carroll 2010). A problem-solving/solution-implementation model, based on clinical decision making for an individual patient is an obviously inadequate analogy for such wide-sweeping, systems-level policy change (Howlett et al. 2009).

A variety of conceptual frameworks are available from policy studies that can generate more nuanced accounts of policy change related to social determinants of health compared to models based on evidence-based medicine. We have shown elsewhere that the *developmental stages framework* of policy making can be a particularly useful heuristic model for advancing KT (Fafard 2008). The framework emphasizes that policy making involves much more than simple decision making. First, an issue or problem has to become part of the government's agenda. Second, the range of possible responses to the policy challenge, including doing nothing, have to be evaluated against a diverse range of criteria, of which scientific evidence is but one such criterion. Third, a decision gets made for almost any complex policy problem, and deciding what to do usually involves a series of decisions by a diverse set of actors over a period of time. Once a decision has been made the preferred course of action is implemented where the substantive content of the decision sometimes gets modified. Finally, in a well-performing policy-making system, policy decisions are routinely evaluated and, as appropriate, changes made (Deleon 1999). Although it is by no means the dominant model of policy making in contemporary policy studies, the stages model does underline the reality that there are multiple points in the policy process when research evidence may be influential, and it helps explain that different barriers to research use may be relevant at different stages (Burton 2006).

Especially important for health equity research, the stages model flags *agenda setting* as the critical first step in policy development. Before research evidence can ever influence a government to solve a problem, there is the prior step of deciding that the problem exists, that it matters and that it can be addressed. Faced with literally thousands of issues that it could focus on, a government selects a platform, or portfolio of target issues, which it believes it has the power, resources and political support to change (Kingdon 2003). Of course, research evidence is but one determinant of the agenda of a government. The ideational and ideological preferences of the governing party, the personal preferences and concerns of individual ministers and public opinion all play a role. However, research can be, and often is, an important influence on the government's agenda. Evidence from social epidemiology could play particularly important roles in the agenda-setting stage of policy change, for example, by presenting normative and empirical arguments as to why, from a population health perspective, it is important to invest in early childhood development, traffic ordinances or community empowerment initiatives. Moreover, the impact of research, including social epidemiologic research on the agenda of a government, is by no means automatic. Here, notwithstanding its limitations, the conventional KT literature does point to potentially useful processes and practices (e.g., plain language summaries, knowledge brokering, etc.). But agenda setting is rarely accounted for in the metrics of conventional KT, which emphasize problem solving and implementation of policy solutions.

13.4.2 Conventional KT Is Concerned with Individual, Not Collective, Action

KT emphasizes the need to identify the key decision maker (or decision-making organization) involved in the policy or practice issue that is being researched and to narrowly tailor the research question and the research findings to address the concerns of, and actions available to, this decision maker. In conventional KT it is routinely asserted that evidence that is not tailored for a target audience is less likely to be reviewed or adopted into use (Graham and Tetroe 2007). Another commonplace assertion is that "linkage and exchange" activities to engage the decision maker directly in the research process will produce research evidence that is more relevant and more likely to be applied in practice. Yet these narrow "target and tailor" approaches emphasize action *within* rather than *across* jurisdictional boundaries, and they are aimed to trigger an *individual* response rather than *collective* action.

Leaving aside the question of whether focusing on a single target audience is a good way to bring about clinical or health system change, it is surely an unpromising approach when it comes to the social determinants of health. Which sector, for example, would be the ideal participant and target audience for research related to mental health among homeless populations? Should researchers foster linkages with representatives in the housing, income assistance and social welfare or health care sectors? In some instances, the relevant government audience for social epidemiology may not exist at all, for example, when researchers look at macro-level issues beyond the reach of the current government (e.g., correlations between infant mortality and types of political regimes) (Coburn 2000). However, results of this type of social epidemiologic research may be of interest to the media and to civil society groups that are influential in the policy-making process, although they are not "decision makers" *per se*.

As these examples suggest, target audiences for social epidemiology research are likely to comprise a wide range of stakeholders working within, across, beyond and sometimes against governments. Effective response to social determinants of health research will almost always require *collective action*, negotiation and coordination that move us quickly into the realm of *politics*. Yet conventional KT, which encourages researchers to narrowly target research findings to guide individual decisions, has relatively little to say about collective action or the political dimensions of decision making. Consequently, it offers limited guidance to social epidemiologists who aim to make their research useful to the diversity of actors with a stake in the social determinants of health.

13.4.3 Conventional KT Assumes Shared, Not Contested, Definitions of Problems

Central to the conventional KT literature is the tacit assumption that researchers and policy stakeholders will agree on the meaning of a common policy problem; that is, they accept the same *framing* of the problem (Dorfman et al. 2005). This discursive agreement is required to generate evidence-based recommendations that are salient to, and executable within, a decision maker's range of action and priorities. A further step is to include government and health system officials directly in the research process either by means of the aforementioned *linkage and exchange* or what some have called *integrated KT* (Gagnon 2011).

When an issue is generally uncontroversial (or it is relatively technical in nature), researchers, policy makers and the wider communities that are affected may share a common definition of the problem. This situation is often the case for some (but certainly not all) clinical or health services issues. However, many social determinants of health problems and most health equity issues are decidedly *not* uncontroversial because they concern unequal distribution of resources across population groups. These kinds of distributive justice problems are complex and informed by social values. They cannot be addressed through technical or administrative changes alone (Daniels 2008). In these cases, researchers and the array of different decision makers and community representatives with a stake in this issue may have widely divergent interpretations of both the *problem* and the salient *solutions*. Contested definitions of social determinants of health issues are particularly vivid when the policy issues are related to stigmatized or illegal health behaviours (e.g., substance use) or marginalized populations (e.g., sex trade workers) (Benoit et al. 2003). For example, there is a multitude of competing ways of framing illicit substance use, including addiction and pathology, criminality, mental illness and self-medication, cultural deprivation, et cetera. These different meaning frames will lead participants to different accounts of what matters in relation to substance use, what needs to be done and who is responsible for doing it.

Importantly, these diverse discourses are not equally authoritative or persuasive. Rather, the authority to name or *frame* a problem and make it stick is a marker of power, and the struggle to challenge, refute and redefine meaning frames through discourse is the stuff of politics (Bevir and Rhodes 2006). In other disciplines, including sociology, communications and critical public health, researchers have used discourse analysis methods to shed light on the ways that policy debates and struggles for social change often coalesce around the authority to name and assign meaning to social phenomena. A discourse analysis approach may be particularly useful for social epidemiologists to draw upon, because it helps to explain tensions that that may arise frequently in relation to contentious health equity research and KT (Bacchi 2008; Murphy and van der Meulen 2008). Here, the goal of close collaboration between researchers and decision makers is a challenging proposition to say the least.

Indeed, important goals of health equity research may be to *resist* how powerful constituencies define issues affecting marginalized populations and to *encourage* stakeholders to understand problems in a new light. For example, social epidemiologists have contributed to a partial shift in the approach to homelessness in Canada by providing evidence that homelessness is a critical *health care* problem in addition to being a social assistance issue (Frankish et al. 2005). Weiss (1979) calls this kind of influence the "enlightenment" model of research use. However, conventional KT provides minimal guidance about how to advance controversial research evidence among decision makers, and, in the same way that it is unconcerned with agenda setting (see above), KT also accords relatively little value to research effects that are reflected in changed attitudes rather than changed actions.

There is ample research that demonstrates how knowledge (including research-based knowledge) can be used to produce, concentrate and exercise discursive power in ways that privilege some definitions of health and social problems and marginalize others. To take but one example, some research on autism emphasizes intensive behavioural interventions to "treat" autistic individuals. Other research focuses on trying to better understand what explains the increased incidence of autism including what some believe to be the cause of autism (e.g., environmental factors and the falsely attributed measles, mumps and rubella (MMR) vaccine). Still other research, often encouraged by autistic adults, sees autism as a form of neurological diversity that, rather than being cured or treated, should be recognized as a legitimate identity. Each of these research endeavours generates knowledge that leads to quite different definitions of the "problem" of autism and what might be the most appropriate "solutions" (Orsini and Smith 2010). Yet the conventional health KT framework tends to assume a naturalistic and uncontested approach to defining policy issues and research questions.

13.4.4   Conventional KT Leaves Little Room for Advocacy

Conventional KT often assumes a strict division between "research" (i.e., the creation of knowledge) and "advocacy" (i.e., making the public case for a preferred policy decision). Researchers including social epidemiologists are expected, of course, to do research, but the conventional model of KT leaves little or no room for subsequent public advocacy. This division partly results from the fact that, in conventional KT, when the value commitments in the research are aligned with those of the decision maker, we call it knowledge translation; when they do not so align, we call it advocacy.

In fact, social and policy change is often the result of disagreement and contestation, if not outright conflict, and public advocacy is sometimes required. Policy choices often involve normative disagreements that are resolved, not by more research, but by public discussion and debate where more or less acceptable compromises are arrived at. Even in those cases where there is little disagreement on the basic epidemiologic research, say for example on the correlation between health status and inequality, there remains considerable room for debate and discussion on what the causal linkage is and, even when this is established, what the optimal policy response might be.

Some social epidemiologists accept, and may even encourage, some or all of the assumptions of conventional KT even when their research has significant policy implications. They are comfortable in the role of researcher separate and apart from the policy discussion. Their preference to not engage in policy advocacy is simply a reflection of the fact that they feel they have neither the training nor the necessary expertise that would allow them to move from research to policy and much less to advocacy.

However, many other social epidemiologists are unwilling to limit their role to that of just research. They are part of the longstanding public health tradition of advocating for social, political and economic change. While on occasion, collaborative work with decision makers may be appropriate and effective, they believe that very often advocacy and public debate are required, particularly when research threatens to disrupt the *status quo*. Thus, some researchers feel an obligation to speak for (or at least with) constituencies affected by health problems that may not have the social capital to champion research findings to influence programs and policy themselves. Indeed, for many, one of the reasons for doing social epidemiologic research in the first place is to foster meaningful change and concerted action on the social causes of health inequality.

Moreover, these are rarely, if ever, solo activities. Policy discussion and debate involves groups of people with differing perspectives on the topical issues of the day who sometimes align themselves to make the case for policy change. Thus, social and political change means becoming part of a more or less organized group or, what political scientists have called, an "advocacy coalition" (Sabatier and Jenkins-Smith 1999). Why should a social epidemiologist join an advocacy coalition? Simply put, advocacy coalitions are a logical response to the nature of policy and program change. Given the sheer complexity of most policy problems (e.g., how to reduce overcrowding in inner city housing) and similarly the complexity of the appropriate response from governments (e.g., social housing, rent controls, increased minimum wage, etc.), not to mention the complexity of government decision making (e.g., how to work with a city council committed to low taxes in order to expand the stock of social housing), advocacy coalitions bring together a range of expertise on how best to define the problem, how to design effective and feasible policy and program responses and, of course, how to most effectively pressure governments to make policy changes.

For some, the goal is not to influence the decision of the government of the day but rather to fundamentally challenge the status quo. This takes us beyond the confines of KT and requires a different way of thinking about the role of knowledge, power and social change that we now wish to sketch, if only briefly.

13.5   KT and Knowledge Constitutive Interests

All told, these examples point to quite a bad fit between the context of research application presupposed in conventional KT frameworks and the actual conditions of health equity policy making that many social epidemiologists will encounter. As a result, many techniques recommended in the KT literature will be difficult for social epidemiologists to execute, and these techniques may be suboptimal or even inappropriate interventions to help increase the practical value and impact of social epidemiology evidence. If it has not already, this impediment threatens to become a serious problem for the discipline, considering not only the urgent need for informed practical action to reduce health inequities but also the increasing likelihood that research funding will be tied to evidence of research impact. Therefore, explaining and resolving social epidemiology's KT obstacles are important.

In the short space remaining in this chapter, we sketch our approach to these challenges. Central to our argument here is the work of Jürgen Habermas (1971), a sociologist of knowledge and political philosopher whose analyses of modernization, communicative rationality and democratization are directly relevant for understanding the discourse on KT. His early research included the elaboration of a conceptual framework for understanding three distinct purposes for (or *interests* in) using knowledge in society. The theory of *knowledge constitutive interests* helps to explain the "bad fit" we find between KT and social epidemiology, and it suggests directions for increasing social epidemiology's chances of having an effect.

Under the knowledge constitutive interests framework, knowledge may be used for *instrumental* purposes (i.e., controlling conditions in the natural world and technical problem solving); *hermeneutical* purposes (i.e., facilitating communication and understanding of the social world); and *emancipatory* purposes (i.e., overcoming domination and rationality). An instrumental interest in knowledge is rooted in the deep-seated desire we have to predict and control natural phenomena. Positivism sees knowledge in these terms; hence, much of what we consider *scientific* research produces what Habermas would call instrumental knowledge. However, he argues that there is a second, equally deep-seated hermeneutical interest in explaining social relationships and improving our capacity for intersubjective understanding. Habermas classifies many of the social sciences and humanities disciplines as belonging to this domain. Finally, there is the emancipatory interest to challenge oppression. Here, we use knowledge to guide critical self-reflection and critical analysis of institutional forces and relationships that limit our options and our capacity for rational action.

Habermas' framework sheds some light on the problems that conventional KT poses for social epidemiology. First, as we have noted, KT was developed to increase the use of research evidence in solving advanced technical problems, particularly in clinical medicine. Despite limited evidence of the comparative effectiveness of different KT strategies in clinical and health care services, systematic reviews of evidence have been used to develop guidelines for treatment of coronary heart disease (Helfand et al. 2009; Mosca et al. 2004); the integrated *knowledge-action cycle* has supported nurses' implementation of best practices in wound care (Graham et al. 2007); and *linkage and exchange* approaches have been associated with increased use of clinical evidence in large health care provider organizations (Lomas 2003). In these and countless other cases, conventional KT strategies have been aimed to support decision makers in addressing biomedical outcomes through technical interventions.

In terms of the knowledge constitutive interests framework, these KT approaches should be understood as supporting instrumental objectives. They were not aimed to advance use of knowledge for hermeneutical (i.e., improving understanding of social relationships) or emancipatory (i.e., advancing rationality and social justice) objectives. That is to say, these KT approaches were not designed to support the practical impact of social epidemiology. Regardless of its positivist methodological principles, social epidemiology is, at least in our reading of it, fundamentally a hermeneutical knowledge project aimed to explain social relationships that affect health. In light of its focus on unequal social relations and health, it also has a strong orientation toward social critique and emancipatory interests. The overwhelming evidence furnished by social epidemiology of the "social gradient in health" is knowledge that explains and provides rational-normative grounds for critiquing the fact that population health differences are *un*natural, complex problems that inequitably limit life chances for some groups. Problems such as these are problems shaped by politics, power and values, and they cannot be resolved through instrumental-technical means alone.

13.6   Taking Politics, Power and Values Seriously in KT

How can social epidemiology respond to these epistemological contradictions with conventional KT and contribute more effectively to equity in social and health policies? We see two potential approaches, both of which are being pursued by social epidemiologists with whom we collaborate around KT approaches, including many of the authors represented in this book. The first involves asking different research questions; the second involves adopting different roles for researchers as actors in policy and social change. Regardless of which path social epidemiologists follow, important revisions to the conventional framework for KT will be required.

On the one hand, researchers can reorient their inquiry and KT projects toward more strategic, technical problem-solving initiatives in order to better support government or service provider stakeholders. Here, social epidemiology aligns more closely with the instrumental approach to KT in clinical and health services research. This might mean, for example, initiating fewer studies to assess correlations between social disparities and health and undertaking more studies to evaluate the relative effectiveness of this or that programmatic intervention under prevailing socioeconomic conditions. A focus on interventions is more likely to have an effect on policy and program choices if only because of the clear link between cause and effect; whereas, studies that emphasize correlations often do not specify the causal pathway in sufficient detail (if at all) to provide guidance for policy and program change.

This approach has recently been described as addressing social versus societal determinants of health (Krieger et al. 2010). It is explored in some detail in other chapters (see Chaps. 1 and 12) in terms of a shift in social epidemiology from problem-focused to solution-focused research.

The other option is to look for alternative KT practices and markers of KT success that may be more consonant with the hermeneutical and emancipatory presuppositions of critical social epidemiology. For example, researchers may seek out more active and engaged roles as public intellectuals by participating in public and social media, speaking out on issues of major importance for the health of marginalized populations and also contributing purposively in advocacy coalitions and other forms of collective action to reform health and social policy. While there are no guarantees that social epidemiologic research will have a greater impact on policy and program choices when researchers take on these roles, this approach does reflect the realities of policy making in a democracy where scientific evidence, however compelling, is rarely the sole impetus for policy change.

Of course, these are roles that some social epidemiologists have traditionally been reluctant to pursue because, as we suggested earlier, they are concerned to protect the privileged status of the research that comes from being rigorously empirical and "untainted" by social and political debate (Weed and Mink 2002; Savitz et al. 1999). However, there are other social epidemiologists who work from the premise that the whole point of understanding the world is to change it and that one of the goals of social epidemiologic research is to foster change that would address the patterns of health inequality that their research reveals. These more public roles are, we argue, essential if social epidemiology is to contribute to the large, complex and multidimensional solutions that are required to address health inequality.

Arguably, there is more than enough room for both solution-focused KT and *engaged scholarship* (Committee on Institutional Cooperation 2005) within social epidemiology. For either approach to strengthen the impact of research evidence in reducing health inequities, however, a significant reconfiguration of the conventional KT account of policy change is required. As we have shown, social epidemiology addresses health and social policy problems that are more complex, more political and more value-laden than what has been described in the conventional KT literature. In this chapter we have aimed to outline what an alternative KT framework, one that is more appropriate for social epidemiology, might look like. Thus, in contrast to the boilerplate KT principles outlined above, which may only be useful from some types of social epidemiologic research, it would appear that social epidemiology also needs an approach to KT that:

- Sees complex policy change in terms of processes, not decisions, and offers researchers a theory of policy change to help explain where, when and why research evidence may (or may not) play an influential role;
- Acknowledges the importance of collective action in advancing social change and does not ignore the role of politics in policy making; and
- Accommodates analyses of power and knowledge relationships and can illuminate roles for research to play in supporting, enriching and also challenging decision makers' understanding of the "problem" of the social determinants of health.

13.7 Conclusions

At the outset we asked why social epidemiology research, in general, and health equity research, in particular, does not play a bigger role in promoting social change. We have tried to answer this question by examining some of the approaches for advancing research's impact that are recommended in the health sciences literature and assessing the relevance of these KT tools for research focused on social determinants of health. Overall, we find that conventional KT is in several respects inadequate to the objectives of social epidemiology as a knowledge project. Drawing on the work of Jürgen Habermas, we have argued that conventional KT emphasizes an *instrumental* (i.e., problem-solving) role for research knowledge in society, while social epidemiology is characterized by its *hermeneutical* (i.e., explanatory) and *emancipatory* (i.e., equity-seeking) goals. These are fundamentally different approaches to research utilization and give rise to different approaches for bridging the gap between research and practice. This discussion allowed us to begin to develop an alternative KT framework that may be more appropriate for significant parts of the social epidemiology and health equity research agenda. This framework takes politics, power and values seriously in efforts to promote social change.

References

Asthana A, Halliday J (2006) What works in tackling health inequalities? Pathways, policies and practice through the lifecourse. The Polity Press, Bristol

Bacchi C (2008) The politics of research management: reflections on the gap between what we "know" and what we do. Health Soc Rev 17:165–176

Benoit C, Carroll D, Chaudhry M (2003) In search of a healing place: aboriginal women in Vancouver's Downtown Eastside. Soc Sci Med 56:821–833

Berkman L, Kawachi I (2000) Social epidemiology. Oxford University Press, New York

Bernal JD (1939) The social function of science. MIT Press, Cambridge

Bevir M, Rhodes R (2006) Governance stories. Routledge, New York

BiomedCentral (2010) About implementation science. http://www.implementationscience.com/info/about. Accessed 9 Aug 2010

Braveman P (2006) Health disparities and health equity: concepts and measurement. Annu Rev Public Health 27:167–194

Burton P (2006) Modernising the policy process. Policy Stud 27:173–195

Buxton M, Hanney S, Jones T (2004) Estimating the economic value to societies of the impact of health research: a critical review. Bull World Health Organ 82:733–739

Carden F (2009) Knowledge to policy: making the most of development research. International Development Research Centre and Sage Publications, Ottawa/London

Chernomas R, Hudson I (2009) Social murder: the long-term effects of conservative economic policy. Int J Health Serv 39:107–121

Coburn D (2000) Income inequality, social cohesion and the health status of populations: the role of neo-liberalism. Soc Sci Med 51:135–146

Commission on Social Determinants of Health (2008) Closing the gap in a generation: health equity through action on the social determinants of health. Final report of the Commission on Social Determinants of Health. World Health Organization, Geneva

Committee on Institutional Cooperation (2005) Resource guide and recommendations for defining and benchmarking engagement. CIC Committee on Engagement, Champaign

Daniels N (2008) Just health: meeting health needs fairly. Cambridge University Press, New York

Deleon P (1999) The stages approach to the policy process: what has it done? Where is it going? In: Sabatier P (ed) Theories of the policy process. Westview Press, Boulder

Dorfman L, Wallack L, Woodruff K (2005) More than a message: framing public health advocacy to change corporate practices. Health Educ Behav 32:320–336, Discussion 355–362

Dunn JR (2002) Housing and inequalities in health: s study of socioeconomic dimensions of housing and self reported health from a survey of Vancouver residents. J Epidemiol Community Health 56:671–681

Evidence-Based Medicine Working Group (1992) Evidence-based medicine. JAMA 268: 2420–2425

Fafard P (2008) Evidence and healthy public policy: insights from health and political sciences. National Collaborating Centre for Healthy Public Policy. http://www.ccnpps.ca/docs/FafardEvidence08June.PDF. Accessed 8 Aug 2009

Frankish CJ, Hwang SW, Quantz D (2005) Homelessness and health in Canada: research lessons and priorities. Can J Public Health 96:S23–S29

Gagnon ML (2011) Moving knowledge to action through dissemination and exchange. J Clin Epidemiol 64:25–31

Graham H (2004) Social determinants and their unequal distribution: clarifying policy understandings. Milbank Q 82:101–124

Graham ID, Tetroe J (2007) How to translate health research knowledge into effective healthcare action. Healthc Q 10:20–22

Graham ID, Harrison MB, Cerniuk B et al (2007) A community-researcher alliance to improve chronic wound care. Healthc Policy 2:72–78

Habermas J (1971) Knowledge and human interests. Beacon Press, Boston

Helfand M, Buckley DI, Freeman M et al (2009) Emerging risk factors for coronary heart disease: a summary of systematic reviews conducted for the U.S. preventive services task force. Ann Intern Med 151:496–507

Howlett M, Ramesh M, Perl A (2009) Studying public policy: policy cycles & policy subsystems, 3rd edn. Oxford University Press, Don Mills

Kingdon JW (2003) Agendas, alternatives, and public policies. Longman, New York

Krieger N (2001) A glossary for social epidemiology. J Epidemiol Community Health 55:693–700

Krieger N, Alegria M, Almeida-Filho J et al (2010) Who, and what, causes health inequities? Reflections on emerging debates from an exploratory Latin American/North American workshop. J Epidemiol Community Health 64:747–749

Lemieux-Charles L, Champagne F (eds) (2004) Using knowledge and evidence in health care: multidisciplinary perspectives. University of Toronto Press, Toronto

Leone R, Carroll BW (2010) Decentralisation and devolution in Canadian social housing policy. Environ Plann C Gov Policy 28:389–404

Limoges C, Schwartzman S, Nowotny H et al (1994) The new production of knowledge: the dynamics of science and research in contemporary societies. Sage Publications, London

Lomas J (2003) Health services research: more lessons from Kaiser Permanente and Veterans' affairs healthcare system. BMJ 327:1301–1302

Lomas J, Fulop N, Gagnon D et al (2003) On being a good listener: setting priorities for applied health services research. Milbank Q 81:363–388

Merton RK (1973) The sociology of science: theoretical and empirical investigations. Chicago University Press, Chicago

Mosca L, Appel LJ, Benjamin EJ et al (2004) Evidence-based guidelines for cardiovascular disease prevention in women. Circulation 109:672–693

Murphy K, Topple R (eds) (2003) Measuring the gains from medical research an economic approach. University of Chicago Press, Chicago

Murphy K, van der Meulen A (2008) What counts, who counts? Research, values, politics and the health of marginalized populations. In: Poster presented at The Summer Institute on KSTE Action, National Collaborating Centres for Public Health, Kelowna

Oakes JM, Kaufman JS (2006) Methods in social epidemiology. Jossey-Bass, San Francisco

Orsini M, Smith M (2010) Social movements, knowledge and public policy: the case of autism activism in Canada and the US. Crit Policy Stud 4:38–57

Pablos-Mendez A, Shademani R (2006) Knowledge translation in global health. J Contin Educ Health Prof 26:81–86

Raphael D (2003) Addressing the social determinants of health in Canada: bridging the gap between research findings and public policy. Policy Options/Politiques. www.irpp.org/po/archive/mar03/raphael.pdf. Accessed 10 Nov 2008

Rose H, Rose S (1970) Science and society. Penguin, Baltimore

Sabatier P, Jenkins-Smith H (1999) The advocacy coalition framework: an assessment. In: Sabatier PA (ed) Theories of the policy process. Westview Press, Boulder

Sackett DL, Strauss S, Richardson SR et al (2000) Evidence-based medicine: how to practice and teach EBM, 2nd edn. Churchill Livingstone, London

Savitz DA, Poole C, Miller WC (1999) Reassessing the role of epidemiology in public health. Am J Public Health 89:1158–1161

Straus S, Tetroe J, Graham I (2009a) Defining knowledge translation. CMAJ 181:3–4

Straus S, Tetroe J, Graham I (eds) (2009b) Knowledge translation in health care: moving from evidence to practice. Wiley-Blackwell, Mississauga

Tibelius K, Stirling L (2007) Research capacity development and knowledge translation at CIHR. In: Presentation at the annual meeting of the Association of Faculties of Medicine of Canada, Victoria

Weed DL, Mink PJ (2002) Roles and responsibilities of epidemiologists. Ann Epidemiol 12:67–72

Weiss CH (1979) The many meanings of research utilization. Public Adm Rev 39:426–431

Wilkinson R, Pickett K (2009) The spirit level: why more equal societies almost always do better. Allen Lane, London

Chapter 14
Community-Academic Partnerships and Social Change

Peter Schafer

Contents

14.1 Introduction 286
14.2 The Role of Social Epidemiologists 290
14.3 Orienting Research to Address the Needs of Public Health Practice 293
14.4 Collaboration Between Social Epidemiologists and Program Planners
     and Policy Makers 297
14.5 Community Participation in Research 300
14.6 Conclusions 303
References 304

Abstract Too often, there is a schism between social epidemiologists who train and work in academic institutions to identify the factors influencing health and program planners and policy makers who work in the field as part of government or non-profit organizations to deliver public health services. Program planners and policy makers need academic partners with scientific expertise to help them make sound evidence-based decisions on the broad array of mechanisms affecting health. The complementary potential of collaborations between the discipline of social epidemiology and the real world service implementation experience of program planners and service delivery staff is vast, but this potential can only be realized if the two cease to work in isolation from one another. From a program planner and policy maker perspective, what is needed from the field of social epidemiology are solution-focused research initiatives – investigating an intervention to understand for whom does it make a difference, in what circumstances does it make a difference and in what respects does it make a difference. In becoming familiar with programs over a period of time, during which technical assistance is provided, knowledge is

P. Schafer (✉)
Community Child Health Research Network, 261 Gates Avenue, Apt. 4A,
Brooklyn, NY 11238, USA
e-mail: peterbschafer328@me.com

P. O'Campo and J.R. Dunn (eds.), *Rethinking Social Epidemiology:*
Towards a Science of Change, DOI 10.1007/978-94-007-2138-8_14,
© Springer Science+Business Media B.V. 2012

gained, trust is built, and social epidemiologists begin to shed the limiting strictures of their formal training. The transfer of knowledge between community and academics becomes unrestricted for the benefit of both parties and for the benefit of the communities whose health problems form their common focus.

Abbreviations

NICHD   National Institute of Child Health and Human Development

14.1   Introduction

Too often, there is a schism between social epidemiologists who train and work in academic institutions to identify the factors influencing health and program planners and policy makers who work in the field as part of government or non-profit organizations to deliver public health services. Program planners and policy makers need academic partners with scientific expertise to help them make sound evidence-based decisions on the broad array of mechanisms affecting health. However, productive community-academic partnerships are too rare in the field of social epidemiology. The purpose of this chapter is to address two questions from the perspective of a community-based health program planner:

1. What kinds of evidence should social epidemiology produce to be of use in community-based practice?
2. What are the relational characteristics of a community-academic partnership that produces actionable evidence for social change?

One of the ongoing frustrations from a policy maker or program planner perspective working within distressed communities to improve health and well-being is that much of health research is focused on describing health problems and associated risk factors in the biomedical tradition; this research does little to inform practice premised on an understanding of health issues that are largely the consequence of socioeconomic and environmental factors. Too often, identified risk factors suffer from their immutable nature (e.g., race viewed as a biological risk factor rather than a social construct) or from a conceptualization of an individual behaviour that pays little regard to the fact that the "problem" behaviour is often significantly influenced by the social and economic parameters of the individual's life (e.g., poor diet as a risk factor) (Dunn 2010).

The limitations of the predominant biomedical model and the appropriateness of a community-focused approach become apparent (if not clearly established through rigorous scientific methods – a schism discussed more fully below) when viewing the geographic clustering of poor health indices, such as poor pregnancy outcomes and other measures of maternal and child health in areas of Baltimore, Maryland. Many unique factors might be contributing to the observed clustering, and from an intervention point of view, the clustering presents an opportunity to deliver services in an efficient manner to those who are in greatest apparent need. A community-focused conceptual framework that seeks to account for the observed geographic clustering of poor outcomes would not only look to commonalities among the community's residents but also at community-level factors. At this junction, the factors that have the greatest potential for intervention in a community may emerge. The fact that communities, at least urban communities in the United States, are often racially segregated and are internally homogenous with respect to socioeconomic status suggests that relationships between residents and the larger society must be accounted for in a conceptual framework describing the mechanisms by which the health of a community's residents are influenced. For example, food insecurity is commonly assessed among individuals and households, but if it is determined also to be a community-level factor (i.e., a factor prevalent across households within a given community determined by a community's disadvantaged geographic, economic or political relationship to the larger society), then possible interventions take on a different shape and scope.

At the other end of the spectrum from approaches that rely on individual characteristics described in biomedical terms, analyses and the resulting prescriptions that would require wholesale change to a society's political and economic systems to address inequities in health are not very helpful in improving the lives of people in the short-term. Such changes in political and economic systems are rare and, to the extent that they do occur, are generally long-term projects and often quite incremental in nature, especially in the United States. Public health and social service practitioners work, and the residents of impoverished communities which suffer the worst health live, in the middle ground where individual biology and behaviour interact with and are influenced by social, environmental and economic structures. It is here that social epidemiology can be most useful in contributing to perspectives, which not only describe health problems but reveal paths to amelioration.

Throughout this chapter I draw upon my experience and that of colleagues, notably Maxine Reed-Vance and Julia Hayman-Hamilton of the Baltimore Healthy Start program, who worked together with Patricia O'Campo in Baltimore. This working relationship was a partnership between a service delivery program and an academic researcher.

The Baltimore Healthy Start program, an infant mortality reduction program in which the American federal government provided funding directly to local communities, began in 1993 as a demonstration project to develop promising approaches to reduce infant mortality. During the development of the Baltimore Project, the predecessor and model program to the Baltimore Healthy Start initiative, the Baltimore City Health Department was fortunate to have technical assistance from the National Institute of Child Health and Human Development (NICHD). Dr. Heinz Berendes, a senior researcher at NICHD, suggested that in order to measure the success of the Baltimore Project it would be critical to create defined geographic areas from which to recruit clients and to establish a goal of high recruitment rates of pregnant women. This approach would ensure that the population served by the project would be representative of the population in the target geographic area. Dr. Berendes explained that most infant mortality reduction programs of the past had achieved penetration rates of less than 50%. Most programs served large catchment areas, making it impossible to determine if apparent program successes, if any, resulted simply from participation of the most motivated or easiest to find women.

This advice to set high recruitment goals within a defined geographic area was applied in the Baltimore Project in 1990 and then carried forward with Baltimore Healthy Start in 1993. Effective recruitment of the eligible population to participate in Healthy Start was critical, both in terms of assessing whether any benefits from Healthy Start participation were actual benefits opposed to an artefact of selection bias and in terms of demonstrating the program's effectiveness for high risk as well as relatively low risk populations and, consequently, its effectiveness in terms of reducing perinatal health disparities for the geographic project area as a whole.

Since the project area communities at large suffered from high rates of poor pregnancy outcomes and since no reliable one-time risk assessment instrument existed that would lead the program to confidently exclude "low risk" women from services, the program attempted to enrol as many women as possible and employed ongoing early identification of risk factors as they emerged as a fundamental strategy to have an impact on community-wide measures. In practice, depending on funding over the years, the enrolment rate ranged from 60% to over 80% of all pregnant women in the community.

An example of the limitations of an individual risk factor approach to targeted interventions is the recommended use of scientifically-validated risk assessments to determine eligibility for, and level and intensity of, case management services that a pregnant woman should receive in order to achieve the program's goal of reducing the incidence of poor pregnancy outcomes. One-time risk assessments at program enrolment, beyond identifying women with a history of prior fetal or infant loss, are poor predictors of subsequent circumstances that could negatively affect pregnancy outcomes, such as eviction or other forms of housing instability or emerging symptoms of preterm labour among women with no history of preterm labour. As a result, the approach taken by Baltimore Healthy Start was to provide case management services with the premise that all clients are potentially high risk in order to be in position to assist with and, if possible, prevent such events. This approach was seen in both the minimum contact standard of bi-weekly contact and monthly home visits and the repeated home visit checklist assessments that were employed, which focused on signs and symptoms of preterm labour, changes in interpersonal relationships and social support and changes in personal economic situation. Many of the circumstances that might have a significant effect on the life of a pregnant woman and influence the course of her pregnancy cannot be reliably predicted for an individual woman at the pregnancy's outset. It was the prevalence of these "hard to predict" destabilizing events, which affected the lives of individuals in certain communities, that led to the intervention design of not excluding women from services on the basis of an assessed one-time, "low risk" status.

The above is an example of a situation where the academic-community partnership provided mutual intellectual and experiential support. The understanding of the limited utility of risk assessments from past research along with the statistical challenge inherent in reliably predicting rare events, coupled with community experience of the often changing circumstances and rapidly emergent stressors in the lives of women, led the academic and community partners to use their shared knowledge to reach a common conclusion. The resulting conceptualization, which recognized environmental and community-level factors, removed interventions from a clinical setting and placed them in a community setting. It recognized community-based interventions working in tandem with formal clinical systems of care as an integral facet of effective clinical care for many marginalized populations. The approach of prioritizing high enrolment rates within the community and employing regular home-based monitoring of emerging needs and perinatal health along with a community-based centre, which allowed women to avail themselves of services when they determined that they need assistance outside of the program-prescribed schedule of home visits (i.e., exercising autonomy with regard to their health and well-being), evolved not from formal research but from program experience.

Originally conceived as a social support and health education program, early program experience led Baltimore Healthy Start case managers to realize that emerging clinical issues, particularly regarding preterm labour, demanded an immediate and coordinated clinical response. The fact that clinical prenatal care services were available to the community from a geographic and health care coverage (i.e., Medicaid) perspective did not obviate the need for a proactive systematic schedule of home-based assessments to identify signs and symptoms of preterm labour. Incorporating such assessments into the regular schedule of home visits – which occurred more often than regular clinical prenatal care visits and were followed by internal nurse review and immediate medical referral for stabilization as indicated – became a key enhancement of the original social support program model. This recognition of the need to coordinate clinical practice with community-based, social support-oriented home visits illustrates the intersectoral nature of both the health problems and the effective means to address those problems. The reason that a program such as Baltimore Healthy Start has a role in making clinical care more effective is the manner in which it compensated for the deficits in other sectors, such as income inequity, poor public transportation, lack of affordable child care, poor education and all the other areas by which poor pregnant women face stressors and demands that both directly contribute to clinical risk and that take their time, focus and energy away from their health and pregnancy. The role of Baltimore Healthy Start in the communities it served is largely one of being a liaison between the community and formal systems of care.

Our academic partners respected what was learned by Baltimore Healthy Start's service providers in the course of providing services, and our service model was adjusted and enhanced in light of this experience. However, the task of evaluating the program and determining which program components contributed to the outcomes of interest was complicated. The dynamic nature of a service demonstration project potentially offered a number of conflicts with an academic researcher trained to control as many variables as possible in order to isolate and discover truth. However, to conduct such analyses entails imposing artificial restrictions on practitioners who are striving to learn from their experiences and apply the lessons that those experiences bring. Rather than stand in the way of these changes, which made their job of evaluation more difficult, program staff were instead buttressed by new data collection procedures that were introduced with the assistance of our academic partners..

14.2   The Role of Social Epidemiologists

Social epidemiologists have the rigorous scientific training for assessing needs and measuring effectiveness of interventions that program planners usually lack. The complementary potential of collaborations between the discipline of social epidemiology and the real world service implementation experience of program planners and service delivery staff is vast, but this potential can only be realized if the two cease to work in isolation from one another.

Of the valuable functions social epidemiologists can offer to the field is movement away from further *describing* the problem of poor health toward *action* to ameliorate the problems of poor health. These functions are rooted in social epidemiologists' research training and experience to: (1) assist community-based programs to develop the tools and institutional capacity to monitor programmatic processes and outcomes, thus enabling programs to identify and promptly address the deficits in their program design and effectively meet the needs of communities they serve; and (2) test, validate and refine the programmatic responses.

With regard to technical capacity to monitor programmatic processes and outcomes, input from social epidemiologists in the development of a data collection system, which serves multiple purposes and constituencies, is key. A number of major purposes each with their respective constituencies must be served by a single data collection system. First, case management staff needs ready access to individual client characteristics and service utilization data to inform and monitor adherence to individual client care plans. Second, supervisory staff needs individual and caseload aggregate client tracking and service utilization data to monitor adherence to program protocol by supervised staff. Third, program planners need aggregate process and outcome data to report progress on goals and objectives to funders. Fourth, program planners and direct service staff need process and outcome data sorted by various client characteristics to understand varying levels of program participation and for whom an intervention makes a difference with respect to outcomes. Finally, independent evaluators need individual-level data across client characteristics and service utilization to conduct more rigorous analyses.

In the case of Baltimore Healthy Start, the development of the Client Tracking System, which served all of the above noted purposes and constituencies, originated from the needs of a social epidemiologist charged with conducting the local independent evaluation. However, unlike in many such scenarios, Patricia O'Campo recognized that the data collection system that she needed for program evaluation also could serve as the data collection system that program planners and operational staff needed to effectively monitor and operate the program. In a very simple and elegant conceptualization of the challenges in collecting quality data, the data collection system development process ensured the participation of the people who would be collecting the data (i.e., the direct service staff). Rather than have a set of data collection requirements imposed on them from an outside entity, the direct service staff, upon whom everyone depended for quality data, determined to a large extent which data the system would collect as a result of what they needed the system to report in order to do their jobs.

Capacity in data management extends beyond the design of the original data system, data collection forms and reports, and should include the capacity to continually modify and improve these systems. This flexibility is necessary to ensure the forms and reports maintain their utility for all parties involved and is fundamental for direct service staff who collect the data. Thus, capacity is not only the hardware and software of a data system, but it is also the human resource capacity to modify and improve the software.

Once this technical capacity is established, ongoing collaboration between social epidemiologists and program staff is needed. This approach might pose challenges to the ideal of scientific objectivity, which is a part of the culture and training of social epidemiologists, but then this whole chapter is intended to be such a challenge (Box 14.1).

Box 14.1

Peter Schafer asked Patricia (Pat) O'Campo to address many of the issues raised in this chapter from her perspective as a social epidemiologist. Excerpts from their conversation follow:

Peter: "You had the evaluation contract for Baltimore Healthy Start, but, unlike a typical scenario where the evaluator came in and imposed a bunch of data collection requirements on a pre-existing operational protocol, you helped to design a system and create the technical capacity within the organization to monitor itself from a very early stage."

Pat: "I think that was a unique feature – that we were all starting together. We were all learning about what we had to collect. Recall that, from a very mainstream perspective, we had this so-called 'minimum data set' required by the federal government. Many of the elements were not useful at all, but because they were required and because the only people who could collect them would be the case managers and outreach workers, they were forced to get involved. In other words, they wouldn't have a future if they didn't collect those data because if you didn't collect the minimum data set then you wouldn't have a program."

(continued)

Box 14.1 (continued)

Peter: "Yeah, the minimum data set was an externally imposed requirement by the national evaluators, not locally generated, and therefore a requirement of the program's federal funding."

Pat: "That's right. So direct service staff got involved in the data collection process. They were in a way forced to participate in research, maybe not in an ideal way, but they were forced to think about the ways in which they collect data and how it could be used for science. They asked a lot of really good questions about the validity of some of the data elements that were in this minimum data set, which we all knew had nothing to do with giving better services to the client. I knew from a scientific perspective that, for example, knowing whether somebody had a tuberculosis test or not was probably not going to make a difference to infant mortality, but feeling like we were all part of a team in shaping the data collection system and commenting on the data elements that we were forced to reply to, I think, helped to empower the local evaluators to give feedback to the national evaluators about the problems with many of the required items. And I think that because there was a view that I was a bit of an open researcher, I wasn't put in the same category as the national evaluators."

Peter: "Well, this is really important here. I want to pursue this. It's important because in terms of the interpersonal dynamics, and the baggage that certain people bring, such as an academic outside evaluator who is naturally seen as someone who is looking – I mean, this is the way it is in programs – an outside evaluator is someone who is looking to find something wrong, things to criticize. But the fact that you were similarly critical and frustrated with the apparent irrelevance of a lot of these national evaluation requirements, which did not conform with what the Baltimore Healthy Start program was about, I think, did a lot to help people view you not as this outside threatening person but as someone who was understanding, and that's important. I mean, this happened in Baltimore and you were from Johns Hopkins..."

Pat: "...which is bad...."

Peter: "...which is a bad thing. [Laughter] I mean, you know?"

Pat: "From the community perspective..."

Peter: "From the community perspective, Johns Hopkins is a bad thing. They [Johns Hopkins] just want to do research on black people and are not really concerned..."

Pat: "...negatively label them..."

Peter: "Negatively label them, and just find out all the things that are wrong with them and blame them for their problems. That's basically the perception, and there are good reasons that that is a perception."

(continued)

Box 14.1 (continued)

Pat: "Having those discussions about whether these data elements were relevant, useful or irrelevant and having the discussions with the staff I think helped engage them in kind of a critical look at research as well so they could then understand that, gee, there are choices here: we could have good research that helps us or we could have not good research that doesn't. And I think it empowered them to comment further on some of the data elements that we ended up liking and retaining going forward."

14.3 Orienting Research to Address the Needs of Public Health Practice

From a program planner and policy maker perspective, what is needed from the field of social epidemiology are solution-focused research initiatives – investigating an intervention to understand for whom does it make a difference, in what circumstances does it make a difference and in what respects does it make a difference.

Multisector programs require multidisciplinary epidemiologic approaches that measure impact across all the areas that a given program aims to affect. In other words, useful social epidemiology does not restrict itself to looking solely at health outcomes; it also considers outcomes in areas such as housing insofar as housing is recognized as a significant factor affecting health. Already, mental health, particularly depression, and substance use are recognized as factors affecting maternal and child health directly, as typically measured, and influencing health care utilization. However, the factors that influence mental health and substance use, like social isolation, community and family violence and unsafe and unstable housing, are generally not examined.

Programs need timely, actionable evidence that provides explications of the underlying mechanisms affecting both program outputs and health outcomes. What programs often need is corroborating evidence to anecdotal observations of changes and new trends, or evidence of changes and new trends absent of any anecdotal observations, so that the programs can respond appropriately and with confidence. The evidence does not need to meet the traditional standards of "evidence" in peer-reviewed scientific journals – it simply has to be "good enough," which is a variable concept dependent upon a variety of factors, including the costs and feasibility of possible interventions and the nature of the leadership within a community organization (Box 14.2).

The type of evidence that is most valuable to programs is information that suggests an enhancement of services or an improved way of delivering services. Community direct service programs are all about doing something about a problem, so further dissections of a problem, which have no practical impact in the realm of

Box 14.2

Peter: "I know that you were frustrated with the reception in the scientific community received by your analysis of the Baltimore Healthy Start program, which was not based on a randomized clinical trial model. Then you talked among your colleagues and said, okay, if that's not going to be accepted then at least the contribution that can come from this, from this experience, is in methods. You were developing new innovative methods to deal with this problem, this predicament, of not wanting to distort the program by applying the standard randomized assignment approach. Instead you applied other scientifically valid methods to evaluate the effectiveness of the program. But even that wasn't well received. So I want you to talk a little bit about, I guess from your perspective as a young professional at that time, how this wasn't paying off in terms of how, I think, an academic young professional would expect it to pay off. You weren't getting stuff published from this, yet you persisted in it. Can you talk about how you dealt with that?"

Pat: "Sure. You make it sound, Peter, like I got the raw end of the deal and that I had to compromise a lot. You're alluding to the fact that I got very few publications from our almost decade long, at that point in time, collaboration. We still collaborate now, which means something, it says something about the partnership. Those markers are often viewed – and I am sorry – maybe they are the only things that are important when you are thinking about promotion, that is, the number of publications. So, it's true, I didn't have a lot of publications to show for all of the work that I did. Healthy Start would take up about 35% of my time, more than a day a week of time, and even a day a week is a lot for a project to take up for me to get, you know, two publications [Laughter]. But I think one thing that is again not talked about in academic training is that what I got out of that partnership was not only good partners to do transdisciplinary research right – and not just social epidemiology research but transdisciplinary research – I also learned what the real priorities of the community were, and I could then go on to have that perspective impact the research that I did afterwards. If I just sat in my office and I looked at the existing literature and I said 'Hmm, what are the problems facing inner city populations?' and if I relied solely on what other researchers who came before me had written about, I would be way off, right?

"So, what I learned was what's written in the literature is very far away from what's actually going on in a community like that, one of the highest risk communities in Baltimore. I learned that approaches that are often talked about in the literature for how to address those issues are way off, so it opened my eyes. I also gained important information about the limitations of, again, the standard measures that are used to measure risk or resilience

(continued)

Box 14.2 (continued)

in a population. So it totally affected my whole research career going forward, and so I rarely ever do research without doing partnerships now because I know that if I rely again on what other mainstream epidemiologists do I would not be helping the population. I would not be characterizing them correctly. I would be wrong and I didn't want to be wrong. So, it's true I didn't gain publications *per se*, but I did gain a new perspective and a new approach to doing research.

"That experience affected the rest of my career. I feel like I am doing better research then I ever did, and I am also about to get more publications out of this new research [Laughter] because I am also smarter about how to do that. I wasn't as smart when we first did CBPR [Community-Based Participatory Research]. I don't know if it was a matter of being inexperienced. I don't know if it was a matter of the timing. But when we did CBPR, it was not widely recognized, so neither were we necessarily encouraged to write about our experiences nor was there any place to publish it even if I did write about our experiences. So if a young person is starting out now, even if they can't get as many publications as they like, I still think it's a worthwhile experience because you learn to do research in a way that is not taught to you when you go to a place like Johns Hopkins for training. The only way I have a chance of improving health in inner city Baltimore with the evidence that I generate is to partner with the community."

Peter: "That's encouraging because I feel bad. The way I am writing this it sounds like I am asking the social epidemiologists to give up a lot, so it's good to hear that."

Pat: "We gain a lot."

---

service delivery at either the operational or strategic (or political or advocacy) level, are not particularly valued.

Such an example of a programmatic intervention based on internal monitoring evidence is the Family Planning Nurse Practitioner component added to the Baltimore Healthy Start case management model. Family planning interconceptional care services – which includes family planning education, individualized counselling and home- and community centre-based contraceptive method prescriptions and method dispensing in accordance with the client's education, employment and family size goals – have been provided to West Baltimore Healthy Start postpartum clients by a certified registered nurse practitioner, who has been fully integrated into Healthy Start case management operations, since 2004.

The intervention was initiated in response to an alarming increase, sustained over 3 years, in the rate of short inter-pregnancy intervals (i.e., <12 months from

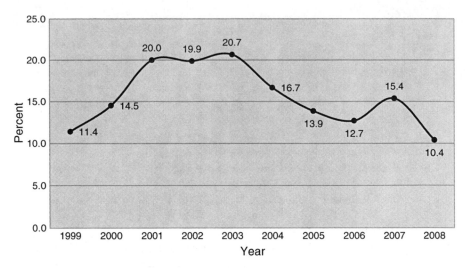

Fig. 14.1 Percent of Baltimore Healthy Start pregnancies with an inter-pregnancy interval of <12 months among clients whose prior pregnancy resulted in a live birth

prior delivery to subsequent conception) among Healthy Start clients in the West Baltimore project area. While internal tracking statistics strongly suggested the extent of the intervention's effectiveness (Fig. 14.1), it also showed that there were still a significant number of pregnant women who continued to have births within short inter-pregnancy intervals.

Those who worked in the program generally believed that some Healthy Start program services, such as the individualized family planning counselling and contraceptive method dispensing included in the intervention, while designed to be effective among all clients, were in actual practice more readily adopted and utilized by the relatively more stable clients (e.g., non-substance users). The result of this practice was that only those relatively low risk pregnancies were being prevented through the intervention, leaving higher risk births to represent a higher proportion of all births. The implication of this underlying phenomena occurred not only at the operational level where direct service staff worked to meet the needs of the clients they served but also at the level of policy and program evaluation where multi-year trends were often analyzed without the benefit of insight that program operational staff (i.e., the community) can provide.

Naturally, funders of programs are very interested in the efficacy of their efforts and dollars spent in improving community-wide health status. How is the effect of a programmatic intervention to be evaluated on the basis of community-wide data without these kinds of underlying influences explicated? The effect of Healthy Start services, in particular the Family Planning Nurse Practitioner intervention, may have had a direct effect on the risk profile of the remaining births as a result because it succeeded in significantly reducing the rate of short inter-pregnancy interval births. In this case, when looking at aggregate statistics at the community level as a measure of program impact, relying on rates of poor outcomes is inadequate because the total number of births may be reduced as a result of the program, and this reduction may have occurred unevenly in terms of the risk status of women. That social epidemiologists have the training and interest to delve into these issues in order to fully understand the underlying dynamics to community-wide health statistics, including the effect of program interventions, is an important contribution to the work of program planners, policy makers and funders.

14.4   Collaboration Between Social Epidemiologists and Program Planners and Policy Makers

The barriers to productive relationships between social epidemiologists and direct service providers often originate in a clash of cultures but not necessarily of values (see Chap. 3). Addressing the culture clash directly, from a common set of values, is the first step toward establishing a transparent and productive relationship. As in many cross-cultural relationships, addressing cultural issues often constitutes a challenge to norms and practices and contributes to the misunderstanding of peers operating under the traditional parameters.

Community-based service programs are often interested in a number of research questions that derive from their experience, with internal monitoring of services and health outcomes providing a focus for those questions. However, programs face an ethical problem in testing programmatic interventions by rigorous scientific methods in that those approaches generally require denying available services to a segment of the population served (i.e., the control group). This approach runs counter to the mission of a community-based organization dedicated to serving its target population. When internal monitoring evidence suggests that a new intervention is effective, a program's natural response is to make it available to all program participants as soon as possible in order to be consistent with its mission to serve.

Resolving the conflict between rigorous scientific research methods (e.g., random assignment to treatment and control groups) and ethical and effective community-based service delivery is, perhaps, the most challenging barrier to collaboration and represents a fundamental difference in cultures between the direct service and scientific research communities. From the point of view of a community-based direct services program, the artificial conditions imposed upon community-based services in order to meet the standards of peer-reviewed research – for example, requiring random assignment of pregnant women into services and not allowing *all* pregnant women to enrol into services in a community when that very practice is integral to the trust built between program and community and, therefore, may be integral to the success of the program – are conditions that act to distort the intervention purportedly being investigated (Box 14.3).

Instead of randomized controlled trials (RCTs), Baltimore Healthy Start relied on evidence generated from "natural experiments," which were generally the product of funding constraints, in order to assess the effectiveness of new intervention designs.

Box 14.3

Peter: "I raise in the chapter the idea of a culture clash between social epidemiologists on one side and program planners and policy makers on the other. What has to happen in order for there to be useful collaboration between the social epidemiologists trained in the academic traditions and program planners out there working in the field?"

Pat: "I think the culture clash stems from the fact that program planners and scientists have very different goals in mind. The scientists' goals and objectives will be to produce work that is scientifically rigorous, and the program planners are interested in evidence that enables them to do their job better and essentially have a successful program. But the two objectives are different, and so the scientists and the program planners are not necessarily working toward the same objectives, and I think that leads to a clash. Some of the culture clash comes from different use of language, but I think the root cause is that they have different objectives.

"The way in which I handled that in our partnership is that, I guess, I kind of threw away what I was trained to prioritize. I was trained to prioritize rigour and methodological aspects toward doing research, and I adopted the goal of trying to ensure that the program was the best program. So my role became to generate evidence, whether it's existing evidence from the literature or trying to ensure that there were good data collection systems as part of the program. But the priorities of all of those activities were consistent with the program planners. It doesn't mean there was perfect alignment, but I did not prioritize scientific rigour.

"The other thing I wanted to say about that is that I believe that training of scientists could take place in a different way to minimize the culture clash you mentioned. Too often the way in which social epidemiologists and epidemiologists are trained is with an emphasis on method, but the context is not mentioned when the method is taught, and epidemiologists aren't trained to understand that methods should be adapted to the context in which they're being applied. So, in a community partnership that is trying to do an evaluation, the methods might be different or modified from how they would do an evaluation, say, in a clinical context where there is a lot more control over both the intervention and the circumstances in which the intervention is being administered. In a community context, especially one that involves home visits like Healthy Start, the context in which you're administering interventions is going to vary. It could be at the centre, it could be on the street corner, it could be in the house."

Peter: "And every house is different…"

Pat: "And every house is different and so you don't have much control over the environment and things that affect the delivery of the intervention. So the fact that methods are often taught without regard to context is really problematic, and it means then that epidemiologists tend to be rigid and inflexible about their methods. They are not encouraged to innovate or adapt to this kind of environment, and I think that contributes to the culture clash."

Such was the case with the Family Planning Nurse Practitioner intervention discussed above, which was introduced in the West Baltimore Healthy Start Project Area in response to a huge upsurge in short inter-pregnancy interval births in West Baltimore. As the intervention was introduced and significant reductions in short inter-pregnancy interval births occurred in West Baltimore, the East Baltimore rates were monitored and remained moderate throughout. Funding priorities were adjusted, and the services were expanded to East Baltimore acting on the evidence of the effectiveness of this new home visit component. While Baltimore Healthy Start would have liked to subject that intervention to rigorous scientific methods to firmly establish its effectiveness, it could not ethically deny services to any subgroup currently not being served if it believed those services were effective. Here is an example, perhaps, of the level of evidence that a program finds sufficient (i.e., internal monitoring of inter-pregnancy interval rates among clients who re-enrol with a subsequent pregnancy) being quite different from what an academic and academic journals would consider adequate evidence of an intervention's effectiveness.

In the future, Baltimore Healthy Start might choose to expand services into new project areas in a limited fashion (e.g., without the Family Planning Nurse intervention) in accordance with funding limitations. Of course, this approach does not utilize random assignment within a community. As alluded to above, programs have concerns that the standard method of scientific research distorts the program purportedly under study by undermining the integral component of trust between the community resident and the program and prefers comparisons of varying services' availability to be conducted between communities rather than within communities. The scientific community views this approach as far from ideal because of the presumed differences between the communities involved. However, this presumption is buttressed by a fallacy derived from aggregate statistics of communities that overlooks the heterogeneity that exists in all communities and that overstates the differences between communities. It is the methodological challenge to the research community to develop scientifically rigorous approaches that do not distort the programmatic intervention being studied, and the failure of the research community to meet the challenge with regard to the design of many community-based programs, that is a potentially fatal obstacle to community-academic collaboration.

Case studies are a promising avenue with which to introduce scientific rigour into how programs often view the evidence available to them, including both qualitative and quantitative experiential evidence. Recent advances in case study methodology designed to address its weaknesses are promising in their potential to bridge the gap between clinically-derived methods, which are best suited to uncomplicated regimented interventions, and methods that embrace and fully account for program complexity as well as those that respect and do not distort the reality of community-based interventions (Yin 2009).

Communities are complex, open systems that are subject to change. This fact needs to be accepted when designing research and accepted and accounted for in analyses of data that will likely result in statistical strength at a lower level than the "gold standard" of biomedical research. In other words, researchers and academic institutions interested in conducting meaningful research that provides evidence to service programs as to which interventions are effective, and why and for whom they are effective, need to reject the biomedical research paradigm. Rather than considering this paradigm as the method by which "truth" is revealed, researchers should consider it to possibly be either not applicable or not useful. In many circumstances, in fact, biomedical research paradigms are the methods by which the "truth" is obscured or overlooked.

With regard to the non-generalizability of results, another oft-cited weakness of non-RCT study design (e.g., case studies, natural experiments or other forms of quasi-experimental design), experience in program planning suggests that the purported generalizability of results from an RCT approach may be illusory. Since the results of an RCT approach derive from a study design that seeks to isolate, through both actual and statistical means, an intervention from the various multisectoral influences that affect the individual lives and communities of the population studied, and through those mechanisms have an impact on the outcome of interest, the real world validity and value of the results need to be scrutinized. Multisectoral influences need to be explicated and understood, not isolated away and controlled for, because in the real world they cannot be set aside. Research based on case studies, natural experiments or other forms of quasi-experimental design might offer conclusions not as statistically strong or methodologically sound as the biomedical tradition, as with an RCT approach, but they may get closer to the truth in that they more fully embrace the real world complexity in which multiple sectors interact on multiple levels to affect health.

The role of differing cultures and career and economic imperatives of the academic and community partners need to be discussed candidly so that conflicts can be addressed openly and strategies jointly developed and pursued that meet both the needs of the social epidemiologist and the program. A fruitful research approach for program planners and policy makers is one that sheds light on the interactions of the multisector influences on a health issue and on possible interventions to address the health issue. One way for social epidemiologists to be informed of these influences is to learn directly from the affected individuals and communities.

14.5   Community Participation in Research

Complementing the social epidemiologist, who reorients research in order to conduct investigations that bridge problem-focused and solution-focused research, are community direct service providers and community residents who take an active role in initiating and shaping research. While many researchers recognize the value of community participation in research implementation – for example, by increasing recruitment and retention rates, reducing reporting bias and reducing measurement error from survey and interview questions that are not culturally aligned with study participants (Cargo and Mercer 2008) – there is less recognition within research institutions of the value of community participation in shaping the purpose and scope of research. Underlying the principles and processes of Community-Based Participatory Research (CBPR) is an implicit recognition that the community context of research has a meaning beyond the setting in which research occurs to also include the community in which the research is designed and conducted (i.e., the community of researchers). To the extent that the community of researchers includes members of the communities that are researched, higher quality and more relevant research will result. A large body of evidence demonstrates that "insider knowledge can enrich academic partners' understandings of the needs, priorities and health concerns of communities, organizations and the public health system and lead to refined and new research questions" and "[e]ngaging with nonacademic partners in shaping the research purpose has the advantage of enhancing contextual readiness for research implementation" (Cargo and Mercer 2008).

Gaining the value of "insider knowledge" through basing and structuring the research process on an equal and collaborative process between community and academic partners, and simultaneously building research capacity within communities typically studied, is a hallmark principle of CBPR. One example of "insider knowledge" might be a greater appreciation of within group differences, opposed to a focus on racial disparities, as the endpoint of investigation and analysis. Community members, and those who work in communities delivering services, are exposed each day to the great heterogeneity among class and racial groups, and it is this heterogeneity that might suggest fruitful areas for solution-focused research (as opposed to reducing a complex system to an oversimplified "racial disparity" in health status). Community participation in research will not only provide the motivation to explore solution-focused research but will also provide insights into how to discover the mechanisms underlying potential solutions (Box 14.4).

Box 14.4

Pat: "I want to add to what you said earlier, because in my opinion Baltimore Healthy Start was more than a cultural liaison. Healthy Start, although it started out in the precursor program going out into the community and telling pregnant women 'You need to get to prenatal care. Let's go!' women often didn't go. Why? Because the program wasn't addressing their top priorities. So the program had to learn that in order to engage this population they had to first address the top priorities of the women. Then there was not only a level of trust built, but also the case managers could give advice and have their clients be responsive to the advice given, some of the advice being that you should go to prenatal care. That enabled the staff to act as cultural liaisons, and I think that's a really important point to make."

(continued)

Box 14.4 (continued)

Peter: "Again I think that's where there is an analogy. The analogy is the program staff wasn't just telling clients that they needed to get to prenatal care, and you weren't telling program staff that they needed to collect this data for the evaluation. You listened to their needs first, just like the program listened to the women's needs first. A real signature aspect of the Baltimore Healthy Start Program is this thing we call emergency needs, and it's assessed at the beginning, at recruitment, through door-to-door outreach. What are those families' emergency needs, in terms of food, in terms of clothing, in terms of shelter, that is, Are they in danger of being evicted? How stable is their housing situation? What type of assistance do they need now? It was recognized that prenatal care and a healthy pregnancy outcome are the program's priorities and not necessarily priorities shared by a woman who's got a lot of other more pressing issues confronting her. And similarly, from a social epidemiologist's point of view, the priorities of finding the 'truth' by following this rigorous scientific method are not the priorities of the program."

Pat: "Yes, so, yes! You read my mind [Laughter]. So I set that up because I was going to say that I think in many ways we can identify commonalities – common interests that the program staff has and that someone like me who has training and privilege and all of that has. As I mentioned before, I had to kind of give up my priorities and adopt the priorities – or at least be on board with the priorities – of the program itself, and then, having done that, we had much more in common. The program staff and I, no matter what colour, no matter what class, no matter what training, no matter what background, had much more in common, and we could move forward together. We could find our common ground, and I think that's really what it boils down to. So to me that suggests, too, that what we identify superficially as racial differences, you know…I think those can kind of disappear if you can identify common ground to work on, and common goals to work toward, and then I think then those other more superficial barriers can just break down."

Peter: "It reminds me of another important point in order to realize that potential, and that is the relationship be an ongoing relationship over time, which includes continuity of partnership and technical assistance. Because part of the presumption about academic researchers is that they're self serving. They just want to publish something. They want to do some research and just publish. They swoop in, get out and are never to be heard from again. You get written about somewhere in some journal that you don't even know about it until you hear someone talk about it later on, about all the

(continued)

Box 14.4 (continued)

bad stuff that was written about you. I mean that's kind of… that's sort of the…[Laughter]"

Pat: "…That's the model."

Peter: "That's the model. So there's this other aspect of what you just said that for it to really work it does require a long term relationship, a long term interest, and I think that that's consistent with an interest of an academic researcher and their career because I mean they invest so much in this project initially upfront that they would hope to – and it's reasonable that they would to be able to – gain something from an intellectual perspective, from a career perspective, from an ongoing relationship. So much of this is interpersonal relationships, interpersonal trust, and breaking down presumptions about where people are coming from and what their priorities are."

14.6 Conclusions

A fruitful partnership between academic social epidemiologists and community-based direct service programs requires a long-term investment in the relationship by both parties. Early and ongoing collaboration can take many forms, including conducting an assessment of a community's needs and strengths as well as its deficits and sources of resilience and community member views of the health problem targeted. It can also include technical assistance, for example, in building a data collection and reporting system that serves client case management, program monitoring and evaluation purposes (and one that also builds capacity in community-based organizations to effectively monitor emerging needs and changing trends and to respond accordingly in a timely manner with appropriate service initiatives). As the partnership collaboratively designs intervention research according to CBPR principles, the social epidemiologist needs to bring a flexible methodological approach that respects the service mission of service delivery programs. Interpretation of findings and involvement in the development of program modifications and enhancements is an area where the benefits of familiarity with a program and with the individuals who operate the program are substantial. In becoming familiar with programs over a period of time, during which time technical assistance is provided, knowledge is gained, trust is built, and social epidemiologists shed the limiting strictures of their formal training. The transfer of knowledge between community and academics becomes unrestricted for the benefit of both parties and for the benefit of the communities whose health problems form their common focus.

References

Cargo M, Mercer S (2008) The value and challenges of participatory research: strengthening its practice. Ann Rev Public Health 29:325–350

Dunn J (2010) Health behavior vs the stress of low socioeconomic and health outcomes. JAMA 303:1199–1200

Yin R (2009) Case study research: design and methods, 4th edn. Sage Publications, Washington, DC

Chapter 15
Producing More Relevant Evidence: Applying a Social Epidemiology Research Agenda to Public Health Practice

David Mowat and Catharine Chambers

Contents

15.1	Introduction	306
15.2	Producing More Relevant Evidence	307
15.3	Understanding Mechanisms	312
15.4	Improving Health Outcomes and Reducing Health Inequalities	316
15.5	Applying Social Epidemiology Research to Public Health Practice	318
15.6	The Role of Partnerships Between Social Epidemiologists and Public Health Practitioners	320
15.7	Conclusions	323
References		323

Abstract To date, social epidemiology research has largely been restricted to the description of health disparities and their association with social gradients. Rarely do social epidemiologists expand upon these general-level associations and begin to examine the causal pathways linking social disparities to health. This research approach presents numerous challenges for public health practitioners who attempt to integrate social epidemiology research into policies and programs, as intervention on the identified social gradients is difficult and may divert efforts from more productive options. Furthermore, social epidemiology research is seldom accessible to public health practitioners in a form that is applicable to practice and adaptable to the local context. In order to generate research that can be translated into action to improve health, social epidemiology must progress from providing descriptions at

D. Mowat (✉)
Peel Public Health, 7120 Hurontario Street, P.O. Box 667, RPO Streetsville,
Mississauga, ON L5M 2C2, Canada
e-mail: David.Mowat@peelregion.ca

C. Chambers
Centre for Research on Inner City Health, St. Michael's Hospital, 30 Bond Street,
Toronto, ON M5B 1W8, Canada
e-mail: chambersc@smh.ca

P. O'Campo and J.R. Dunn (eds.), *Rethinking Social Epidemiology:*
Towards a Science of Change, DOI 10.1007/978-94-007-2138-8_15,
© Springer Science+Business Media B.V. 2012

the general level and begin to understand mechanisms leading to health outcomes. The purpose of this chapter is to discuss how social epidemiologists can produce such evidence and ensure that their research is more relevant to public health policy and practice. This chapter will also examine the challenges associated with integrating social epidemiology research into practice and offer guidance for how a social epidemiology research agenda can be implemented.

Abbreviations

CHSRF   Canadian Health Services Research Foundation
CIHR   Canadian Institutes of Health Research
SGA   small for gestational age

15.1   Introduction

The branch of epidemiology referred to as social epidemiology is often equated with research that describes social group membership and its impact on health outcomes. Since its inception, social epidemiology has firmly established that there are a number of social characteristics, particularly socioeconomic status, which are correlated with a variety of health outcomes, including risk factor prevalence and morbidity and mortality rates. This conclusion is undisputed. However, much of the discussion around social determinants of health has repetitively described the same associations between social gradients and health outcomes, and social epidemiologists have rarely moved beyond the description of these associations at the general level. Although social epidemiology may attempt to delve deeper into understanding the specific contexts and mechanisms between social determinants and health outcomes, for example when multiple levels of influence are examined, there is not always consistency in the strength or sometimes even the direction of these associations. Understandably, public health practitioners often have difficulty in translating this, at times, contradictory knowledge into policy and practice.

There can be little doubt about the value of social epidemiology in demonstrating relationships between the social determinants of health and health outcomes as well as in starting to explain mechanisms leading to various states of health. However, if an integral role of social epidemiology is to meet the needs of public health practitioners, then it must provide knowledge that can be translated into action to improve health. Not only must this knowledge be readily accessible to public health practitioners, it must be accessible in a form that is both applicable to practice and adaptable to a variety of contexts. In order to generate such knowledge, social epidemiology must progress from providing descriptions at the general level and begin to understand mechanisms leading to health outcomes. Additionally, it must move beyond detecting simple associations to revealing complex causal pathways between social inequalities and their associated health outcomes, and it should ultimately point toward potential interventions for ameliorating poor health outcomes and reducing social inequalities. This chapter will discuss how social epidemiologists can produce such knowledge and ensure that social epidemiology research is relevant to public health policy and practice. It will examine the challenges associated with applying a social determinants of health perspective toward public health practice and offer guidance for how this research agenda can be implemented. Finally, this chapter will discuss how partnerships between public health practitioners and social epidemiologists can help accomplish this research agenda and how training programs for new social epidemiologists can help ensure applicability to public health practice.

The content of this chapter is based on the writings of and discussions with Dr. David Mowat, the Medical Officer of Health for the Region of Peel in Ontario, Canada. Interspersed within this chapter are excerpts from an interview with Dr. Mowat that was held in July 2010 with researchers at the Centre for Research on Inner City Health in Toronto, Canada. In this role as the Medical Officer of Health, Dr. Mowat is responsible for protecting and promoting the health of more than one million people in the Region of Peel. During his extensive career, Dr. Mowat has gained invaluable experience working in public health and collaborating with researchers through positions held at local, provincial and national levels. Prior to joining the Region of Peel in February of 2007, Dr. Mowat was Deputy Chief Public Health Officer at the Public Health Agency of Canada. In this role, he had particular responsibilities for strengthening public health practice, including surveillance systems, knowledge translation, workforce development and public health information policy, privacy, law and ethics, and participated in many federal, provincial and territorial committees as well as national initiatives. Dr. Mowat joined Health Canada in 1998 and moved to the newly created Public Health Agency of Canada in 2004. Previous appointments also include Consultant in Maternal and Child Health in the Public Health Branch of the Government of Newfoundland, Medical Officer of Health for Kingston and area and Chief Medical Officer of Health for Ontario.

15.2 Producing More Relevant Evidence

Historically, a major focus of the study of the social determinants of health has been on health disparities and socioeconomic status, particularly income. An emphasis on income as the pre-eminent determinant of health has been apparent in much of the literature (Lynch et al. 2004a, b; Ross et al. 2000). Although income is relatively easy to measure and has been widely and persistently found to be related to a broad range of health outcomes, thinking about income as being more fundamental than other determinants (e.g., Link and Phelan 1995) is not always helpful in practice. Furthermore, the evidence about the exact nature of the relationship between income and health disparities is inconsistent; both the shape and the slope of the income gradient of health vary within different contexts and according to additional factors (e.g., age, sex, immigrant status) (Box 15.1). In the Region of Peel, for example,

Box 15.1

What types of social epidemiology research have been particularly useful to your public health practice?

During my years of teaching at the graduate level, I often remarked that we always find an association between income gradients and health outcomes. It seemed that the income gradient of health was always present. However, when we went to prepare a health status report for the Region of Peel, the gradient was not there! There was no association between the percent of households below the low-income cut-off in each census tract and mortality rates. We went back to the data and changed the analysis to examine median incomes by census tract and still found no association. Peel, like much of the Greater Toronto Area, has a large proportion of recent immigrants. According to the 2006 Canadian census, 49% of Peel residents are immigrants (Statistics Canada 2009). For this reason, we thought our findings would have something to do with immigrants, so we repeated the analysis separately for Canadian-born and foreign-born persons. By working with Statistics Canada, we were able to stratify our analysis by immigrant status and use household-level income rather than median income by census tract. What we found was a very slight association between low income and life expectancy for immigrants. In contrast, the non-immigrant curve showed a gradient across quintiles followed by a large drop in health status in the lowest income quintile. In all quintiles, large differences in mortality were observed between Canadian-born and foreign-born persons, with consistently lower mortality rates among immigrants. For example, remaining years of life at age 25 was 8.6 years shorter for Canadian-born men compared to immigrant men in the lowest income quintile. Importantly, this enormous difference was observed not *between* income groups but *within* an income group.

New immigrants generally have better health and have a slightly higher educational status than non-immigrants (i.e., the healthy immigrant effect) but, at least initially, have lower incomes. Over time, the health status of immigrants tends to become more like that of other residents (Region of Peel Public Health 2008). When we were examining the population as a whole, the expected relationship between income and health was being obscured by the different socioeconomic circumstances of the 49% of residents who were not born in Canada. This finding provides a good example of how relationships between selected determinants and health outcomes can vary on a number of other factors, for example immigrant status. This kind of information directly impacts the design of programs within public health. Further investigation into life expectancy among Canadian-born men in the lowest income quintile will help us to identify potential ways in which to intervene.

there is a modest association between income and self-reported health in multivariate analyses (Table 15.1). However, for other outcomes, for example obesity rates, the association between income and health status is non-significant or varies in magnitude and/or direction according to an additional factor, in this case sex (Fig. 15.1). Obviously, the picture is more complicated and dynamic than these simple associations suggest, even when multiple risk factors or potential confounders and interaction terms are accounted for in statistical models.

Table 15.1 Binomial logistic regression analysis for the association between fair or poor self-reported health and the determinants of health and related predictors, Region of Peel, 2000/2001 to 2007/2008, n = 7,347

Variable	Percent reporting fair or poor general health	Adjusted odds ratio (95% confidence interval)
Determinants of health		
Age	–	*1.05 (1.04, 1.05)
Sex		
Male	10.5	*0.74 (0.59, 0.93)
Female	14.4	1.0
Household income level		
Lowest to middle	25.0	1.30 (0.84, 2.02)
Upper-middle	15.2	1.0
Highest	7.5	*0.61 (0.48, 0.77)
Educational level of respondent		
Less than secondary	23.6	*1.54 (1.18, 2.00)
Secondary graduate	14.0	1.18 (0.93, 1.51)
Other post-secondary	10.8	0.98 (0.66, 1.45)
Post-secondary graduate	9.6	1.0
Ethnicity		
White	13.1	1.0
Black	13.2	1.04 (0.66, 1.62)
East/Southeast Asian	10.8	1.37 (0.85, 2.18)
West Asian/Arab	8.9	0.83 (0.33, 2.07)
South Asian	11.3	1.37 (0.91, 2.07)
Latin American	11.8	1.32 (0.62, 2.82)
Other	12.0	0.97 (0.59, 1.59)
Immigrant status		
Recent immigrant	8.3	1.02 (0.65, 1.60)
Long-term immigrant	16.5	1.16 (0.93, 1.46)
Non-immigrant	10.9	1.0
Marital status		
Now married/common law	11.8	1.0
Divorced/separated/widowed	21.2	1.00 (0.76, 1.31)
Single	9.0	*1.47 (1.08, 2.02)

(continued)

Table 15.1 (continued)

Variable	Percent reporting fair or poor general health	Adjusted odds ratio (95% confidence interval)
Sense of belonging to local community		
Very strong/somewhat strong	10.2	1.0
Somewhat weak/very weak	15.5	*1.58 (1.27, 1.97)
Self-perceived life stress		
Quite a bit/extremely	10.3	*2.85 (2.29, 3.55)
Not at all/not very/A bit	18.6	1.0
Employment status in past week		
At work last week/absent last week	7.5	1.0
No job last week	18.5	*1.30 (1.03, 1.65)
Other predictors		
Weekly alcohol consumption		
Yes	9.4	*0.72 (0.57, 0.90)
No	14.7	1.0
Smoking status		
Current smoker	13.9	*1.85 (1.35, 2.52)
Former smoker	13.6	*1.41 (1.07, 1.87)
Never smoker	11.2	1.0
Physical activity level		
Active	5.9	1.0
Moderate	8.9	1.00 (0.71, 1.40)
Inactive	16.0	*1.47 (1.13, 1.91)
BMI		
Underweight	18.0	*2.46 (1.41, 4.30)
Overweight	11.7	1.23 (0.97, 1.56)
Obese	23.5	*2.65 (2.05, 3.41)
Normal	9.0	1.0

Source: Canadian Community Health Survey (2000/2001, 2003, 2005, 2007/2008)
Analysis excludes respondents under 18 years of age
*Indicates statistically significant findings ($p < 0.05$)

Despite improvements in life expectancy over time, largely resulting from better physical and work environments and advances in sanitation and nutrition, disparities in the health status of the more and the less advantaged parts of the population still persist (Syme 2008). The influence of income on these health disparities is both important and pervasive. However, as social epidemiologists begin to explore the details of the relationship, the consistency and the certainty of these associations start to diminish. For example, in much of the social epidemiology literature, a debate exists about the importance of absolute versus relative income measures (Marmot 2005; Wilkinson 1997) and the corresponding material deprivation and psychosocial explanations of the association. At one point, there was a strong consensus that, at least in developed countries, relative income was more important. This proposition would be consistent with the psychosocial theory, which suggests differences in health are caused by perceived differences in social status. While this

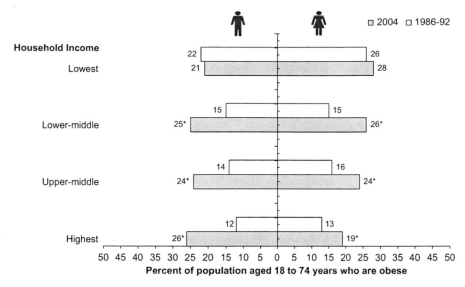

Fig. 15.1 Prevalence of Obesity by Sex and Household Income, Canada, excluding territories, 1986–1992 and 2004. *Significantly higher than estimate for 1986–1992 (p<0.05). Source: Canadian Heart Health Surveys (1986–1992); Canadian Community Health Survey (2004): Nutrition. For each sex/household income group, the estimate based on the Canadian Heart Health Survey was age-standardized using the distribution of the corresponding 2004 CCHS population (Adapted from Statistics Canada publication (2006))

explanation certainly seems to be a plausible mechanism when studying occupational rank (Marmot et al. 1984), recent systematic reviews of the literature (Lynch et al. 2004b; Subramanian and Kawachi 2004) found no association between income inequality and life expectancy when comparing countries using relative income.

These inconsistencies present obvious challenges for public health practitioners when designing programs or interventions to ameliorate health inequalities. From a public health perspective, academic debates around the influence of absolute versus relative income on health are immaterial; rarely are public health interventions capable of increasing the average income within a population or reducing the size of the income gradient, nor are they intended to. Furthermore, if we acknowledge that income – or, broadly speaking, socioeconomic status – is, in fact, merely a proxy measure for other influences (e.g., social status, power relations, poverty, etc.) that are causally linked to health outcomes, then income gradients in and of themselves become less pragmatic targets for public health action (see Chap. 5). In order to be more relevant to a public health practice, social epidemiologists must expand their research beyond demonstrating the existence of income gradients and their associations to health inequalities and begin to provide research on factors that are more amenable to change as well as offer realistic strategies for action. As will be discussed later in the chapter, the identification of these factors and strategies will require further insight into the complex mechanisms linking social determinants to health inequalities.

Apart from an improved understanding of mechanisms, social epidemiologists must also consider how the local environment may influence these relationships. Research on social determinants from a neighbourhood-level perspective shows that there is an independent effect of neighbourhood characteristics on health outcomes (Lemstra and Neudorf 2008; Pampalon and Raymond 2000; Ross et al. 2004), which is at least partially attributed to the physical environment (e.g., poor infrastructure, facilities and amenities, etc.). However, certain influences remain even after accounting for a neighbourhood's material deprivation, suggesting that other influences, for example social interaction, can also impact health at this level (Pampalon and Raymond 2000) and should be accounted for when designing public health programs and interventions. Although a conceptual basis is lacking, these geographically-based studies are useful as indicators of the need for services and for communicating the needs of specific areas. They may also serve to indicate populations with multiple social and economic disadvantages together with multiple risk factors.

From a policy-making perspective, the clustering of risk factors in disadvantaged populations may indicate the need to address the more distal determinants (i.e., upstream socioeconomic factors) rather than attempting to influence risk factors directly. However, continuing debate in the literature exists about the relative importance of proximal versus distal determinants (Kaplan 2004; Rothman et al. 1998; Susser and Susser 1996). As we move toward more distal social determinants, the solutions are rarely well-defined, feasible or effective. While there is often more certainty about proximal risk factors and their association with health outcomes, more distal social determinants potentially have equivalent, if not greater, influence on a wide range of health conditions. In order to be useful in practice, social epidemiologists should not restrict their research to the study of distal social determinants alone (Kaplan 2004) and should begin to consider all elements, both proximate and intermediate, which connect causally to health outcomes. Interactions with other determinants and contextual factors must also be considered, as these factors (as well as policies aimed at these factors) can buffer the effects of income inequalities (Lynch et al. 2000; Ross et al. 2000).

15.3   Understanding Mechanisms

Throughout history the most effective public health interventions have been those directed towards social determinants; however, continued progress in improving overall health status will require a better and fuller understanding of social determinants, behavioural and biological risk factors, health outcomes and their interrelationships. Often social epidemiologists attempt to develop a single model of causation and focus on understanding the components of a single model in more detail. By examining these "pieces of the puzzle," social epidemiologists can begin to draw sound conclusions about the causes of social determinants and their impacts on health outcomes. However, in order to be more useful to public health practice, a larger, multilevel comprehensive explanation is required – a task which is far from complete (Box 15.2). One challenge for putting these findings together into an understandable whole is the plethora of models used to help us think about causes. Rarely do these models provide answers about causation, and no one "right" model can exist for all health issues (Bhopal 2008).

In public health practice, social epidemiology research is often presented as competing models of disease causation. These models can be briefly summarized as follows. The *biomedical* model of disease asserts that disease results from disruption of normal biological and physiological functioning, without any consideration of the social, psychological or behavioural factors that may contribute to poor health (Engel 1977). The *behavioural* model of disease, in contrast, considers the individual-level influences on health-related actions and decisions. This model is particularly concerned with the identification and modification of risk factors (i.e., the health behaviours that are proximally related to health outcomes) (Rosenstock et al. 1988). However, this model still fails to consider the social and contextual factors within which these behaviours occur. The *social determinants of health* is a term introduced in the 1970s as part of an argument that too much attention was being devoted to individuals at the expense of understanding population-level influences. This concept reflected a realization that the greatest improvements in health status

---

Box 15.2

As a public health practitioner, does the impact factor of a journal matter to you?
We all have our own prejudices and our own patterns of reading. Impact factors are not always kept in mind! I usually look for the names of the authors. I think a lot of people would look at who wrote the paper rather than the journal. Epidemiology journals *typically* have limited material on social epidemiology. Journals such as *The Lancet*, the *BMJ* (*British Medical Journal*) and the *Journal of Epidemiology and Community Health*, however, generally do include some social epidemiology research, as do some others. That being said, we often consult information specialists to assist with our research. Nothing beats the help of an experienced librarian when attempting to investigate specific research questions. Social epidemiology research in academic publications doesn't present to public health practitioners as part of one great universal model of everything. It appears as little pieces. All of the information is in there but rarely is it synthesized to a point where it becomes applicable to the public health practitioner. For example, how do we get a school food policy right? What are we going to do about this health problem among immigrant groups? Everything is in there, but it presents to public health practitioners as these discrete associations between risk factors and outcomes separate from their causal pathways. In order for social epidemiology research to become more useful, social epidemiologists must continue moving beyond simply describing associations to building a consistent and understandable whole.

over the previous century had been due less to medical care, or even clinical prevention, than to improvements in social conditions (Graham and Kelly 2004). While there is no universally accepted list of determinants, income, education and employment, housing, child development and the physical environment, as well as social connectedness and social capital, are usually included.

There is a considerable body of evidence to suggest that socioeconomic determinants exert a direct effect upon health outcomes such that social determinants are fundamental causes of disease (Graham and Kelly 2004). While there is some evidence to suggest that risk behaviours are a key influence independent of social determinants on outcomes, for example in cardiovascular disease research (Lynch et al. 2006), more often health behaviours vary by socioeconomic status, suggesting the presence of a common pathway (Syme 1996). Thus, for some health outcomes, socioeconomic status influences health status directly, while for other outcomes the pathway from social determinants to health occurs indirectly through health behaviours (Dunn 2010). Social epidemiologists should consider testing for these potential mediation factors in statistical models, as appropriate public health programming will likely depend on which pathway is operating. Further studies are needed in this area.

Although one cannot choose among competing models of causation as being the "right" one, one can certainly eliminate some approaches as being entirely unhelpful. The *biomedical*, *behavioural* and *social determinants* approaches, taken individually, fall into this category. These approaches are often presented as competing models; however, in reality, they represent only partial models of the same health phenomenon. In order to be more relevant to a public health practice, social epidemiologists should consider biomedical and behavioural risk factors and social determinants together within a single model of causation. This model should acknowledge both proximal and distal components of social determinants, including measures of relative social status and socioeconomic disadvantage as well as the more fundamental social structures such as economic and social welfare systems (see Chap. 9). Furthermore, empirical evidence suggests that there are factors that influence health, which do not fall easily into these fairly simple categories, but which should be included in models of causation. One example is the built environment, a higher-order concept that incorporates features of the physical environment and urban form but also encompasses issues such as social structure, transportation policy, economic policy and urban planning, to name a few. Ethnocultural identity could be considered as another higher-order concept, incorporating such diverse issues as health behaviours, socioeconomic position, social support and others.

Following the identification of pathways between social determinants and health outcomes, social epidemiologists should then consider how these pathways are connected. Take, for example, the association between education and health status. A simple linear explanation going from education through health literacy to health status is sometimes quoted; however, this pathway has obvious limitations, including the inability to explain the extension of the relationship beyond the threshold at which literacy ceases to be an issue. Michael Marmot describes three types of causal linkages: social causation, health selection and indirect selection (Marmot et al. 1997).

One might also term these direct (A causes B), reverse (B causes A) and indirect (something else causes both A and B) causation, respectively. In reality, all three causal linkages are found, to some degree, in any causal model that accurately represents the empirical evidence.

Although we have stressed the necessity of building a comprehensive model of causation to evaluate relationships and pathways, the purpose is not to develop a single grand solution to all of our health problems. In practice, we are looking to identify, on the basis of good evidence, points that are most promising for intervention. These points of intervention will vary greatly depending upon the disease process, the population affected and the context (Box 15.3). Public health practitioners require practical tools and standards for measuring health disparities and identifying promising points of intervention. Some helpful tools have been developed, such as the Health Inequalities Intervention Tool of the London Health Observatory (2010); however, further work is required in this area. These tools

---

Box 15.3

Can you provide an example of social epidemiologic research being effectively (or ineffectively) applied to a public health practice?
One example is the identification of points of intervention for cervical cancer. To address inequalities in the incidence of cancer of the cervix, behavioural approaches that attempt to reduce risk behaviours would seem futile, and action to change the socioeconomic structure of society (i.e., a social determinants approach) would be both challenging and not proven to produce the desired effect. A biomedical approach that includes a universal free program of immunization against human papilloma virus combined with an organized universal free program of cervical screening would clearly affect the occurrence of disease at all levels of socioeconomic status and would probably reduce absolute (if not relative) disparities in incidence and mortality as well (Gupta et al. 2009). However, cervical cancer screening rates differ across age groups, income level and recent immigrant status even within systems of universal health care. In Ontario, for example, older, low-income and immigrant women are less likely to be screened (Lofters et al. 2010). For this reason, a biomedical approach must be expanded to also consider the individual behaviours for seeking health care as well as the social determinants that influence access to services. In general, universal free access to medical care has not resulted in a reduction of health disparities, and clinical prevention services, for example cervical screening, continue to be less utilized by disadvantaged groups. Provision of universal access to immunization and screening programs may ensure decreased rates among non-immigrant, high income women; however, alternative approaches will be required among immigrant and low-income groups to address the economic, social and cultural barriers to accessing health care.

should be developed and used to identify and prioritize public health interventions that will have the greatest impact on improving health outcomes and, at the same time, improving health inequalities.

15.4 Improving Health Outcomes and Reducing Health Inequalities

Rose (1992, 1985) has distinguished between the causes of disease at the individual level and the causes of disease incidence at the population level, while Graham and Kelly (2004) have distinguished between the determinants of health and the determinants of inequality. These distinctions imply that priorities for action at the population level may be quite different from those that would improve health at the individual level. It also implies that the unequal distribution of determinants should be the basis of efforts to tackle inequalities in health outcomes. The implications for public health agencies is that all programs and services should have two explicit goals: (1) maintaining and improving the average health status of the population; and (2) reducing inequalities between advantaged and less advantaged portions of that population.

Local public health practitioners have long pondered the relative merits of universal versus targeted approaches. To what extent should we aim to "shift the curve to the left" and to what extent aim to reduce its spread? Marmot (2010) coins the term "proportionate universalism" to describe the strategy of actions which are universal but proportionate to the level of disadvantage. In some cases, targeting an intervention towards the most deprived groups will potentially affect only a small portion of the burden of disease within the total population. In other approaches, small reductions in risk may occur over large groups of people, resulting in a substantial overall benefit to the population. It is unlikely that one theory or strategy will apply to all circumstances. However, a thorough analysis of the issues within the local context followed by a careful design of policies and programs to take determinants and inequalities into account will provide for effective public health practice that not only improves the average health status of the population but also reduces social disparities.

Take, for example, two public health programs that aimed to reduce socioeconomic disparities: fluoridation of municipal drinking water and campaigns to reduce the prevalence of tobacco smoking. These two universal programs, while both designed to improve the overall health status of the population, produced opposite effects on socioeconomic disparities. Fluoride supplementation has been shown to reduce the prevalence of dental caries and tooth decay in both children and adults (Centres for Disease Control and Prevention 2011). In general, children of low socioeconomic status have poorer dental health relative to children in higher income brackets (Al-Jewair and Leake 2010; Edelstein 2002; Edelstein and Chinn 2009), due in part to lower use of fluoride products (e.g., oral supplements, topical gels and varnishes and toothpaste) compared to higher income families (Mansbridge and

Brown 1985; Steele and Lader 2004). It is generally accepted that fluoridation of municipal drinking water reduces inequalities in dental health across the income gradient. Specifically, universal fluoridation programs provide fluoride to low-income groups who do not receive it topically but who are otherwise at risk for more dental caries and who may be more likely to drink municipal water.

In contrast, the example of smoking cession demonstrates a universal public health program that exacerbated socioeconomic inequalities. The reduction of tobacco smoking rates in Canada is regarded as one of public health's greatest successes. Through a variety of universal interventions, mainly policies, mass media campaigns and changes in the social environment, smoking rates have fallen steadily. However, simply examining these rates does not provide a clear picture, as these aggregate-level data obscure the differences in rates by sex, age, ethnicity, income and education. Evidence from the United Kingdom shows that the prevalence of smoking has fallen in all income groups over the last several decades, but more so in higher income groups, resulting in an augmentation of the pre-existing socioeconomic disparities (Stellman and Resnicow 1997).

Taken together, these findings highlight the need for social epidemiologists to investigate the specific mechanisms linking determinants and health outcomes as well as to improve our understanding of the effect of local contexts. Efforts to improve health through changes in health behaviours, particularly through education, have been shown to be initially more effective among populations with better education and higher incomes (Davis et al. 1995), due in part to the greater availability of resources and higher health literacy among well-off groups. Consequently, educational-based interventions may function, at least temporarily, to increase in socioeconomic differences in health. Ischaemic heart disease is an example. Earlier in the twentieth century, heart disease was more prevalent among higher socioeconomic groups, but since that time the rates in the upper classes have fallen and the disparities between high- and low-income groups have increased, even though disease incidence and mortality rates among all income groups decreased over time (Jemal et al. 2008; Mackenbach et al. 2003; O'Flaherty et al. 2009).

Over the last few decades in Canada, the overall health status of all income groups has improved without a meaningful reduction in disparities. There are two ways of looking at this phenomenon. First, the differences in health status are inequitable, and our values would compel us to take action to reduce them. Second, the health status of the most privileged group represents a state that should be achievable by all. Thus, the observed differences in health status represent a burden of disease that is potentially avoidable. There is no simple answer to achieving a balance between effectiveness and equity or prioritizing aggregate improvement versus reduced inequality. Even the ways in which inequalities and changes in inequalities are measured (e.g., absolute versus relative changes) involve value judgments (Harper et al. 2010). At a minimum, these issues should be identified, measured and discussed with input sought from public and governing bodies (see Chap. 3 for a discussion on values in social epidemiologic research).

15.5   Applying Social Epidemiology Research to Public Health Practice

What are the necessary factors required for public health to incorporate social epidemiology research into practice? At present, public health programs may incorporate features related to determinants and inequalities, but too often these programs are short term, small scale or limited to new funding, leaving the bulk of resources and activities untouched. Gilles Paradis (2009), Scientific Editor of the Canadian Journal of Public Health and a Professor at McGill University, has the following view of the social determinants of health agenda for public health practice in Canada:

> The social determinants agenda lacks clear direction. …This stems in part from a public health system that lacks the capacity to integrate social determinants in program and policy planning. Professionals lack knowledge about social determinants and about interventions to influence these determinants. The need for increased research on effective policies to reduce inequities and improve population health is acute and urgent.

In other words, in order to move forward with this agenda, the products of social epidemiology must be rendered more relevant to public health and knowledge about social determinants must be put more readily into action. These challenges in advancing a social determinants agenda to the stage at which its findings can be widely applied in practice clearly call for increased collaboration between social epidemiologists and public health practitioners in both research and knowledge translation activities (as will be discussed later in this chapter).

The public health community's current engagement with the social epidemiology knowledge base has been criticized for its seeming inability to progress beyond the proclamation of high-level associations between determinants and health outcomes. Only a small portion of the literature on social determinants discusses feasible actions to improve health or reduce disparities through determinants. So far, many of these recommendations for action have been too general to meaningfully effect change (Lemstra and Neudorf 2008; Public Health Agency of Canada 2010). These actions include "an integrated strategy" of targets, monitoring, collaboration and priority areas that promote engaging with other sectors "in the development of structures and mechanisms" and emphasize strengthening of research and knowledge exchange. Others have recommended specific social policies, including changes to benefits, taxation and rules for social assistance and unemployment benefit, particularly aimed at the reduction of child poverty (Lemstra and Neudorf 2008). However, there has been little success using findings from social epidemiology to change policies in the desired direction. Broad policy interventions (e.g., income redistribution) may also have a role to play in securing better health for all, but these interventions do not constitute a complete answer to addressing this issue and present obvious feasibility challenges. Action by public health agencies at the local level might include advocacy for policy changes along these lines, but they should not be limited to these strategies.

Members of governing bodies may be strongly oriented to the delivery of services and to visible, short-term results. However, addressing the social determinants of health and reducing social disparities demands more long-term solutions and will require financial and political commitments for program planning at all levels of government. In order to achieve continued action on this issue, public health leaders must endeavour to impart an understanding of the determinants of health throughout health care organizations. To the extent possible, attention to determinants in terms of improving health status and reducing disparities should be incorporated into an organization's priorities, objectives and reports.

Social epidemiologists have an important role to serve in increasing the awareness of social determinants and their impact on health outcomes among not only politicians and health care administrators but also the public. In this sense, social epidemiologists can play an "agenda setting" role in policy making (see Chap. 13). Particularly, social epidemiologists can increase the awareness of social determinants among these groups, particularly if examples of selected social determinants and their impacts on health outcomes are illustrated using local data and accompanied by implications for action (Bhopal 2008). Many public health departments will use this knowledge of the distribution of social determinants locally to modify or target programs to disadvantaged groups (Ontario Public Health Association and Association of Public Health Agencies 2010). Public health departments can also engage in advocacy, either directly or as part of a coalition, about distal social determinants (e.g., poverty reduction). In reality, however, we know little about how these departments are incorporating action on social determinants of health directly into programs and policies to influence change. Although there has been more emphasis on the social determinants as causes of health inequalities than on the social determinants as determinants of health, both are important for implementing population-based strategies that improve health status for all parts of society as well as those which reduce inequalities.

There are also important constraints that should be considered on the ability of epidemiologists, public health practitioners and others to bring about change on the more distal determinants of health, as often these social influences lie outside of the health sphere. Public health practitioners typically must adopt a strategy of mitigating social inequalities and their impacts on health outcomes rather than directly intervene on distal social determinants. One exception, however, may be the incorporation of *Health in All Policies*, a government strategy in which multiple health and non-health sectors are involved in improving population health such that the reduction of social inequalities moves to the forefront of political agendas to improve health (Shankardass et al. 2010). Although public health practitioners can make the case for action on a particular determinant, planning and advocating for specific policy changes may be beyond the competence of public health practitioners (Rothman et al. 1998). Forming coalitions with individuals who possess the requisite knowledge, skills and connections to produce meaningful change in the appropriate political arenas is, therefore, advisable.

Social epidemiology, in practice, is dependent upon information infrastructure. Access to data at a sufficient level of detail and in a timely manner is required without undue restrictions or limitations. Good linkage of records, particularly between health and other databases from other sectors such as education, labour and social services, is available in some parts of Canada (e.g., British Columbia and Manitoba) but not everywhere. In some jurisdictions, the quality and timeliness of vital statistics data could also be improved (Public Health Agency of Canada 2008). Although there are few data sources available for chronic disease research in Canada, some databases have provided good quality data and their methodology could be expanded to other diseases and conditions. The Canadian Diabetes Surveillance System and the Canadian Cancer Registry are two examples of such databases. In addition, there is a need for easily accessible synthesis of research in social epidemiology, for example meta-analyses, as well as a process for routinely incorporating updates of recent social epidemiologic findings. The recently announced decision to cancel the mandatory Canadian Long Form Census in favour of a voluntary system is a major loss for researchers, policy makers and public health practitioners to formulate policies and programs based upon reliable, unbiased evidence. This decision will have numerous short-term (e.g., program planning and resource allocation within a fiscal year) and long-term (e.g., comparability to other census years to investigate trends over time) consequences for public health in Canada.

15.6 The Role of Partnerships Between Social Epidemiologists and Public Health Practitioners

Public health decisions are often made in the absence of complete data and without rigorous evaluation methods and, possibly, without a solid theoretical base. Public health practitioners must rely on the "best available evidence" at the time of decision making and use this evidence to determine how generalizable knowledge applies to their local community. In this way, public health practitioners employ *evidence-informed decision making*. Sometimes when reliable evidence is lacking, further research is required to better to understand the local context and its impact on health outcomes. However, this investment in additional research is usually prohibitive in terms of time and cost constraints. When decisions must be made in the absence of reliable or appropriate evidence, the role for partnerships between public health practitioners and social epidemiologists becomes more apparent.

Public health is a field in which the transfer of knowledge through "push" and "pull" activities should be augmented by the co-production of evidence (see Chap. 13). Partly as a result of encouragement by funding agencies, such as the Canadian Institutes of Health Research (CIHR) and the Canadian Health Services Research Foundation (CHSRF), public health practitioners are increasingly becoming involved as "decision-making partners" in academic research *knowledge translation* programs. These partnerships aim to produce "actionable evidence" (i.e., evidence that is amenable to application in public health practice), which will further improve the collaboration between social epidemiologists and providers.

In the Region of Peel, for example, our partnerships focus on evidence: how to acquire it; how to appraise it; and how to use it. In general, we use evidence that is already available from the academic literature. Often times, however, we must adapt this evidence such that it is applicable to the local context. The association between the income gradient and health is a good example (Box 15.1). We were unable to find an association between income and mortality in Peel until we took into account the large population of recent immigrants who were obscuring the trend among non-immigrant residents. Public health departments need to further develop competencies in acquiring and interpreting evidence as well as create infrastructure for incorporating social epidemiology research into practice. Such approaches could and should include forming partnerships with skilled information specialists and academic researchers (Box 15.4) as well as providing tools to assess the quality and applicability of evidence.

In Peel, we have committed resources to conducting reviews (e.g., systematic reviews, realist reviews) for the health problems that are relevant to our community. As a large department, we find this work to be feasible but only through forming partnerships with academic researchers. Some smaller organizations may not have the resources available to conduct this amount of research. Through our partnerships, our public health staff developed the needed skills to both appraise existing systematic reviews and update them with the current literature. These partnerships enabled us to review the evidence on topics related to the built environment, child

---

Box 15.4

Can you provide an example of a successful partnership between social epidemiologists and public health practitioners?
Low birth weight (less than 2.5 kg at birth) is a determinant of infant health, survival and development. When we were looking at our birth outcomes for a health status report in Peel, we found that our prevalence of low birth weight was clearly elevated above the average rate for Ontario. The first thing we did was to determine if our low birth weights were the result of preterm births or small for gestational age (SGA) births. Preterm births refer to babies who are born less than 37 weeks gestational age (a normal, full-term pregnancy is 40 weeks); whereas, SGA births are those infants whose birth weight is below the tenth percentile for that particular gestational age. By separating preterm from SGA births, we found that the higher rate of low birth weight in Peel was entirely due to infants being born SGA rather than preterm.

Given that a large proportion of our population in Peel are recent immigrants, particularly from South Asian countries, we suspected that ethnicity might explain some of our findings (at least partially). We discovered a small pilot study at St. Michael's Hospital in Toronto, which showed that birth weights varied by ethnicity. We worked with our research partner at St. Michael's to plot the birth weights for all the births in Peel over a 5-year period by gestational age and sex and stratified these plots by birthplace of mother (as a proxy for ethnicity). This analysis gave us intra-uterine growth charts by ethnicity and showed that each ethnicity had a different growth curve, with South Asian male and female births being lighter by 220 and 189 g, respectively. That's a good example of how an epidemiologist helped us figure out a public health issue. Most importantly, the implications for action were significantly altered as a result of our further investigation.

development, breastfeeding and others as well as to participate in research on health issues of our residents of South Asian origin, as an example (Box 15.4). Furthermore, partnerships with social epidemiologists can help us develop conceptual models for the more complex health issues that we, as public health providers, must tackle. This commitment to making evidence-informed decision making a priority is outlined in our Strategic Plan, and we have been fortunate in being able to develop partnerships with social epidemiologists in academic settings.

Finally, there is an important role for universities and educators to ensure that public health concepts are appropriately integrated into epidemiology training programs and course curriculums. This approach could include instruction at the classroom level but also could encompass field placements within public health settings. By improving training programs for social epidemiology students, we can begin to ensure social epidemiology research becomes more relevant to public health practice for the next generation of researchers and practitioners (Box 15.5).

Box 15.5

If you were teaching a group of social epidemiology students, what do you think they would need to know about your work in terms of producing more relevant evidence?

There are three things they should know. One, we work with the data we have. This doesn't preclude going out and collecting more data – we do that – but there are limits on what is feasible. For example, we do a major health survey in our schools once every 5 years. It takes a lot of effort. It's not feasible for us to conduct these projects more frequently or on a larger scale. So mainly you work with the data that you have. We have to work with the best available evidence, and often times there are problems with the quality or relevance of evidence in the literature. Two, they must understand the context for their findings because the context will differ from setting to setting. Of course, the general-level associations apply, but you need to know the specifics in order to effectively and appropriately implement public health programs in the community. Three, they have to realize that they (academics) live in a world of disproving hypotheses, but we (public health practitioners) live in a world of trying to solve problems. The evidence and the data are never perfect. Although it's always a good thing to do more research, practical decisions need to be made now. Too often our conclusion is that "no good quality evidence exists" or "the evidence is inconsistent." As a general component of our public health practice, we do descriptive epidemiology, and we often identify remarkable trends or patterns that need more research. For example, we found no income gradient of health (Box 15.1) and noticed an increase in low birth weights (Box 15.4). We then took these curious findings and worked with epidemiologists to figure out what was going on. That's the way we work in practice. We describe the trends and then determine why these trends are occurring.

15.7 Conclusions

In order to produce evidence that is more relevant to public health practice, social epidemiologists must begin to consider the full range of determinants that can affect health outcomes. In particular, the concept of social determinants of health must be broadened from a focus on socioeconomic disparities and income gradients to include other underlying social factors that are amendable to change. In order to advance the social determinants research agenda in the field of public health, an improved understanding of the mechanisms and casual pathways through which the social determinants of health affect health outcomes is required. These mechanisms should encompass biomedical and behavioural risk factors and social determinants of health within a single model as well as include higher-order concepts such as the built environment. Public health practitioners also have a role to play in incorporating social epidemiology research into practice. Health departments should have an explicit mandate to both improve the overall health status of the population and to reduce disparities in health status. Action on the social determinants of health is required to achieve both these goals and will require greater advocacy by social epidemiologists to promote an understanding of the social determinants of health amongst clinicians, politicians, governing bodies and the public. Finally, increased partnerships between public health practitioners and academic researchers are required in order to advance social epidemiology to the stage at which its findings can be widely applied in practice.

References

Al-Jewair TS, Leake JL (2010) The prevalence and risks of early childhood caries (ECC) in Toronto, Canada. J Contemp Dent Pract 11:1–8

Bhopal R (2008) Causes in epidemiology: the jewels in the public health crown. J Public Health 30:224–225

Centres for Disease Control and Prevention (2011) Community water fluorination. http://www.cdc.gov/fluoridation/. Accessed 31 Jan 2011

Davis SK, Winkleby MA, Farquhar JW (1995) Increasing disparity in knowledge of cardiovascular disease risk factors and risk-reduction strategies by socioeconomic status: implications for policymakers. Am J Prev Med 11:318–323

Dunn JR (2010) Health behavior vs the stress of low socioeconomic status and health outcomes. JAMA 303:1199–1200

Edelstein BL (2002) Disparities in oral health and access to care: findings of national surveys. Ambul Pediatr 2:141–147

Edelstein BL, Chinn CH (2009) Update on disparities in oral health and access to dental care for America's children. Acad Pediatr 9:415–419

Engel GL (1977) The need for a new medical model: a challenge for biomedicine. Science 196:129–136

Graham H, Kelly MP (2004) Health inequalities: concepts, frameworks and policy. Health Development Agency, London

Gupta S, Sodhani P, Sharma A et al (2009) Prevalence of high-risk human papillomavirus type 16/18 infection among women with normal cytology: risk factor analysis and implications for screening and prophylaxis. Cytopathology 20:249–255

Harper S, King NB, Meersman SC et al (2010) Implicit value judgments in the measurement of health inequalities. Milbank Q 88:4–29

Jemal A, Ward E, Anderson RN et al (2008) Widening of socioeconomic inequalities in US death rates, 1993–2001. PLoS One 3:e2181

Kaplan GA (2004) What's wrong with social epidemiology, and how can we make it better? Epidemiol Rev 26:124–135

Lemstra M, Neudorf C (2008) Health disparity in Saskatoon: analysis to intervention. Saskatoon Health Region, Saskatoon

Link BG, Phelan J (1995) Social conditions as fundamental causes of disease. J Health Soc Behav 35:80–94

Lofters AK, Moineddin R, Hwang SW et al (2010) Low rates of cervical cancer screening among urban immigrants: a population-based study in Ontario, Canada. Med Care 48:611–618

London Health Observatory (2010) Department of Health. Welcome to the health inequalities intervention toolkit. http://www.lho.org.uk/LHO_Topics/Analytic_Tools/HealthInequalities InterventionToolkit.aspx. Accessed 31 Jan 2011

Lynch JW, Davey Smith G, Kaplan GA et al (2000) Income inequality and mortality: Importance to health of individual income, psychosocial environment, or material conditions. BMJ 320:1200–1204

Lynch J, Davey Smith G, Harper S et al (2004a) Is income inequality a determinant of population health? Part 2. US national and regional trends in income inequality and age and cause specific mortality. Milbank Q 82:355–400

Lynch J, Davey Smith G, Harper S et al (2004b) Is income inequality a determinant of population health? Part 1. A systematic review. Milbank Q 82:5–99

Lynch J, Davey Smith G, Harper S et al (2006) Explaining the social gradient in coronary heart disease: comparing relative and absolute risk approaches. J Epidemiol Community Health 60:436–441

Mackenbach JP, Bos V, Andersen O et al (2003) Widening socioeconomic inequalities in mortality in six Western European countries. Int J Epidemiol 32:830–837

Mansbridge JN, Brown MD (1985) Changes in dental caries prevalence in Edinburgh children over three decades. Community Dent Health 2:3–13

Marmot M (2005) Social determinants of health inequalities. Lancet 365:1099–1104

Marmot M (2010) Fair society, health lives: strategic review of health inequalities in England post-2010. The Marmot review, London. http://www.marmotreview.org/. Accessed 31 Jan 2011

Marmot MG, Shipley MJ, Rose G (1984) Inequalities in deatt: specific explanations of a general pattern? Lancet 323:1003–1006

Marmot M, Ryff CD, Bumpass LL et al (1997) Social inequalities in health: next questions and converging evidence. Soc Sci Med 44:901–910

O'Flaherty M, Bishop J, Redpath A et al (2009) Coronary heart disease mortality among young adults in Scotland in relation to social inequalities: time trend study. BMJ 339:b2613

Ontario Public Health Association and Association of Public Health Agencies (2010) Activities to address the social determinants of health in Ontario Local Public Health Units. Summary Report. Joint OPHA/alPHa Working Group on Social Determinants of Health, Sudbury

Pampalon R, Raymond G (2000) A deprivation index for health and welfare planning in Quebec. Chronic Dis Can 21:104–113

Paradis G (2009) Social determinants of health: so what? Can J Public Health 100:164

Public Health Agency of Canada (2008) Canadian perinatal health report, 2008th edn. Public Health Agency of Canada, Ottawa

Public Health Agency of Canada (2010) Creating a healthier Canada: making prevention a priority. Declaration on prevention and promotion from Canada's ministers of health and health promotion/healthy living. Public Health Agency of Canada, Ottawa

Region of Peel Public Health (2008) A picture of health. A comprehensive report on health in Peel, 2008. Region of Peel Public Health, Brampton

Rose G (1985) Sick individuals and sick populations. Int J Epidemiol 14:32–38

Rose G (1992) The strategy of preventative medicine. Oxford University Press, New York

Rosenstock I, Strecher V, Becker M (1988) Social learning theory and the health belief model. Health Educ Q 15:175–183

Ross NA, Wolfson MC, Dunn JR et al (2000) Relation between income inequality and mortality in Canada and in the United States: cross sectional assessment using census data and vital statistics. BMJ 320:898–902

Ross NA, Tremblay SS, Graham K (2004) Neighbourhood influences on health in Montreal, Canada. Soc Sci Med 59:1485–1494

Rothman KJ, Adami HO, Trichopoulos D (1998) Should the mission of epidemiology include the eradication of poverty? Lancet 352:810–813

Shankardass K, Solar O, Murphy K et al (2010) Health in all policies: a snapshot for Ontario. Results of a realist-informed scoping review of the literature. In: Getting started with health in all policies: a resource pack. Report to the Ministry of Health and Long-Term Care (Ontario). Centre for Research on Inner City Health, St. Michael's Hospital, Toronto. http://www.stmichaelshospital.com/knowledgeinstitute/search/details.php?id=18218&page=1. Accessed 12 May 2011

Statistics Canada (2009) Immigration and citizenship highlight tables, 2006 census. Statistics Canada, Ottawa. http://www12.statcan.gc.ca/census-recensement/2006/dp-pd/hlt/97-557/Index-eng.cfm. Accessed 31 Jan 2011

Statistics Canada publication (2006) Health reports, Catalogue 82-003, 17(3):57. http://www.statcan.gc.ca/studies-etudes/82-003/archive/2006/9279-eng.pdf

Steele J, Lader D (2004) Children's dental health in the United Kingdom, 2003. Social factors and oral health in children. Office for National Statistics, London

Stellman SD, Resnicow K (1997) Tobacco smoking, cancer and social class. IARC Sci Publ 138:229–250

Subramanian SV, Kawachi I (2004) Income inequality and health: what have we learned so far? Epidemiol Rev 26:78–91

Susser M, Susser E (1996) Choosing a future for epidemiology: II. From black box to Chinese boxes and eco-epidemiology. Am J Public Health 86:674–677

Syme SL (1996) Rethinking disease: where do we go from here? Ann Epidemiol 6:463–468

Syme SL (2008) Reducing racial and social-class inequalities in health: the need for a new approach. Health Aff (Millwood) 27:456–459

Wilkinson RG (1997) Socioeconomic determinants of health: health inequalities: relative or absolute material standards? BMJ 314:591–595

Chapter 16
Conclusions

James R. Dunn and Patricia O'Campo

Contents

16.1 Introduction 328
16.2 Theory 328
16.3 New Approaches to Methods 330
16.4 Training and Education 332
16.5 Conclusions 333
References 333

Abstract In this volume, we challenge the evolving field of social epidemiology to rethink the goals, desired impacts, assumptions and practices that currently dominate the discipline. We attempt to steer the development of social epidemiology towards a science that has direct relevance and makes important contributions to formulating solutions to the pressing contemporary social issues that impact population health. We seek to raise questions, provide examples of an expanded social epidemiology, and spark discussion and debate as to whether and how the *status quo* should change. To address the complex problems of macro- and multi-level determinants of health, we should move away from a focus on single studies as a means of advancing knowledge and consider conceptualizing and designing research agendas that address solutions to social determinants, utilizing a range of new and innovative research methods. There is a need for new theories; for example, social epidemiologists should adopt explicit Marxist, feminist, constructivist

J.R. Dunn (✉)
Department of Health, Aging and Society, McMaster University, Kenneth Taylor Hall 226,
1280 Main Street West, Hamilton, ON L8S 4L8, Canada
e-mail: jim.dunn@mcmaster.ca

P. O'Campo
Centre for Research on Inner City Health, St. Michael's Hospital, 30 Bond Street,
Toronto, ON M5B 1W8, Canada
e-mail: O'CampoP@smh.ca

P. O'Campo and J.R. Dunn (eds.), *Rethinking Social Epidemiology:*
Towards a Science of Change, DOI 10.1007/978-94-007-2138-8_16,
© Springer Science+Business Media B.V. 2012

or behaviourist theoretical approaches to inform their work. Finally, we cannot proceed in isolation. By partnering with policy makers, program planners, members of affected communities and scientists from other disciplines, we can ensure that social epidemiology becomes a science of change.

Abbreviations

ACHIEVE	Action for Health Equity Interventions
CIHR	Canadian Institutes of Health Research
CRICH	Centre for Research on Inner City Health
HiAP	Health in All Policies

16.1 Introduction

As with all other health fields, social epidemiology is continuously changing. Our goal in writing this book is to raise questions about the progress of our field and to steer its development towards a science that has direct relevance to the pressing contemporary social issues that impact population health. Social epidemiology, as we and the contributing authors in this book have argued, should be a science that informs solutions to the problems of the day. Movement towards a "science of change" is not only an exciting prospect but has begun to take hold and is illustrated by the research being undertaken by the authors in this volume. We have not laid out a single path forward; scientific advancement is not linear. Rather, the questions we have raised here should challenge us to rethink the goals, desired impact, assumptions and practices that currently dominate our discipline. We have argued that there should be room for multiple types of social epidemiology and an explicit acknowledgement within our science of the values we hold that inform our research as well as our ability to directly impact the policies and programs we seek to change. In this volume, we have provided examples of principles and methods that an expanded discipline might include. Consistent with the goals of critical epidemiology (see Chap. 1 for definition), we have sought to raise questions and spark discussion and debate as to whether and how the *status quo* should change. In this last chapter, we briefly highlight and build upon themes that have consistently emerged across the chapters.

16.2 Theory

One of the recurrent themes throughout this volume has been a call for more attention to theory in social epidemiology. There are a number of factors that are in fundamental tension with such a call, not the least of which is that epidemiology tends to be a very empirically-oriented discipline, owing to its roots in positivism, a philosophy of science described in Chap. 2. We are not the first to call for more theory in social epidemiology (Wainwright and Forbes 2000; Forbes and Wainwright 2001; Krieger 1994, 1999, 2001, 2011; Muntaner 2004). The meaning of the term "theory" is widely taken as self-evident, but the realist perspective unpacks this in a way that provides helpful guidance for the future of social epidemiology.

According to Sayer (1992), there are three notions of the term that are common and worth highlighting. First, there is the notion of theory as a hypothesis or unproblematic explanation; for example, the association between eating and hunger is positive because eating fills a person's stomach. Typically this notion involves very functional explanations that simply convey the relationship between variables where the variables are taken as unproblematic representations of real phenomena. Theories of this type are common in social epidemiology. The second notion of "theory" is an "ordering framework" that allows for observations and data to be classified into thematic categories, possibly for constructing models. This kind of theorizing is also common in social epidemiology and often appears as a conceptual model. These first two kinds of theory share the assumption of an unproblematic relationship between variables and their real world referents, as well as the use of variables as relatively thin concepts, not complex, real world phenomena. The third notion of theory refers to conceptualization, where theorizing involves explicitly advocating or prescribing a particular conceptualization of a phenomenon. This notion of theory conflicts with positivism and many current working assumptions within epidemiology because positivism insists on value-neutrality and objectivity of science. Yet, in most of the social sciences, it is widely acknowledged that such objectivity is an illusion and that all science is value laden (Burawoy 2004; see also Chap. 3).

In order for social epidemiology to become a science of change, it will need to embrace this third notion of theory more fully. So, for example, social epidemiologic studies need to take a more explicitly Marxist, feminist, constructivist or behaviourist theoretical approach and examine a particular phenomenon from that approach. Without such explicit theorization, or theory as conceptualization, change is impossible. Social epidemiologic research questions merely reflect the existing common sense and unexamined conceptualizations held by the researcher and the audience. Moreover, in theorization as conceptualization, the protagonists need to be real world phenomena, not variables (as is often the case in the hypothesis and the ordering framework versions of theory) because the question of how the real world phenomena behave is quite separate from how they are measured.

In other words, as Albert Einstein said, "it is the theory that decides what can be observed" (Hickey 2005), and therefore, theory is the key ingredient to a science that examines new levers for change. As we argued in Chap. 2, this is also reflected in the realist perspective, where, according to Sayer (1992), "part of 'the facts' about human existence is that it depends considerably on societies' self-understanding, that it is socially produced, albeit only partly in intended ways, and that changes in this self-understanding are coupled with changes in society's objective form."

16.3   New Approaches to Methods

One of the questions that may emerge from this book is how individual scholars in social epidemiology should conduct their research programs differently based on what has been presented. Our current practice in this field is to focus on single studies. But if we are to embrace the complexity and broad health impacts of adverse social exposures, we must begin to conceptualize our studies differently. Instead of designing single studies, we should consider conceptualizing and designing research agendas on social determinants and their solutions. In particular, Chap. 2 described how some modest changes are needed, like more recognition for books and more outlets for longer articles that tackle deeper conceptualization and retroduction. That chapter also suggested that academic institutions have to give more credit for such research, and that the focus on the number of publications and the impact factor of the publication venue is a barrier. Another barrier is the current funding structures for academic positions for epidemiologists and social scientists. Since, increasingly, social epidemiologists work wholly or partly in "soft money" positions and have to raise funds for their own salary, the possibilities for risk taking and depth of analysis are impacted. In other words, if an individual scholar's output is going to be measured annually by the number of papers published, and ongoing funding for their position depends on quantifiable scholarly output (number of publications and impact factor of the journals in which they are published), then this is going to be a barrier to that scholar publishing books and longer articles that involve deeper, more theoretically informed and contextually aware analysis. Assuming that these kinds of barriers could be addressed, what would we recommend that scholars do differently?

We believe that there are implications for both training and for individual scholars' career paths. Considering the career path of individual scholars first, we believe that a different approach is needed to individual studies. When writing a paper, most scholars in social epidemiology are usually seeking to publish a definitive study in a high-impact journal. The realist perspective would suggest that an individual journal article is unlikely to be definitive because it only presents a thin slice of understanding of the phenomenon of study. Instead, each individual study, if it is an empirical study, should describe the relationship between variables at the level of events (see Fig. 2.1), but it will still be necessary to engage in retroduction to identify the mechanisms and structures that are responsible for those events and to sort out the necessary and contingent relations that are responsible for the findings. To do all of this, theoretical and/or synthesis research may be needed. This, however, may raise more questions that must be addressed empirically, which may involve more (apparently) traditional epidemiologic research, as well as qualitative or even (quasi-)experimental research, either from primary data or secondary sources. In other words, the activities outlined in Fig. 2.1 could be considered those that a scholar engages in over his or her entire career.

One of us, James Dunn, has pursued a path similar to that conveyed in Fig. 2.1 for over 15 years. For example, Dunn investigates the relationship between housing and health. This sounds simple enough, but housing is actually a complex phenomenon with multiple attributes that may have some causal powers related to health (e.g., physical, psychological, etc.) and that are bound up in the unfolding of both biological developmental processes (e.g., epigenetic expression of atopic phenotypes due to environmental exposures and stress processes) and social ones (e.g., childhood, independent household formation, ageing) that unfold over the life course. Early in his research in this area, Dunn focused on conceptualizing the relationship between housing as a complex phenomenon and health. Specifically, he conceptualized material, meaningful and spatial aspects of housing as important (Dunn et al. 2006), and he sought to establish whether these were associated with general and mental health outcomes (Dunn 2002). Latterly, he explored whether there was a gendered effect to this relationship (Dunn et al. 2004). Now he is engaged in quasi-experimental research on the effect of receiving subsidized housing on adult mental health and healthy child development, as well as in a study of the effect of receiving newly constructed housing in a redeveloped social housing neighbourhood (Regent Park in Toronto) on the health of long-term social housing residents. In both of these studies, the complexity of the interventions raises questions about *how* effects occur, and not just about *whether* they occur. As such, Dunn (2010) is engaged in examining public housing redevelopment as a de-stigmatization strategy using both theoretical and empirical research at the same time as he conducts a large, quasi-experimental study of the impact of the redevelopment on the health of residents so that he can gain an understanding of the mechanisms at work and the contextual features that shape the operation of those mechanisms (similar to the principles employed in Chap. 12).

Another example of knowledge generation emerging from a research agenda comprised of concrete and abstract research, generalizations and syntheses (versus from an individual study or series of studies) in the area of macrosocial determinants is our work on Health in all Policies (HiAP), led by Patricia O'Campo. Designed by several cross-disciplinary scientists at the Centre for Research on Inner City Health (CRICH), we are undertaking work on the subject of whether and how HiAP improves overall population health and whether, in particular, it reduces health inequities. HiAP is a government-led strategy that seeks to improve population health by implementing coordinated strategies across health and non-health sectors. HiAP can be applied at any level: country, province or state, county or city. While the literature on HiAP includes population-based (extensive) and descriptive case (intensive) studies, our team seeks to use this information to develop the theory around the mechanisms involved in HiAP as well as conduct in-depth, explanatory case studies (Shankardass et al. 2010a, b). We are also undertaking realist syntheses of HiAP to examine the question of whether, how and in which contexts HiAP works. This research project is a transdisciplinary effort involving social epidemiologists, economists, physicians and knowledge brokers. It is an example of policy epidemiology (see Chap. 1), as the original idea to undertake a synthesis came from the Ontario Ministry of Health and Long-Term Care, where program planners who had plans to initiate HiAP in Ontario were seeking to build upon a strong evidence base. Researchers from CRICH had refined and advanced several such research methods to pursue this research agenda, including employing realist synthesis and multiple, explanatory case study methodologies. Fortunately, mainstream funders such as the Canadian Institutes of Health Research (CIHR), an organization committed to a strong population research agenda, provided funding for this innovative research agenda through multiple grants.[1,2] While this agenda started out as a classic example of policy epidemiology (see Chap. 1), we are also providing an opportunity to take the information public, as components of this agenda, namely the database of case studies of intersectoral action, will be publically available online. As interest in HiAP and intersectoral action increases, the World Health Organization has proposed a partnership with CRICH to create a user-friendly, interactive database of evaluative cases for use by policy makers, program planners and researchers. Online users can update their own cases and contribute to a discussion about barriers and facilitators for HiAP or intersectoral action. We see this as an additional opportunity to gain knowledge from those who actually carry out these programs about how well HiAP and other similar intersectoral efforts do or do not work in various settings.

16.4   Training and Education

With respect to training, there is an unfortunate focus in almost all graduate-level epidemiology programs on training students to become professional epidemiologists. The key activity is training in the proper execution of the standard quantitative methods, including study designs, measurement, statistical analysis and standardized synthesis methods. In part, the concern is that people who are going to go out into the world and call themselves epidemiologists should have a high level of competency in the complete toolkit of epidemiologic methods. The concern is really one of professionalization, rather than education. While it is perfectly valid and necessary to train people to be public health epidemiologists, for example, it is insufficient training for a social epidemiology aimed at reducing health inequalities. Such training would include an exposure to and the opportunity for pursuing other types of epidemiology and not just professional epidemiology. Coursework, internships and continuing education would provide opportunities to excel in policy or popular epidemiology in addition to professional epidemiology (see Chap. 1). Moreover, to ensure scholarly competence, programs would have to provide education about the principles and philosophical underpinnings of different methodological approaches and about the importance of theory.

One current example of post-doctoral training that provides a range of learning options for methods, topics and competencies consistent with this vision is the ACHIEVE (Action for Health Equity Interventions) program. The ACHIEVE

---

[1] Knowledge Synthesis Grant funded by the Canadian Institutes of Health Research (O'Campo 2010).

[2] Knowledge Synthesis Grant funded by the Canadian Institutes of Health Research (Laupacis and O'Campo 2009).

program has adopted a realist philosophical approach to its education and focuses on generating evidence to promote social change through reducing health inequities. The methods taught in the ACHIEVE program focus on conceptualizing and measuring how interventions succeed (or fail). A central feature of the program is engaged partnership building between program Fellows and a range of stakeholders, including community agencies, health care providers, policy makers and advocacy organizations in order to advance the use of research evidence.

Another mechanism that could be helpful in promoting scholarly education would be an accreditation system like that which exists for professional geoscientists (e.g., Association of Professional Geoscientists of Ontario). The courses in graduate programs can be used as part of achieving professional designation, but the professional designation by the association remains separate from the degree-granting function of academic institutions, allowing for uniform quality control of training and more freedom, on the part of university-based programs to pursue an overlapping, but distinct function.

16.5   Conclusions

Like many before us (e.g., Syme 2008; Shy 1997; Kaplan 2004; Berkman 2004; Cassel 1964), we seek to engage social epidemiologists in critical assessment of our field. We seek to challenge the field of social epidemiology to become a science of change. By "science of change," we refer to both the need for social epidemiology to generate evidence that is used by program planners and policy makers in their efforts to ameliorate health inequities, and to the need for our discipline to evolve and respond with new methods and approaches to achieve this goal. The good news is that we have willing partners who see the unique value in social epidemiologic research. By partnering with policy makers, program planners, members of affected communities and scientists from other disciplines we can accelerate the process of realizing this goal.

References

Berkman LF (2004) Seeing the forest and the trees: new visions in social epidemiology. Am J Epidemiol 160:1–2

Burawoy M (2004) Public sociologies: contradictions, dilemmas, and possibilities. Soc Forces 82:1603–1618

Cassel J (1964) Social science theory as a source of hypotheses in epidemiological research. Am J Epidemiol 54:1482–1488

Dunn JR (2002) Housing and inequalities in health: a study of socio-economic dimensions of housing and self-reported health from a survey of Vancouver residents. J Epidemiol Community Health 56:671–681

Dunn JR (2010) Is "socially-mixed" public housing redevelopment a de-stigmatization strategy? A preliminary analysis. In: Proceedings, responses to discrimination and racism: comparative perspectives. Center for European Studies, Harvard University, Cambridge

Dunn JR, Walker J, Graham J et al (2004) Gender, socio-economic attributes of housing, and self-rated health. Rev Environ Health 19:1–19

Dunn JR, Hayes MV, Hulchanski JD et al (2006) Housing as a socio-economic determinant of health: findings of a national needs, gaps and opportunities assessment. Can J Public Health 97:S11–15

Forbes A, Wainwright SP (2001) On the methodological, theoretical and philosophical context of health inequalities research: a critique. Soc Sci Med 53:801–816

Hickey TJ (2005) History of twentieth-century philosophy of science, 2nd edn. Thomas J. Hickey, New York

Kaplan GA (2004) What's wrong with social epidemiology, and how can we make it better? Epidemiol Rev 26:124–135

Krieger N (1994) Epidemiology and the web of causation: has anyone seen the spider? Soc Sci Med 39:887–903

Krieger N (1999) Embodying inequality: a review of concepts, measures, and methods for studying health consequences of discrimination. Int J Health Serv 29:295–352

Krieger N (2001) Theories for social epidemiology in the 21st century: an ecosocial perspective. Int J Epidemiol 30:668–677

Krieger N (2011) Epidemiology and the people's health: theory and context. Oxford University Press, New York

Laupacis A, O'Campo PJ (Principal Investigators) (2009) Health in All Policies: a scoping review. http://webapps.cihr-irsc.gc.ca/cfdd/db_results_submit

Muntaner C (2004) Commentary: social capital, social class, and the slow progress of psychosocial epidemiology. Int J Epidemiol 33:674–680

O'Campo PJ (Principal Investigator) (2010) A realist synthesis of initiation of Health in All Policies (HiAP): intersectoral perspectives. http://webapps.cihr-irsc.gc.ca/cfdd/db_results_submit

Sayer A (1992) Method in social science: a realist approach, 2nd edn. Routledge, London

Shankardass K, Solar O, Murphy K et al (2010a) Health in All Policies: a snapshot for Ontario. Results of a realist-informed scoping review of the literature. In: Getting started with Health in All Policies: a resource pack. Report to the Ministry of Health and Long-Term Care (Ontario). Centre for Research on Inner City Health, St. Michael's Hospital, Toronto. http://www.stmichaelshospital.com/knowledgeinstitute/search/details.php?id=18218&page=1. Accessed 12 May 2011

Shankardass K, Solar O, Murphy K et al (2010b) Results of a realist-informed scoping review of the literature. Appendix 1. Detailed methodology of five stage scoping review and the identification of Health in All Policies cases. In: Getting started with Health in All Policies: a resource pack. Report to the Ministry of Health and Long-Term Care (Ontario). Centre for Research on Inner City Health, St. Michael's Hospital, Toronto. http://www.stmichaelshospital.com/knowledgeinstitute/search/details.php?id=18218&page=1. Accessed 12 May 2011

Shy CM (1997) The failure of academic epidemiology: witness for the prosecution. Am J Epidemiol 145:479–484

Syme SL (2008) Reducing racial and social-class inequalities in health: the need for a new approach. Health Aff 27:456–459

Wainwright SP, Forbes A (2000) Philosophical problems with social research on health inequalities. Health Care Anal 8:259–277

Index

A

AARP. *See* American Association of Retired Persons (AARP)

Aboriginal, 8, 71, 73, 75, 76, 79, 80, 82, 96. *See also* Ethnicity; First Nations; Indigenous peoples; Inuit; Métis

Absolute income, 139, 310, 311, 315

Academic audience, 7, 62

Academic institutions, 14, 60, 87, 218, 286, 330, 333

Academic journals. *See* Peer-reviewed literature

Academic partners. *See* Partners

Access

to health care, 68, 121, 178, 181, 221, 238, 315

to resources, 87, 101, 121, 129, 148, 162, 163

to services, 68, 76, 168, 219, 221, 236, 238, 297, 315

Acquired immunodeficiency syndrome (AIDS). *See* HIV/AIDS

Actionable evidence. *See* Evidence

Action for Health Equity Interventions (ACHIEVE) program, 328, 332, 333

Action-oriented research, 69

Activity space, 170

Advocacy, 5, 44, 59, 60, 75, 106, 158, 171, 209, 269, 272, 276–277, 280, 295, 318, 319, 323, 333

Advocacy coalitions, 269, 277, 280

Affirmative approach, 23, 25

to health inequalities research, 23–25

African American. *See* Black; Ethnicity

African American Health Initiative Planning Project, 82

Agency, 8, 68, 72, 75, 76, 82, 88, 121, 143, 145, 162, 163, 207, 208, 210, 218, 219, 223, 224, 270, 307, 318, 319. *See also* Conflict theory

Agenda setting, 273, 274, 276, 319

A-historicism, 191–193

Air pollution, 124, 126, 140, 142, 145, 148

Allostatic load, 119, 120, 130

Allostatic overload, 119, 126, 127, 130

American Association of Retired Persons (AARP), 171

American College of Epidemiology, 47

Analysis

comparative analysis, 190, 192–194

discourse analysis, 275

hierarchal modelling, 138

interaction, 12, 61, 105, 169, 309

meta analysis, 184, 232, 235, 320

multilevel modelling, 140, 146–147

multivariate analysis, 193, 218, 220, 309

random effects models, 249, 294

regression, 190, 191, 193, 194, 309

stratification, 13, 98, 163

time series, 183, 190–193, 195

APGO. *See* Association of Professional Geoscientists of Ontario (APGO)

Association, 3, 5, 31–33, 39, 54, 56, 69, 96, 100, 123, 142, 150, 159, 168, 170, 171, 178, 180, 184, 187, 188, 193, 195, 196, 210, 211, 216–218, 220–222, 225, 226, 236, 306, 308–314, 318–320, 322, 329, 333

in statistics, 308, 309

Association of Professional Geoscientists of Ontario (APGO), 333

Asthma, 124, 126, 142, 147, 150, 160, 161
    in childhood, 141, 143, 145
Attitudinal discrimination. *See* Discrimination
Audience, 5–7, 45, 62, 79, 271, 274, 329

B
Baltimore, 14, 79, 163, 286–292, 294–297,
    299, 301, 302
Baltimore City Health Department, 287
Baltimore Healthy Start program, 14, 287,
    292, 294, 302
Baltimore Project, 287, 288, 296
Behaviour
    behavioural intervention, 207, 218, 276
    behaviour change, 222, 223, 239
    risk behaviour, 207, 211, 222, 314, 315
    social cognitive theory (*see* Theory)
Behavioural model. *See* Models of causation
Bell Curve, The, 74. *See also* Herrnstein, R.J.;
    Murray, C.
Bentham, J., 52
Berendes, H., 287
Bias, 27, 57, 60, 95, 102, 182, 193, 216,
    288, 300
Biological model. *See* Models of causation
Biological plausibility, 217
Birth outcomes, 73, 80, 121, 321
Birthweight
    by education, 103, 104
    low birthweight, 103, 104
    preterm birth, 321
    by race, 103, 104
    by race and education, 103, 104
    small for gestational age (SGA), 321
Black. *See* African American; Ethnicity
BMJ. *See* British Medical Journal (BMJ)
Bourdieu, P., 61, 161, 224
Brant Castellano, M., 70
Bridge sciences, 48
British Medical Journal (BMJ), 313
Built environment. *See* Environment
Burawoy, M., 5–7, 45, 60, 62

C
California Endowment, The, 158
Canada, 8, 14, 44, 54, 68, 71–73, 75, 76, 79,
    80, 82, 88, 96, 97, 218, 219, 250, 269,
    270, 276, 307, 308, 311, 317–320
Canadian Cancer Registry (CCR), 320
Canadian Community Health Survey (CCHS),
    76, 310, 311
Canadian Diabetes Surveillance System, 320

Canadian Health Services Research
    Foundation (CHSRF), 306, 320
Canadian Institutes of Health Research
    (CIHR), 2, 8, 71, 73, 268, 270, 306,
    320, 328, 332
Canadian Journal of Public Health, 318
Cancer, cervical, 315
Capability approach. *See* Ethics
Capitalism, 61, 179, 182, 188
Cardiovascular disease, 98, 115, 314
Case study. *See* Research methods
Cattell, V., 169, 170, 172
Causal pathways, 189, 210, 211, 222, 279,
    306, 313
Causation
    direct causation, 315
    indirect causation, 314, 315
    models (*see* Models of causation)
    reverse causation, 315
Causes of the causes. *See* Fundamental
    causes
CBPR. *See* Community-based participatory
    research (CBPR)
CCHN. *See* Community Child Health
    Research Network (CCHN)
CCHS. *See* Canadian Community Health
    Survey (CCHS)
CCR. *See* Canadian Cancer Registry (CCR)
CD. *See* Chronic disease (CD)
CDC. *See* Centers for Disease Control and
    Prevention (CDC)
Census
    census dissemination area, 159
    census tract, 159, 308
Census data, 129, 139, 146
Census of Canada, 88, 308, 320
Center for Health and Place, 158
Centers for Disease Control and Prevention
    (CDC), 71, 158, 164
Centre for Research on Inner City Health
    (CRICH), 307, 328, 331, 332
Chicago, 144, 151, 160, 161, 164, 165, 167,
    168, 171, 172
Chicago School, 144
Chronic disease (CD), 12, 113–130, 139, 149,
    159, 319
CHSRF. *See* Canadian Health Services
    Research Foundation (CHSRF)
CIHR. *See* Canadian Institutes of Health
    Research (CIHR)
Class. *See* Social class
Clement, T., 54
Client tracking systems, 290
Clinical epidemiology. *See* Epidemiology

Cognitive model, of rational choice, 222
Cohort, 73, 190, 211, 215, 219
Cohort study. *See* Study design
Coleridge, S.T., 76
Collaboration. *See* Partnerships
Collective efficacy, 140, 161, 168
Commission on Social Determinants of
    Health, 2, 3, 10–12, 68, 89, 139, 181,
    268. *See also* World Health
    Organization
Communitarianism. *See* Ethics
Community, 6–8, 14, 46, 53, 58, 59, 61, 62,
    67–89, 97, 99, 100, 123, 128, 142, 145,
    149–151, 158, 160, 163, 165, 209, 218,
    219, 234, 238, 239, 251, 257, 258, 271,
    274, 275, 285–303, 310, 311, 313, 318,
    320–322, 333
Community-based participatory research
    (CBPR), 8, 73, 295, 301, 303
Community-centric approach, 81–84, 87
Community Child Health Research Network
    (CCHN), 68, 79, 86
Community engagement, 72–73, 84
Comparative analysis. *See* Analysis;
    Macro-comparative analysis
Comparative study. *See* Study design
Complete Streets policy, 171
Complex adaptive system, for chronic disease
    and stress, 125
Complex health intervention. *See* Intervention
Compositional effects, 139
Comte, A., 26
Concept mapping, 74, 84, 129
Conceptual framework, 10, 114–116, 125,
    127, 211, 273, 278, 287
Conceptualization, 5, 50, 82, 86, 128, 129,
    189, 195, 224, 286, 289, 291, 329, 330
*Condition of the Working Class in England,
    The*, 179. *See also* Engels, F.
Conflict theory. *See also* Theory
    agency, 162, 163
    hegemony, 163, 165
    ideology, 163–165
    political economy, 163–165
    structure, 162, 163
Confounders, 126, 127, 158, 195, 249, 309
Confounding, 32, 125, 127, 142, 147, 184,
    192, 220, 225, 233
Consequentialist ethics. *See* Ethics
Context, 14, 34, 36, 37, 40, 46, 48, 52, 53, 55,
    57, 59, 62, 69, 74, 75, 77, 78, 81, 84,
    88, 89, 97–102, 104, 114, 115, 120,
    121, 126, 127, 138, 139, 142, 144–147,
    150, 160, 166, 169, 177–179, 191, 192,

206–208, 214, 216–218, 221–224, 233,
    235, 239, 242, 243, 249–251, 253,
    255–260, 278, 298, 301, 306, 307,
    315–317, 320, 322, 331
Contextual effects, 14, 139, 140, 232, 233
Control group, 260, 297
Coping, 75, 95, 116, 118–127, 129, 130,
    219, 220
Counterfactual, 31, 32, 260
CRICH. *See* Centre for Research on Inner City
    Health (CRICH)
Crime, 123, 124, 126, 138, 140, 145, 151, 158,
    160, 164, 167, 258
    rate, 142, 143, 165, 177–178
Critical epidemiology. *See* Epidemiology
Critical realism. *See* Realism
Critical theory. *See* Theory
Crossdisciplinarity. *See* Transdisciplinarity
Cross-sectional study. *See* Study design
Cultural determinants of health, 275
Culture, 32, 47, 75, 80, 82, 86, 177, 220, 226,
    291, 297, 298, 300

D
Data
    access to, 70, 88, 319
    administrative data, 129, 159
    analysis (*see* Analysis)
    collection, 13, 59, 69–72, 75–76, 80, 216,
        219, 225, 290–292, 298, 303
    "data insults," 71
    gatekeepers, 70, 72, 77
    governance, 13, 68, 69, 71, 80–82, 84, 242
    individual-level data, 78, 290
    ownership, 8, 70, 88
    population-level data, 316
    as a social resource, 13, 69, 75, 87
    uses of, examples, 190, 220, 242
Database, 13, 88, 138, 139, 182, 234, 319,
    320, 332
Data systems, 13, 68–89, 291
Decision making
    decision events, 272
    decision maker, 5–7, 15, 45, 51, 55, 59,
        60, 62, 170, 248, 250, 258, 271–277,
        279, 280
    decision-making partner, 320
    evidence-informed decision making,
        320, 322
Democracy, 164, 180, 182, 184–187, 189, 190,
    195, 280
Demographics, 32, 94, 99, 121, 161, 164
Dental caries, 316, 317

Deontological ethics. *See* Ethics
Deportation, 211, 221–222, 225
Deprivation amplification, 140, 147
Determinants
   cultural determinants (*see* Cultural
      determinants of health)
   distal determinants, 312, 319
   environmental determinants (*see*
      Environmental determinants of health)
   proximal determinants, 12
   social determinants (*see* Social
      determinants of health)
Diagnostic and Statistical Manual of Mental
      Disorders (DSM), 68, 84, 95
Discourse, 12, 99, 114, 115, 122, 123, 163,
      165, 167, 216, 219, 275, 278
Discourse analysis. *See* Analysis
Discrimination
   attitudinal discrimination, 101, 102
   institutionalized discrimination, 101, 102
   structural discrimination, 101
Disparities. *See* Health inequities
Dissemination, 70–72, 74–75, 79, 81,
      159, 271
   of scientific research (*see* Knowledge
      translation)
Distributive justice. *See* Justice
Downtown Eastside, Vancouver, 219
Downward drift, 98
Drinking water, municipal, fluorination of,
      316, 317
DSM. *See* Diagnostic and Statistical Manual
      of Mental Disorders (DSM)
Dunn, J.R., 12, 14, 330, 331
Durkheimian sociology, 179, 180

E
Economic environment. *See* Environment
Economy, 12, 32, 148, 163–165, 170,
      178–182, 189–191, 194–196, 208, 210,
      218, 223, 226
Education, 3, 4, 25, 68, 72, 75, 79, 80, 82, 94,
      99–101, 103–105, 124, 128, 187, 188,
      190, 194, 249, 289, 295, 314, 317, 319,
      332–333
Egalitarianism, 45, 178
Ego dystonic homosexuality, 95
Einstein, A., 329
Empirical study. *See* Study design
Employment
   as a health indicator, 74, 184, 188, 190
   opportunities, 101, 105, 163, 262
   policies, 82, 99, 101, 163, 209

training, 68, 99
unemployment rate, 32
Empowerment, 13, 67–89, 100, 105, 221,
      222, 274
Enabling environment, 208, 209, 221
Engaged scholarship, 269, 280
Engels, F., 179, 197
England. *See* Great Britain
Environment(s)
   built environment, 50, 56, 122, 123, 144,
      225, 314, 321, 323
   economic environment, 2, 210
   macrosocial environment, 12
   natural environment, 123, 144, 215, 217
   physical environment, 122, 149, 162,
      312, 314
   political environment, 2, 124, 138, 143,
      144, 163, 166, 210, 226
   psychosocial environment, 310
   risk environment, 205–227
   social environment, 123, 124, 144, 160,
      166, 211, 287, 317
   structural environment, 123,
      205–227
Environmental determinants of health, 80
Epidemiologists
   critical epidemiologists, 62
   public epidemiologists, 62
   social epidemiologists, 2, 4, 5, 8–10,
      12–15, 39, 40, 46, 62, 63, 68, 70, 89,
      94, 95, 99, 102, 105, 120, 124, 125,
      128–130, 138–140, 142, 145–148, 150,
      158, 170, 190, 232, 243, 249–254, 261,
      262, 268–270, 275–280, 286, 290–293,
      295, 297–300, 302, 303, 306, 307,
      310–314, 317–323, 330, 331, 333
Epidemiology
   clinical epidemiology, 74, 143,
      248, 249
   definition of, 44
   policy epidemiology, 7, 331, 332
   political epidemiology, 45, 177, 178,
      194–197
   professional epidemiology, 7, 8, 332
   public epidemiology, 8
   social epidemiology, 2–10, 12–15, 24–29,
      31, 32, 38–40, 44–51, 54–58, 60–63,
      68, 69, 89, 94, 95, 98, 100, 101, 117,
      127–130, 137–152, 175–197, 205–227,
      233, 242, 243, 247–262, 267–281, 286,
      287, 290, 293, 294, 305–323, 328–330,
      332, 333
   training programs, 10, 307, 322
Epistemology, 24, 25, 191, 250

Equity, 56, 84, 85, 279, 317
  in health, 70, 76–80, 89, 138, 144, 149,
      256, 257, 261, 262, 268, 269, 273, 275,
      276, 278, 281, 328, 332
Essentialism, 97–98
Ethics
  capability approach, 13, 53–55
  communitarianism, 13, 44
  consequentialist ethics, 51–52
  deontological ethics, 13, 51, 56
  Kantian ethics, 51
  rights theory, 13, 52
  utilitarianism, 52
  virtue ethics, 13, 52–53, 55, 56
Ethnicity. *See also* Race
  African American, 74
  Black, 76, 309
  and inequality, 76
  and inequity, 106
  Latino, 161, 162
  South Asian, 309, 321
  stratification, 13, 94, 101
  White, 74, 76, 106, 121, 161, 309
Ethnocultural identity, 314
Ethnography. *See* Research methods
Euclidean space, 149
Evaluation, 4, 13, 14, 32, 55, 59, 73, 83, 94,
      95, 159, 178, 232, 233, 236, 237, 241,
      242, 247–262, 290–292, 296, 298, 302,
      303, 320
Everyday violence, 213, 219, 220
Evidence
  actionable evidence, 14, 286, 293, 320
  in decision making (*see* Evidence-
      informed decision making)
  in research, 268, 272–274, 276, 278,
      280, 333
Evidence-informed decision making,
      320, 322
Evidence synthesis, 13, 258
Explanation, 9, 13, 14, 59, 61, 78, 85, 95–100,
      114, 116, 127, 140, 141, 143, 146, 147,
      150, 151, 177, 181, 190–194, 215, 217,
      234, 259, 268, 310–312, 314, 329
  using realist approach, 23–40, 233
Explanation sketch. *See* Narrative sketch
Extensive research, 34–36, 40, 140
Extrajudicial practices, 212

F
Fallibility, of knowledge, 39
Family planning, 295, 296, 299
Fascism, 192

Feminist theory. *See* Theory
"Fight or flight" response, 118, 119
First Nations. *See* Aboriginal
First Nations Regional Longitudinal Health
      Survey (RHS), 79, 82
Fluoridation, of drinking water, 316, 317
Forbes, A., 24, 25
Foucault, M., 57, 69, 70, 223
Framework, 6, 8, 10–14, 24, 44–49, 51–57,
      59, 60, 62, 69, 74, 82, 106, 114–117,
      125–128, 143, 146, 149, 161, 166,
      179, 189, 195–197, 208, 211, 217,
      219, 222, 223, 235, 237, 248, 254,
      256, 258–259, 269, 271–273, 276,
      278–281, 287, 329
Frankfurt School (of philosophy), 61
Freudian psychology, 38
Fundamental causes, 29, 141–146, 149,
      152, 314

G
Gender, 4, 13, 34, 68, 94, 96, 97, 104, 105,
      162, 181, 188, 208–210, 214, 216–218,
      221–225
Gendered violence, 216
Generalizability, 15, 36, 39, 259, 300
Geographic cluster, 220, 286, 287
Geographic Information System (GIS), 114,
      130, 138, 140, 148, 149, 206, 220
Geography
  emotional geography, 121, 130, 150
  physical geography, 149, 169
  time geography, 121, 150
Giddens, A., 223
GIS. *See* Geographic Information
      System (GIS)
Globalization, 182, 184–189, 195, 197
Government, 6, 9, 34, 50, 75, 123, 140, 160,
      165, 170, 177, 178, 180–182, 187–191,
      250, 252, 273–275, 277, 279, 286, 287,
      291, 307, 319, 331
Gradient. *See* Income gradients
Great Britain. *See* England
Gunaratnam, Y., 97, 98

H
Habermas, J., 14, 268, 269, 278, 281
Habitus formation, 224
"Hard to reach" populations, 82
Harm reduction, 13, 44, 50, 54–57, 60, 62,
      209, 220
Harvard University, 195

HCV. *See* Hepatitis C virus (HCV)
Health Canada, 79, 307
Health care
    access to, 68, 121, 178, 181, 221, 238, 315
    delivery, 49, 271
    providers, 238, 252, 279, 333
    screening, 235–241, 315
    unmet needs, 79, 253, 254
Health care system, 101, 102, 268, 271
Health equity. *See* Equity
Health in All Policies (HiAP), 319, 328,
    331, 332
Health inequalities, 3, 4, 10, 12, 15, 23–40, 45,
    48, 59, 74, 102, 125, 138, 143, 148,
    151, 152, 177–181, 185, 187–190,
    195–197, 277, 280, 311, 315–317,
    319, 332
Health Inequalities Intervention Tool, 315
Health inequities, 4, 9, 12–15, 69–78, 83, 84,
    87, 95, 96, 98–102, 106, 139, 140, 181,
    248–257, 262, 268, 269, 278, 280,
    331, 333
Health status, 2, 4, 13, 24, 25, 29, 31, 38, 39,
    59, 76, 128, 139, 188, 273, 277, 296,
    301, 308–310, 312–314, 316, 317, 319,
    321, 323
Healthy Bodegas Initiative, 139, 149
Heart disease, 25, 142, 159, 161, 278, 317
*Heat Wave: A Social Autopsy of Disaster in
    Chicago. See* Klinenberg, E.
Hegemony. *See* Conflict theory
Hempel, C.G., 192
Hepatitis C
    and injection drug use, 211, 215–218
    seroconversion, 215–218
    serostatus, 225
    and sexual intercourse, 215, 217
Hepatitis C virus (HCV), 206, 211,
    215–218, 225
Herrnstein, R.J., 74
Heterogeneity, 13, 96–98, 102–106, 121, 145,
    184, 299, 301
HiAP. *See* Health in All Policies (HiAP)
Hierarchal modelling. *See* Analysis
Higher-order concept, 314, 323
Hill, A.B., 144
HIV/AIDS, 12, 32, 36, 119, 130, 151, 185,
    205–227
HIV risk
    among injection drug users, 205–227
    among sex workers, 220
    gender differences, 210, 225
    and migration, 211, 222
    and social inequalities, 210

Homeostasis, 119
Homerton University Hospital, 124
Home visit, 288, 289, 298
HOPE IV program, 159, 160
Housing, 101, 144, 159, 165, 168, 171, 209,
    277, 288, 314, 330
    and health, 3, 4, 68, 80, 82, 83, 160,
    169, 196, 234, 238, 273, 274, 293,
    302, 331
HPV. *See* Human papilloma virus (HPV)
Human papilloma virus (HPV), 315
Hunter, M., 32, 36, 39, 151

I
Idealist philosophy, 27
Ideology. *See* Conflict theory
IMF. *See* International Monetary
    Fund (IMF)
Immigrant
    and asthma risk, 124
    healthly immigrant effect, 308
    and life expectancy, 308
    mortality rates, 164, 308
    and neighbourhoods, 124, 129, 164
Immigration
    in Canada, 96
    historical differences between Canada and
    the United States, 96
Immunization
    against human papillomavirus, 315
    measles, mumps, rubella (MMR)
        vaccine, 276
    program, 185, 187
Implementation science. *See* Knowledge
    translation
Income
    absolute income, 139, 310, 311, 315
    and employment, 99, 138, 209, 314
    and health, 188, 307–309
    as a health indicator, 188, 190
    high/low income countries, 3, 182
    high/low income neighbourhoods, 101,
    129, 147
    and inequality, 139, 177, 179–181,
    187, 311
    measurement of, 188, 190
    relative income, 310, 311
    stratification, 94, 95, 100
Income assistance, 83, 274
Income gradients, 307, 308, 311, 317, 320,
    322, 323
Income quintiles, 308
Income redistribution, 318

Indigenous peoples
   communities, 70
   and data, 70
   health, 70
   knowledge systems, 70
   scholars, 70
Individualism, 52
Individual level, 12, 58, 78, 83, 98–99, 105,
        114, 115, 120, 123, 130, 138, 140, 142,
        143, 146, 150, 166, 167, 184, 186, 189,
        206, 207, 220, 222, 224, 225, 260, 290,
        313, 316
Infant, 76, 80, 86, 94, 106, 124, 184–188, 274,
        287, 288, 292, 321
Informed social control, 161, 219
Injection drug use, 208
Injection drug users, 12, 130, 205–227
Institute for the Study of Labor
        (IZA), 102
Institutionalization, 238
Institutionalized discrimination. See
        Discrimination
Instrumental knowledge. See Knowledge
Integrated strategy, for public
        health action, 318
Intellectual property, 242
Intelligence quotient (IQ), 74
Intensive research, 34–36, 142, 151, 152
Interaction. See Analysis
Interactionist theory, 12, 162, 166–168.
        See also Theory
International Monetary Fund (IMF), 186,
        189, 196
Intersectoral action, 178, 253, 332
Intervention
   complex health intervention, 241, 249,
        250, 256–258, 261
   evaluation, 4, 13, 14, 55, 83, 94,
        95, 232, 233, 241, 250, 257,
        259, 260
   harm reduction, 44, 50, 54, 55,
        60, 209
   and policy, 7, 178, 318
   and public health, 56, 222, 311,
        312, 316
   realist reviews of, 234, 235, 240, 241
   and values, 47, 54–56, 60, 278, 279
Intimate partner violence (IPV), 13, 209, 215,
        216, 232, 234–243
Inuit. See Aboriginal
IPV. See Intimate partner violence (IPV)
IQ. See Intelligence quotient (IQ)
IZA. See Institute for the Study
        of Labor (IZA)

J
Johns Hopkins University, 292, 295
Journal of Epidemiology and Community
        Health, 313
Justice
   criminal justice system, 212
   distributive justice, 49, 275
   market justice, 49, 50
   social justice, 48–49, 57–59, 62, 100,
        178, 279

K
Kant, I., 51
Key informant interview.
        See Research methods
Klinenberg, E., 12, 151, 160, 162,
        164–167, 172
Knowledge
   instrumental knowledge, 6, 45, 278
   knowledge broker, 274, 331
   knowledge user, 332
   practically adequate knowledge, 27, 30,
        37, 116
   reflexive knowledge, 6, 7, 45
   technically rational knowledge, 6, 7
Knowledge constitutive interests
   emancipatory knowledge, 278–279
   hermeneutical knowledge, 279
   instrumental knowledge, 278
Knowledge production, 8, 57
Knowledge translation (KT)
   knowledge-action cycle, 278
   linkage and exchange activities, 274
   partnerships (see Partnerships)
   political knowledge translation, 59
   in public health, 307, 320
   "push" and "pull" activities, 320
   in social epidemiology, 259, 268, 270,
        272–277
   strategies, 14, 269–272, 278, 279, 318
   "target and tailor" approach, 274
   and values, 14, 59, 60, 62, 269, 279
Krieger, N., 5, 48, 59, 208

L
Labour, 3, 5, 9, 83, 97, 99, 165, 178, 179, 188,
        193, 194, 196, 288, 289, 319
Labour market, 97, 165, 178, 179, 188
Lacks, H., 71
Lancet, The, 116, 313
Late democracy, 192
Latino. See Ethnicity

Latino paradox, 124
"Left wing" political orientation, 178, 189
Lewontin, R.C., 195
Liberalism, 53
Life course perspective, 128, 129
Life expectancy, 184–186, 188, 308, 310, 311
Little Village, Chicago, 161, 162, 164, 165, 167
Lived experience, 207, 211, 219
Logistic inertia, 218
London Health Observatory (LHO), 315
Longitudinal study. *See* Study design

M
Macro-comparative analysis, 191, 194
Macro level, 99, 130, 167, 181, 191, 219,
        222, 274
Macrosocial level, 9, 10, 12, 13, 138, 147,
        190, 195, 249, 331
Mäori peoples, 85
Marginalization, 3, 68–72, 74–75, 84
Marginalized populations, 12, 75, 76, 269,
        275, 276, 280, 289
Market justice. *See* Justice
Marmot, M., 143, 314, 316
Marxism, 37
Marx, K., 162
Material deprivation, 310, 312
Maternity Experiences Survey (MES), 75
McGill University, 318
Means of production, 162
Mechanisms, 4, 12–14, 25, 27–34, 36, 38–40,
        68, 75, 84, 94, 95, 100, 102, 105, 116,
        117, 126, 128, 138–147, 150–152, 158,
        160, 166, 168–170, 179–181, 189, 191,
        194, 196, 212, 220, 225, 226, 233–237,
        240, 242, 249–251, 253, 255, 257–260,
        286, 287, 293, 300, 301, 306, 311–318,
        330, 331
Meso level, 166, 219
Meta analysis. *See* Analysis
Métis. *See* Aboriginal
Mexico, 73, 206, 211, 221, 222, 224
Micro level, 219, 222
Mill, J.S., 52
Mincome guaranteed income experiment, 83
Ministry of Health, Ontario, 331
Mixed methods. *See* Research methods
Models of causation
        behavioural model, 313
        biological model, 9, 313
        disease-specific models, 9, 190
        social determinants of health (*see* Social
            determinants of health)

Morbidity, 10, 85, 142, 179, 236, 306
        morbidity rate, 142, 236
Mortality
        among immigrants, 308
        cause of, 10, 98, 166
        in children under five, 184, 188
        disease specific, 9, 115
        in infants, 80
        mortality rate, 76, 158, 164, 185, 188
        premature, 119, 179
Mowat, D., 14, 305, 307
Multicollinearity, 194
Multidisciplinarity, 210
Multilevel modeling. *See* Analysis
Multisector, 293, 300
Multivariate analysis. *See* Analysis
Murray, C., 74

N
Narrative sketch, 192
Narrative synthesis, 241
National Institute of Child Health and Human
        Development (NICHD), 286, 287
National Library of Medicine (NLM), 123
"Natural" disasters, 3, 160, 166
Natural environment. *See* Environment
Natural experiments. *See* Research methods
Neighbourhood
        administrative definition of, 129, 159
        disorder, 12, 122, 167–170
        effects on health, 123, 144
        and immigrants, 124, 129, 164, 308
        neighbourhood-health research, 12,
            158–160, 170–171
        neighbourhood-level influences, 12, 32,
            122, 123, 144, 159, 163, 165, 170
        and place, 12, 16, 17, 120–124, 128, 129,
            138, 142, 147, 148, 151, 158–172
        planning, 123, 128, 139, 144
        and poverty, 32, 128, 129, 140, 148, 158,
            159, 161, 164, 169
        resources, 100, 101, 121–124, 128, 129,
            140, 146–149, 158, 161–163, 165, 170
        safety, 117, 124, 145, 164
        and segregation, 139, 140, 147, 170
        and social class, 144
        stress, 12, 101, 114, 117, 119, 121–125,
            128, 129, 140, 142, 143, 145, 149, 150,
            159, 331
        and violence, 12, 121, 123, 124, 142, 143,
            145, 150, 163, 164, 215
        walkability, 100, 123, 124
Neo-Durkheimian approach, 179

Neo-liberalism, 196
Neo-Marxism, 179
New Mexico Partnership for Healthier
    Communities (NMPHC), 73
New York City, 139, 149
New Zealand, 84, 85
New Zealand Health Information Service
    (NZHIS), 85
New Zealand Health Survey, 85
Non-profit organizations, 285, 286
North Karelia, Finland, 142
North Lawndale, Chicago, 161, 162, 164,
    165, 167
Nurse practitioner, 295, 296, 299
Nussbaum, M.C., 54
Nuu-chah-nulth First Nation, 71

O
Obesity, 13, 44, 50, 54, 56–57, 59, 103, 104,
    113, 115, 149, 158, 309, 311
Objectivity, 5, 47, 48, 53, 58–61, 190,
    291, 329
O'Campo, P., 1, 13, 14, 67, 93, 175, 231, 287,
    290, 291, 327
OCAP. See Ownership, Control, Access and
    Possession
Occupational rank, 311
O'Connor, A., 9
Ordering framework, 329
Organization for Economic Cooperation
    and Development (OECD), 176, 184,
    188, 190
"Other" category, 97, 217
Outbreak
    HIV, 212
    typhus, 179
Ownership, Control, Access and Possession
    (OCAP) (of data), 8, 81, 82

P
Panel study. See Study design
Paradis, G., 318
Participant observation.
    See Research methods
Participatory action research, 58, 73.
    See also Community-based
    participatory research
Partners
    academic partners, 14, 86, 285–303
    community partners, 6, 8, 78, 79, 81, 258,
        288, 289, 298, 300
    decision-making partners, 320

Partnerships
    advocacy coalitions (see Advocacy
        collations)
    community-academic partnerships, 14, 86,
        285–303
    in knowledge translation, 14, 320
    in public health, 14, 209, 286, 287,
        320–323, 332
    in research, 6, 8, 14, 73, 77–79, 81, 84,
        86–89, 217, 218, 254, 286, 288, 294,
        295, 298, 302, 303, 307, 320–323, 333
Pathways. See Mechanisms
Pawson, R., 255
Pearlin, L.I., 116, 117, 120, 127, 128
Peel, Region of, 14, 307–309, 320
Peer education, 124
Peer-reviewed literature, 235, 236
Philosophy, 13, 23–40, 61, 70, 232, 233, 329.
    See also Positivism; Realist
    philosophy
    in science, 32
Physical disorder, 12, 139, 158,
    168–170
Physical environment. See Environment
Place. See also Neighbourhood
    geographic notion of, 12, 80, 101, 149,
        158, 287, 288
    physical insidedness, 171
    place attachment, 170, 171
    place-based stress (see Stress)
Police (or policing), 209, 211–214,
    219, 220
Policy
    evidence base, 44, 45, 55, 56, 286, 331
    and health, 14, 45, 46, 178, 180, 198,
        204, 307
    neo-liberal policy, 49, 196
    policy maker, 5, 14, 50, 72, 73, 75, 77–83,
        106, 158, 254, 275, 286, 293, 297, 300,
        320, 328, 332, 333
    policy making, 6, 151, 159, 268, 270, 271,
        273, 274, 278, 280, 312, 319
    in public health, 14, 45, 209,
        306, 307
    social policy, 77, 88, 130, 269, 280
    and values, 47, 49, 52, 54, 60, 62, 268,
        269, 275, 279, 297, 318, 328
Policy change
    advocacy (see Advocacy)
    developmental stages model, 273
    and knowledge translation, 14, 59–60, 62,
        259, 268–281, 307, 318, 320
Policy epidemiology. See Epidemiology
PolicyLink, 158

Politics
    democracy, 180, 182, 184, 186, 189,
        195, 280
    and knowledge translation, 14, 59–60, 62,
        259, 268–281, 307, 318, 320
    political economy
        (*see also* Conflict theory)
    political epidemiology (*see* Epidemiology)
    political parties, 187, 194, 196, 197
    political science, 190, 270
    political sociology, 181, 190
    political tradition, 178, 181, 182, 184–190,
        195, 196
    polity scores, 186
    social democracy, 164, 180, 182, 184–187,
        189, 190, 195, 280
Population health, 6, 9, 12, 13, 44, 47, 67, 69,
        121, 125, 128, 140, 151, 176–184,
        187–190, 194–197, 267, 268, 270, 273,
        279, 318, 319, 327, 328, 331
Positivism, 6, 13, 23, 24, 26–29, 37, 40, 47,
        61, 278, 329
Post-colonial theory, 70
Post-World War II period, 188, 190
Poverty, 2, 3, 9, 10, 32, 44, 54, 56, 68, 69, 83,
        97, 99, 128, 129, 140, 148, 158, 159,
        161, 164, 169, 177, 181, 208, 210, 311,
        318, 319
Poverty knowledge, 9
Power. *See also* Conflict theory
    discursive power, 223, 276
    power relations, 194
    and race, 4, 94, 95, 97, 100, 101, 105, 162,
        166, 217
    and social class, 25, 98, 100, 104, 116,
        144, 179, 188, 194, 195, 197
    in statistics, 72, 75, 88, 96, 97, 184, 226,
        296, 299, 308, 311, 319
Pregnancy, 73, 106, 286, 288, 289, 295, 296,
        299, 302, 321
Preterm birth. *See* Birthweight
Preterm labour, 288, 289
Priorities, 316, 319
    in research, 82–84, 86, 87, 216, 271, 275,
        294, 298, 299, 301–303
Problem-focused research, 3–5, 69
Professional epidemiology. *See* Epidemiology
* Program, 2, 29, 50, 72, 99, 124, 139, 158,
        177, 209, 232, 250, 268, 286, 307
Program evaluation, 251, 290, 296

Proportionate universalism, 316
Proximity, geographic
Psychoneuroimmunology, 114, 117
Psychosocial theory. *See* Theory
Public epidemiology. *See* Epidemiology
* Public health, 2, 44, 68, 96, 117, 140, 164,
        177, 207, 236, 250, 275, 286, 305
Public Health Agency of Canada (PHAC), 68,
        75, 79
Public intellectuals, 44, 269, 280
Putnam, R.T., 98, 161

Q
Qualitative methods. *See* Research methods
Quantitative methods. *See* Research methods
Quasi-experimental methods.
        See Research methods
Questionnaire, 88, 211, 215, 219, 220

R
Race. *See also* Ethnicity
    and discrimination, 95–97, 101, 102, 105
    and health, 4, 13, 68, 84, 88, 94–98, 100,
        101, 103–105, 161, 162, 217, 249, 286
    as a health indicator, 74
    and inequality, 10, 38, 58, 72, 76, 125, 139,
        151, 163, 177, 179–181, 187, 210, 222,
        224, 252, 268, 277, 280, 311, 317
    measurement of, 84, 94–96, 102
    racial discrimination, 95, 208, 223
    racial identity, 97
    stratification, 13, 94–96, 98, 100, 101
Random assignment, 40, 297, 299
Random effects models. *See* Analysis
Randomized controlled trials (RCT).
        See Study design
Realism, 14, 25, 27–28, 32, 35, 37, 233, 250.
        See also Realist philosophy
Realist philosophy
    in evaluation, 13, 32
    and health inequalities, 13, 25, 27, 32
    and social epidemiology, 13, 25, 27, 32
    in systematic literature reviews, 12, 13, 181
Realist review. *See* Research Methods
Reductionist model, 210
Reference group, 71, 72
Reflexive knowledge. *See* Knowledge
Reflexivity, 59, 61, 62

Where there is an * the terms have occurred more than 200 times. The page numbers given are first
occurrences from each chapter.

Regent Park, Toronto, 331
Regression. *See* Analysis
Relative income, 310, 311
Research agenda, 14, 242, 281, 305–323
Research methods
    case study, 210–222
    ethnography, 36, 211
    key informant interview, 242
    literature review, 12, 13, 181–183, 186, 236
    mised methods, 33, 34, 130, 210, 211, 218,
        225, 226
    natural experiments, 40, 142, 171, 297, 300
    participant observation, 211, 215
    qualitative methods, 10, 61, 172, 192, 206,
        207, 226
    quantitative methods, 6, 27, 34, 40, 159,
        193, 332
    quasi-experimental methods, 300, 330, 331
    realist review, 79, 231–243, 321
    systematic review, 4, 33, 231–243, 278,
        311, 321
Research question, how to frame, 36, 49,
    57–58, 86, 100, 158, 169, 211, 219,
    226, 234, 274, 276, 279, 297, 301,
    313, 329
    Research utilization. *See* Knowledge
        translation
Resolution 62.14, 89. *See also* World
    Health Assembly
Resource
    environmental resource, 122, 123, 127
    neighbourhood resource, 100, 101,
        121–124, 128, 129, 140, 146, 148, 149,
        158, 160–163, 165, 170
    personal resource, 118
Resource-hazard conflict, 124
Retroduction, 30, 33, 36, 38, 330
Rights theory. *See* Ethics
"Right wing" political orientation, 190,
    192, 196
Rime of the Ancient Mariner, The, 76.
    See also Coleridge, S.T.
Risk
    of essentialism, 97–98
    high-risk populations, 206
    for HIV (*see* HIV risk)
    risk behavior, 160, 314, 315
    risk environment (*see* Environment)
    risk factor, 3, 4, 9, 10, 32, 73, 75, 98,
        114, 115, 119, 139–143, 150, 161,
        192, 210, 221, 286, 288, 306, 309,
        312–314, 323
    risk reduction, 219, 220

Roman, C., 100
Rose, G., 32, 140, 181, 270, 316
Rowles, G., 170
Russia, 130, 211–213, 224, 225

S
Saint-Simon, H., 26
Sample size, 84, 184, 186, 190, 218
    "Small N" problem, 191, 193–194
Sampling
    purposive sampling, 219
    snowball sampling, 215
    targeted sampling, 218
San Francisco, 211, 215, 225
Sayer, A., 25, 27–38, 61, 95, 116,
    147, 329
Screening
    case-finding approach, 236, 239
    for cervical cancer, 315
    for HIV, 219
    for intimate partner violence, 13,
        209, 215, 216, 232, 239–241,
        324–236
    universal approach, 236–238, 241, 243
Segregation, 101, 105, 139, 140,
    147, 170
Self-determination, 8, 70
Self-perceived health, 184, 186
Self-Sufficiency Project, 83
Selye, H., 117–119
Serbia, 211–214, 224, 225
Seroconversion
    for hepatitis C virus, 211
    seroconverter, 217
    seroincidence, 216
Service provider, 80, 161, 165, 238, 279, 289,
    297, 300
Sexual orientation, 68
Sexual violence, 219
Sex work, 208, 209, 215, 216, 218–221
Sex workers, 130, 205–224
Small for gestational age (SGA). *See*
    Birthweight, low
Smoking, 56, 74, 75, 115, 119, 123, 126, 127,
    192, 234, 249, 310, 316
Social capital, 11, 12, 124, 139, 143, 145,
    147–149, 151, 160, 161, 163, 167–170,
    177, 194, 277, 314
Social change, 5, 10, 13, 14, 38, 44, 47,
    48, 57, 58, 68, 69, 87, 193, 243,
    268, 269, 275, 277, 279–281,
    285–303

Social class, 11, 25, 98, 100, 104, 116, 144, 179, 188, 194–195, 197
Social cognitive theory. *See* Theory
Social cohesion, 11, 124, 161, 168, 169, 180, 181, 220
Social control, informed. *See* Informed social control
Social democracy, 184
Social determinants of health, 2–4, 7, 9–12, 49, 58, 68, 83, 89, 104, 139, 144, 158, 177, 181, 253, 268, 269, 273–275, 280, 281, 306, 307, 313, 318, 319, 323
Social environment. *See* Environment
Social epidemiologist, 2, 4, 5, 8–10, 12–15, 39, 40, 46, 62, 63, 68, 70, 89, 94, 95, 99, 102, 105, 124, 125, 128–130, 138–140, 142, 145–148, 150, 158, 170, 190, 196, 232, 243, 249, 250, 252–254, 261, 262, 268–270, 275–280, 286, 290–293, 295, 297, 298, 300, 302, 303, 306–307, 310–314, 317–322
Social epidemiology
  data and data systems, 13, 68–72, 75–79, 81, 82, 84, 85, 87, 89
  definition of, 44
  knowledge translation (*see* Knowledge translation)
  methods (*see* Research methods)
  and politics, 12, 175–197, 266–2810
  and public health (*see* Public health)
  and realist philosophy (*see* Realist philosophy)
  theory (*see* Theory)
  and values, 13, 43–63, 317
Social exclusion, 13, 68–69, 71, 78, 83, 86, 88, 89
Social justice. *See* Justice
Social mapping, 211, 219
Social status. *See* Social class
Social structure
  plausibility, 115, 217
  production of risk, 207
Social support, 105, 106, 119, 121, 123, 124, 243, 288, 289, 314
Social theory. *See* Theory
Social values, 11, 46–48, 275
Socioeconomic position (SEP). *See* Socioeconomic status, Social class
Socioeconomic status (SES), 24, 101, 115, 126, 129, 139, 144, 249, 287, 306, 307, 311, 314–316
Sociospatial disparities, 114–116, 127–129

Solution-focused research, 2–4, 8, 10, 69, 102, 103, 158, 160, 171, 234, 250, 269, 280, 293, 300, 301
South Africa, 32, 36, 151
Southern California, 142, 143, 145, 148
Stakeholders, 73, 77–79, 82, 88, 234, 255, 258, 259, 274–276, 279, 333
Statistics, 72, 75, 76, 88, 96, 97, 184, 226, 296, 297, 299, 308, 311, 319
Statistics Canada, 72, 76, 88, 96, 97, 308, 311
Status Indian, 80
St. Michael's Hospital, 321
Strategic plan, 322
Stratification. *See* Analysis
Stress
  acute stress, 118–119, 125
  chronic stress, 12, 78, 101, 115–117, 119–120, 122–130, 142, 143, 145, 150
  and health, 12, 75, 101, 106, 114–117, 119–129, 142, 143, 145, 150, 208, 315, 331
  and neighbourhoods
  place-based stress, 12, 113–130
  stress process, 116, 117, 120, 121, 128, 331
Stressors, 117–130, 140, 149, 222, 289
Structural confounding, 32, 147
Structural discrimination.
    See Discrimination
Structural violence, 12, 205–227
Structural vulnerability, 12, 205–227
Structuration, 208, 211, 212, 223, 224
Structure, 26, 28–30, 34, 36, 38–40, 57, 60, 61, 78, 82, 85, 88, 101, 120, 121, 129, 144, 145, 149, 150, 162–164, 167, 169, 177, 192, 196, 197, 206, 208–210, 215, 222–224, 239, 256, 287, 312, 314, 315, 318, 330. *See also* Conflict theory
Structured conceptualization, 129
Study design
  cohort study, 211, 215
  comparative study, 191
  cross-sectional study, 184
  empirical study, 330
  longitudinal study, 86
  panel study, 160
  randomized controlled trial (RCT), 74, 233, 249, 297
Subjectification, 210, 223–225
Surveillance, 69, 70, 76, 79, 80, 88, 212, 307, 320

Survey, 35, 36, 75, 76, 79, 81, 82, 85, 86, 88,
    160, 168, 170, 172, 184, 186, 211, 215,
    217, 221, 300, 310, 311, 322
Symbolic interactionism.
    See Interactionist theory
Symbolic violence, 164, 219, 223
Synergistic effects
    of policies, 104, 233, 254
    between variables, 104, 105
Systematic review. *See* Research methods
Systems view, 12, 113–130

T

TANF. *See* Temporary Assistance for Needy
    Families (TANF)
Targeted intervention (or program), 288
Temporary Assistance for Needy Families
    (TANF), 10
Terris, M., 177
Thatcher, Margaret, 49
Theory
    conflict, 12, 162–166
    critical, 13, 44, 48, 61
    feminist, 61, 216
    going beyond, 9–14
    interactionist theory, 12, 162,
        166–168
    psychosocial theory, 310
    social cognitive theory, 239
    in social epidemiology, 10, 12, 13, 24, 25,
        31, 32, 38, 51, 138, 139, 148, 149, 151,
        180, 195, 211, 242, 250, 251, 255–261,
        280, 328, 329
    social theory, 9–14, 26, 69, 157 172, 310
Tijuana, 221, 224, 225
Time–activity patterns, 145
Time series. *See* Analysis
Tobacco. *See* Smoking
Traffic, 124, 126, 140, 142, 145, 148, 150,
    158, 209, 274
    related to air pollution
        (*see* Air pollution)
Training programs, 10, 99, 307, 322
Transactional model, 120, 126
Transdisciplinary, 211, 242, 254,
    294, 331
Trust, 8, 54, 81, 86, 124, 139, 161, 168, 169,
    286, 297, 299, 301, 303
Truth, 27, 28, 37, 39, 69, 100, 289,
    300, 302
    in science, 27, 28, 37
Tuskegee experiments, 71
Typhus outbreak (or epidemic), 179

U

United States, 9, 44, 45, 49, 59, 74, 76, 83, 86,
    96, 97, 103, 104, 123, 150, 158, 159,
    161, 164, 171, 178, 211, 217, 221, 222,
    224, 287
Universities, 2, 88, 322
University of California
    Santa Barbara, 9
Unnatural Causes, 159
Utilitarianism, 52. *See also* Ethics

V

Values
    cognitive values, 47
    cultural values, 13, 57, 59–61, 224,
        275, 297
    in knowledge translation, 14, 59–60, 62,
        267–281
    in social epidemiology, 5, 9, 13, 14,
        27, 43–63, 140, 178, 195, 268–270,
        275, 276, 278–280, 306, 317, 328,
        329, 333
    social values, 46–48, 275
Vancouver, 54, 55, 211, 218, 219,
    224, 225
Variables, 6, 12, 13, 31, 39, 94–98, 100,
    101, 104, 105, 150, 158, 162, 178,
    182–184, 186, 187, 190, 191,
    193–196, 217, 218, 220, 225, 226,
    289, 293, 309, 310, 329, 330
Victim blaming, 50, 62, 207, 222
Violence
    everyday violence, 208, 211–214, 216,
        219, 220, 223, 224
    gendered violence, 209, 211, 215–218,
        220, 225
    intimate partner (*see* Intimate partner
        violence)
    and neighbourhoods, 12, 121, 124,
        142, 143, 145, 150, 163, 164, 209,
        211, 215
    and stress, 12, 121, 123, 124, 126, 142,
        143, 145, 150, 208
    structural violence, 12, 123, 150, 163,
        205–227
Virchow, R.L.K., 179, 226
Virtue ethics. *See* Ethics
Visible minority, 96

W

Wainwright, S.P., 24, 25, 329
Ward, R., 96

Welfare
    governance, 189
    regime, 12, 179–184, 187–190, 192,
        194–196, 274
    state, 12, 74, 83, 178–182, 184–188,
        190–192, 195–197
    system, 83, 179, 196, 274
White. *See* Ethnicity
Whitehall Study, 194
WHO. *See* World Health
        Organization (WHO)
*Why Place Matters: Building the Movement
    for Healthy Communities*, 159

Women, 10, 32, 35, 49, 73, 74, 85,
        103–106, 121, 124, 161, 215–217,
        225, 287–289, 296, 297,
        301, 315
World Bank, 189, 196
World Health Assembly, 89
World Health Organization (WHO),
        10–12, 89

Y
Yen, I.H., 6, 8, 12, 123, 124, 144, 148,
        157–172

CPSIA information can be obtained at www.ICGtesting.com
Printed in the USA
LVOW070250230812

295569LV00006B/20/P